*The publisher and the University of California Press
Foundation gratefully acknowledge the generous support of the
Lisa See Endowment Fund in Southern California History
and Culture.*

Health as Property

AMERICAN CROSSROADS

Edited by Earl Lewis, George Lipsitz, George Sánchez, Dana Takagi, Laura Briggs, and Nikhil Pal Singh

Health as Property

RACIAL CAPITALISM AND SEXUAL
LIBERALISM IN LOS ANGELES

Nic John Ramos

UNIVERSITY OF CALIFORNIA PRESS

University of California Press
Oakland, California

© 2026 by Nic John Ramos

All rights reserved.

Library of Congress Cataloging-in-Publication Data

Names: Ramos, Nic John author
Title: Health as property : racial capitalism and sexual liberalism in Los Angeles / Nic John Ramos.
Other titles: American crossroads 75.
Description: Oakland, California : University of California Press, [2026] | Series: American crossroads ; 75 | Includes bibliographical references and index.
Identifiers: LCCN 2025012369 (print) | LCCN 2025012370 (ebook) | ISBN 9780520404120 cloth | ISBN 9780520404137 paperback | ISBN 9780520404144 ebook
Subjects: LCSH: Academic medical centers—California—Los Angeles County—History—20th century | Medical care—California—Los Angeles—History—20th century | Racism—California—Los Angeles—History—20th century | Equality—California—Los Angeles—History—20th century | Los Angeles (Calif.)—Race relations
Classification: LCC RA982.L67 R36 2026 (print) | LCC RA982.L67 (ebook) | DDC 362.1109794/94—dc23/eng/20250611
LC record available at https://lccn.loc.gov/2025012369
LC ebook record available at https://lccn.loc.gov/2025012370

GPSR Authorized Representative: Easy Access System Europe, Mustamäe tee 50, 10621 Tallinn, Estonia, gpsr.requests@easproject.com

35 34 33 32 31 30 29 28 27 26
10 9 8 7 6 5 4 3 2 1

*For my parents, Nicanor and Rosalinda
and grandparents, Artemio, Potenciana, Venancio, and
Eufrosina*

CONTENTS

List of Illustrations viii
Acknowledgments xi

Introduction: Free Market Healthcare, In Full Color 1

1 · Profiting from Black Sickness 29

2 · A New Lease on Black Life 72

3 · The Psychological Wages of Blackness 110

4 · Profiting from Working Poverty 145

5 · An Asylum Without Walls 184

6 · Profiting from Violence 215

Epilogue: "A Pessimist, If I Am Not Careful" 252

Notes 267
Bibliography 317
Index 337

LIST OF ILLUSTRATIONS

FIGURES

1. Dr. M. Alfred Haynes, 1982 *102*
2. Training at Drew Medical School, 1976 *104*
3. A megalopolis broken into "bite-size pieces," with downtown being "the biggest bite of them all" *153*
4. Johnnie Tillmon, 1968 *155*
5. Tom Bradley, 1973 *173*
6. City center, Los Angeles *200*
7. Policing through new community norms *207*
8. Ambulance services, 1958 *226*
9. Bringing wartime medicine home, 1972 *234*

MAPS

1. Spatial overview of Los Angeles *14*
2. Housing segregation in 1930s Los Angeles *45*
3. Black Los Angeles, 1930 *62*
4. Black Los Angeles, 1960 *63*
5. Los Angeles hospital service areas, 1965 *66*
6. Dr. Sol White's proposed hospital district *67*
7. Hospitals in and near to Watts *89*
8. Constructing Black mental wellness in LA *111*

9. Anchoring working poverty *175*
10. Skid Row's relationship to Black, Asian, and gay neighborhoods *185*
11. The containment and mitigation policy *193*
12. The county's two paramedic demonstration projects *228*
13. Race, false advertising, and emergency rooms, 1981 *243*
14. Safety net hospitals in Los Angeles *249*

ACKNOWLEDGMENTS

An entire community helped me write this book. I am lucky to have grown up knowing and being cared for by both sets of my grandparents. Artemio (Tonyong) and Potenciana (Enciang) Dilan Fajardo and Venancio (Ben) and Eufrosina (Celing) Gangano Ramos were, without a doubt, my first teachers. I am also a fortunate and proud product of public education. I am no doubt the result of attentive educators who spent more time investing in me than I perhaps had the good sense to invest in myself when I was younger.

Among many great professors I had as an undergraduate at the University of California at Irvine, I am especially indebted to Linda Vo, Dorothy Fujita-Rony, Fred Moten, and Katherine Tate. They inspired me to look at academia and scholarship through the lens of the community from which I came and to look back at my community through the critical eyes of an activist-scholar. These practices of looking, learning, and hearing have served me well in my approaches to campus, community, and labor organizing, particularly in the six years I spent organizing healthcare and city workers with various locals of the National Union of Healthcare Workers (NUHW) and the Service Employees' International Union (SEIU).

I want to thank the leadership of NUHW, the Committee of Interns and Residents-SEIU, and those who worked and led United Healthcare Workers-West before 2009 for the lessons I learned in forging community in what continue to be difficult and complex times for healthcare workers and patients. Among organizers and workers, I learned firsthand that new kinds of communities and new types of futures are possible both because of, and in spite of, the differences that divide society.

It was an honor to work alongside so many inspiring rank-and-file leaders in healthcare. I learned so much from Dr. Nailah Thompson, Dr. Opal

Taylor, Denise Rollins, Sandra Rodriguez, David Mallon, and Jim Clifford, and from committed leaders such as Amy Hall, Eric Scherzer, Michael Phelan, Barbara Lewis, Gary Guthman, Michael Krivosh, Glenn Goldstein, Ralph Cornejo, and Sal Roselli. There are countless times that I have come to depend on the sage advice and comforting words of Kelly Gray, Grace Regullano, Luis Bocaletti, Francisco Cendejas, Abid Yahya, and Brian McNamara as both fellow organizers and very close friends. I hope the healthcare workers and labor organizers I have worked with and alongside recognize this book as both a joyful praise and respectful critique of the work and courage it takes to organize for new futures.

Although the observations that sparked me to write this book have origins in my experience as a union organizer, I could not have written it without the academic community that helped me hone the skills and methods to turn thought into research and research into writing. The Department of American Studies and Ethnicity at the University of Southern California served as an amazing starting point. I am thankful for Laura Pulido, Juan De Lara, Andrew Curtis, Andrew Lakoff, Dorinne Kondo, George Sanchez, Jack Halberstam, John Carlos Rowe, Manuel Pastor, Karen Halttunen, Karen Tongson, Maria Elena Martinez, Nayan Shah, Phil Ethington, Robin Kelley, Sarah Gualtieri, Sarah Banet-Weiser, Simeon Man, Suzy Woo, and Viet Nguyen. I certainly could not have finished this dissertation without smiles, advice, cheering, and friendly reminders from Kitty Lai, Jujuana Preston, and Sonia Rodriguez. I had a dream committee of scholars led by Nayan Shah that included George Sanchez, Juan De Lara, Jack Halberstam, and Bill Deverell.

Especially after a long period of time working outside of academia, the Department of American Studies and Ethnicity provided life-giving space and community to belong and contribute to that was both sustaining and nourishing. I want to thank Jih-Fei Cheng, Emily Raymundo, Emmett Harsin Drager, Quinn Anex-Reis, Sarah E. K. Fong, Cristina Faiver, Rosanne Sia, Bekah Park, Jenny Hoang, Crystal Baik, Genevieve Carpio, Celeste Menchaca, Ryan Fukumori, Umayyah Cable, Jessie Young, Sophia Azeb, Colby Lenz, Christina Heatherton, Kai Green, Analena Hope, Treva Ellison, Jessi Quizar, Huibin Amee Chew, Priscilla Leiva, Sriya Shrestha, David Stein, Deb Al-Najjar, Sabrina Howard, Joshua Mitchell, Flori Boj Lopez, Jess Lovaas, Laura Fugikawa, Mark Padoongpatt, Anjali Nath, Divana Olivas, Jennifer Tran, Alvaro Marquez, Jed Samer, Micha Cardenas, Christian Paiz, David-James Gonzales, Max Felker-Kantor, and Alicia Gutierrez-Romine. Joseph Bernardo, Jennifer Nazareno, Precious Singson,

Mark Pangalingan, Mark John Sanchez, Emily Raymundo, Genevieve Clutario, and James Zarsadiaz have also played an important role in helping me stay connected to my first academic passion—Filipino and Filipino American Studies. All of you have continued to support my work despite distance in time and space.

Brown University's Center for the Study of Slavery and Justice, Cogut Institute for the Humanities, and the Department of Africana Studies was a perfect space for me to deepen my understanding of the long-lasting impact of slavery on the history of medicine. I want to thank Tony Bogues, Amanda Anderson, and Brian Meeks for their leadership during my time as the Mellon Postdoctoral Fellow of Race and Science in Medicine. I am also grateful for support from Maiyah Gamble-Rivers, Shana Weinberg, Diane Straker, and Catherine Van Amburgh. I cherish the friendships I developed with Zachary Sell, Crystal Nicole Eddins, and Laura Garbes. While living in Providence, Felicia Bevel, Felicia Denaud, Bedour Alagraa, Emma Amador, Matthew Guterl, Francoise Hamlin, Debbie Weinstein, Naoko Shibusawa, Daniel Rodriguez, Leticia Alvarado, Elena Shih, Keisha-Khan Perry, Leon Hilton Jr., Jasmine Johnson, Christine Mok, and Sarah Wilbur were incredible champions for my scholarship. Without Lundy Braun, this project would never have been completed. I am eternally grateful to Lundy for taking a chance on supporting my scholarship.

My time at Drexel University was incredibly formative in the creation of this book. I am thankful for the leadership of David Brown, Kelly Joyce, Norma Bouchard, Tiago Saraiva, Jonathan Seitz, Amy Slaton, Abioseh Porter, Jennifer Yusin, Chloe Silverman, and Kristene Unsworth for leading the dizzying array of appointments and affiliations that I am fortunate to have been a part of. The entire place would not be able to run without the expertise of Irene Cho, Khushi Patel, Sharon Eichelberger, Jessica Greene, Jackie Rios, Liz Heenan, Sharde Johnson, Jennifer Thorndike-Gonzales, Melissa Johnson, and Kate Hughes. Debjani Bhattacharyya, Adam Knowles, Gabriel Rocha, and Alden Young welcomed me to Drexel with open arms. Scott Knowles, Don Stevens, Lloyd Ackert, Jesse Ballenger, Sharonna Pearl, Scott Hanson, Jonson Miller, Toni Pitock, Ros Remer, and Kathy Steen have all been amazing colleagues in the History Department. I am eternally grateful for my fellow interdisciplinary colleagues in Africana Studies (Jakeya Caruthers, Tasneem Siddiqui, Sonia Vaz Borges), Gender and Sexuality Studies (Liz Polcha and Mercer Gary), the Center for Science, Technology, and Society (Alberto Morales), and at the Ubuntu Center (Sharelle Barber,

Jennifer Ware, and Tanisha Barnes). I cherish my friendships with Meg Guliford, Ayden Scheim, Linda Kim, Amy Auchincloss, Francis Tanglao Aguas, Sue Bell, Mary Ebeling, Nada Matta, Kelly Underman, Amelia Hoover Green, Cara Scharf, Alexis Schulman, and Rebecca LeFevre.

I am blessed to have had the opportunity to spend time at the University of Pennsylvania as a Ford Postdoctoral Fellow in the Program on Race, Science, and Society. Hafeeza Anchrum, Maddie Johnson, Karen Tani, Jasmine Harris, Sebastian Gil-Raino, Susan Lindee, Beth Linker, Beans Velocci, Sam Schrivar, Zehra Hashmi, and Gavriel Cupita-Zorn have made Penn a second home. Dorothy Roberts is legendary and I cannot thank her enough for her lasting support for my scholarship. A whole host of great people—Lauren Gutterman, Steve Hoelscher, Stephanie Kaufman, Alex Beasley, Iván Chaar López, Lina Chhun, Cary Cordova, Janet Davis, Randy Lewis, Stephen Marshall, Julia Mickenberg, Sage Ponder, Shirley Thompson, Eric Tang, Abena Osseo-Assare, and Cathy Schlund-Vials—have welcomed me in as a colleague at the University of Texas at Austin. I am excited to finish this book and launch the next project at such an intellectually rich space.

There are a host of archivists and special collections staff who have not only helped me with this book but have helped me teach elements related to it in the classroom. Peter Blodgett of the Huntington Library; Russell Johnson at UCLA's Darling Biomedical Library; Brian McNerney and Allen Fisher of the LBJ Presidential Library; Masoud Farajpour, Yuriy Shcherbina, Susan Hikida, and Daniel O'Brien of USC's Special Collections; Kendra Gonzalez at Cal State Northridge's Tom and Ethel Bradley Center; John Anderies and Bob Skiba of the William Way LGBT Center's John Wilcox, Jr. Archives; Loni Shibuyama and Bud Thomas of the ONE Archives at USC; Matt Herbison at Drexel University's Legacy Center; Matt Lyons, Simon Ragovin, and Matthew Sherman of Drexel University's Special Collections; Raul Pizano of UCSB's Special Collections; Lisa Marine of the Wisconsin Historical Society; and Sye Gutierrez and Christina Rice of the Los Angeles Public Library, have all been helpful in the making of this book.

A humbling number of folks have offered feedback and their time at various stages of writing this book. I want to thank Christina Hanhardt, Adria Imada, Cindy I-Fen Cheng, Jane Hong, Mari Yoshihara, Daniel HoSang, Regina Kunzel, Chandan Reddy, Nancy Tomes, Kathleen Jones, Alyosha Goldstein, Natalia Molina, John McKiernan-Gonzales, Alexandra Stern, Douglas Haynes, Laura Barraclough, Elliott Powell, Darius Bost, Cathy Cohen, Stephen Colbrook, Rebecca Davis, David Helps, Scott Larsen, Lina-

Maria Murillo, and Natalie Lira. The book was particularly enriched by invited talks initiated by Kirsten Ostherr, Ileen Devault, Paul Ortiz, Lauren Gutterman, Randy Lewis, Stephanie McCormick, Bonnie Lucero, Jenny Reardon, Mark Jerng, Andrew Karhl, Deborah McDowell, Fiona Vernal, Carolyn Calloway-Thomas, Jeffrey McCune, Alden Young, Dietrich Neumann, Jeffrey Hegelson, Benny Andres, and Danielle Egan. I cannot thank Emily Hobson, Myrl Beam, Katie Batza, and Salonee Bhaman enough for our collective "BIAD" writing group. Zach Sell, Sam Schotland, and Christian Paiz a million thanks for reading various drafts of this book multiple times.

There are a number of people in the fields of history of medicine and science for whom I am extremely thankful. These folks include Janet Golden, Nancy Tomes, Kathleen Jones, Susan Reverby, Beatrix Hoffman, Ted Brown, Harold Braswell, Mical Raz, Debbie Doroshow, Naomi Rogers, Joanna Radin, John Warner, Jeremy Greene, Christopher Crenner, Dennis Doyle, Jason Chernesky, Laura Hirschbein, Jacob Steere-Williams, Christy Slobogin, Alex Parry, Scottie Buehler, Allison Law, and Ben Schneider. I must give particular thanks to those who share my interest in the overlap between race and medicine. I am lucky to be in the company of folks like Ayah Nuriddin, Antoine Johnson, Abena Osseo-Assare, Dierdre Cooper Owens, Samuel Roberts, Jr., Carolyn Roberts, Christopher Willoughby, Rana Hogarth, Adam Biggs, Jason Glenn, Keith Wailoo, George Aumoithe, Merlin Chowkwanyun, Aishah Scott, Richard Mizelle, Pablo Gomez, Tali Ziv, and Matthew Edwards.

It has been a personal goal of mine to bridge the gap between the work of clinicians and the work of medical humanities scholars. Dannie Ritchie, Ry Garcia-Sampson, Steven Rougas, Joe Diaz, and Sara Skeels at Brown University's Alpert School of Medicine and School of Public Health; Shamser Samra, Matthew Hing, Daniel Kennedy, Marcia Meldrum, and Philippe Bourgois at UCLA's Medical School and Medical Humanities Program; Jeremy Greene, Alexandre White, Maggie Cogswell, and Marian Robbins at Johns Hopkins University; Alyssa Basmajian at Columbia University's Mailman School of Public Health; Devon Golaszewski and Gideon Manning at Cedars-Sinai Medical School; Matthew Edwards at Stanford's School of Medicine; Mical Raz and Christy Slobogin at the University of Rochester's Corner Society; and Dorothy Roberts and Hafeeza Anchrum at University of Pennsylvania Program in Race, Science, and Society have all been critical to facilitating conversations with clinicians. I hope to continue these conversations in the future.

I have been lucky to have had a long line of brilliant students who have contributed their thoughts to this book and have enriched my journey during their time in my classroom. I want to thank Lyle Cherneff, Bethlehem Desta, Tali Ginsburg, Stefanie Lyn Kaufman-Mthimkhulu, Shio Lim, Lily Meyersohn, Andy Pham, Rowan Potter, Brooch Solomon, Edward Tie, Yema Yang, Erin West, Dominick Armato, Summer Benbrook, Hunter Cheng, Anaya Cherry, Cameron Collar, Violet Collins, Izzy Curtin, Trinity DuBois, A.J. Easterday, Rim Es-Sagar, Athina Filipos, Nathaniel Ferrari, Stephanie Garcia, Cameron Glowacki, Marie Goulis, Kim Gui, Mia Hernandez, Cole Hunt, Charlotte Ingram, Emma Johnson, Miranda Johnston, Em Krajc, Blue Koenig, Ava Koloseike, Stephen Lang, Victoria Lang, Zack Levy-Dyer, Robin Lumbard, Faizan Malik, Claire Manigo-Bizzell, Jada Mapp, Chelsea Martin, Luke Matheson, Bailey Michalak, Madison Mies, Emory Morgan, Nathan Nazario, Gabby Olivares, Michael O'Neill, Nora Pav, Macie Perry, Ryan Pomales, Brooke Quigley, Victoria Rodriguez, Izzy Sangaline, Sol Seales, Jack Schruender, Ange Seak, Arjun Sethi, Anna Shetler, Abby Tinzberg, Faya Tekyane, Ken Turner, Lauren Warda, Cianni Williams, and Bug Wylie-Chaney. I am particularly indebted to Yala Tippett, who read the final manuscript in its entirety and provided critical feedback. I am proud to not only call Alex Burnett, a former mentee of mine, a coauthor but also a fellow scholar.

In addition to the research support of the Mellon and Ford Foundations, this book also received significant support from the Consortium of History of Science, Technology, and Medicine, the Huntington Library, and the John and Randolph Haynes Foundation. The project also benefited from grant support from the Lyndon Baines Johnson Presidential Library, the Darling Biomedical Library at UCLA, USC Graduate School, USC Department of American Studies, USC Center for Law, History, and Culture, USC Transpacific Studies Center, and USC Dornsife College of Arts, Letters, and Sciences. Significant support for copyediting, map generation, and obtaining image permissions and releases came from Drexel University's College of Arts and Sciences and the University of California Press's First Gen Program. I am particularly indebted to the editorial and indexing expertise and cartographic eye of Paula Dragosh, Mark Mastromarino, and Tyler Munn. The fruits of all that support include several article prizes that appear in this book in adapted forms. I thank the prize selection committees for the *Journal of History of Medicine and Allied Science*'s Stanley Jackson Prize, the Western History Association's Ray Allen

Billington Prize, the Committee of LGBT Historians' Audre Lorde Prize, and the American Studies Association's Wise-Sussman Prize.

I have been supported since graduating by a number of legendary mentors who have supported me in amazing ways. I want to particularly thank Nayan Shah, Dorothy Roberts, Nancy Tomes, Martin Summers, Regina Kunzel, Jack Halberstam, Sam Roberts, William Deverell, Amanda Anderson, and Christina Hanhardt for their willingness to support my scholarship in the most crucial ways. Nayan, in particular, has been an unwavering champion for my scholarship and I am convinced that the best parts of this book can be attributed to his mentorship and friendship. It is a dream to have my book published in the American Crossroads series. I believe the book is one hundred percent better because of the mentorship and critical feedback given to me by George Lipsitz, Laura Briggs, and the anonymous reviewers who read earlier versions of this book. The staff at UC Press has been amazing. Thanks to Niels Hooper, Nora Becker, Chad Attenborough, Raina Polivka, Catherine Osborne, Teresa Iafolla, and Francisco Reinking.

I know that this entire project would not have been possible without the faith and support of my parents, Nicanor and Rosalinda; my older brother, Neal, and his wife, Damaris, and their children, Dany and Jade; and my little brother Norman. Since meeting Michael, my family has grown to include the love and support of Larry, Jackie, Karen, Tim, Roger, Deb, Carver, Joe, JT, Tucker, Lauren, and Maeve. In addition to my family, I cannot express how grateful I am for my chosen family. Jollene Levid, Hans Dumayag, and Charlene Manalo have been with me in this journey from the very beginning. Without them, and the love and time they have given me, this project would not have been possible.

This project is what it is because of Michael Carver. No one has ever seen me as vulnerable and as strong as he has seen me. He encouraged me to continue with the book and with this career when I was not sure I would ever finish it.

Introduction

FREE MARKET HEALTHCARE, IN FULL COLOR

I FIRST SET FOOT on King-Drew Medical Center's main campus in the summer of 2005. As a staff member for the largest intern and resident physicians' union in the nation, I was sent there by union leadership to help King-Drew's resident physician members submit testimony to protest the Los Angeles County Board of Supervisors' decision to close the center's acute obstetric and gynecological services. King-Drew's resident physician leaders argued that the consequences of closing the hospital's obstetrical and gynecological services were a simple matter of life and death for a majority of LA's poorest people of color, many of whom lived within a ten-mile radius from the center. In a region where an estimated 2.5 million people were uninsured, King-Drew not only tended to the poorest and sickest patients in Los Angeles County but also served those most vulnerable to police harassment and deportation as Black and Brown people and undocumented immigrants.

Many resident physician leaders, however, framed the consequences of ending services for pregnant and recently pregnant people in terms that they believed the supervisors would find more compelling. Instead of focusing on the personal crises and individual consequences facing poor and undocumented people of color, several doctors argued that shutting down the hospital's services would have a dire impact on the operation and profitability of LA's *for-profit* healthcare system. As one physician argued, private hospitals surrounding King-Drew depended on its existence because, as he phrased it, their physicians "are not familiar nor are they excited, to put it nicely, about serving King-Drew patients."[1] By appealing to King-Drew's economic identity as a containment and management system for sickness and poverty, these physicians appealed to the Board of Supervisors' identity as trustees of the region's taxpaying voters and guardians of the region's reputation as a business-friendly destination for those seeking health and sunshine. According to these doctors, the burden of taking care of the poorest and most expensive patients would soon, like contagion, overwhelm and close private hospitals outside and on the border of King-Drew's health service area.

Such a sobering analysis of the political-economic relationships between public and private hospital care starkly contrasted with the Board of Supervisors' decision, nearly forty years prior, to designate King-Drew as an economic development engine to eradicate poverty in the city's Black neighborhoods. The decision to build the medical center was as a direct response to the 1965 Watts Uprisings, a weeklong rebellion in "the late, hot summer of 1965."[2] Initially sparked by an incident of police brutality on the evening of August 11, 1965, involving Marquette Frye and his mother, Rena Price, the uprisings drew national attention to the problem of economic racism and police brutality after an estimated ten thousand protestors took to the streets to cause nearly $40 million in property damage.

After the uprisings, the fear of more violence prompted LA's leaders to experiment with novel ways to govern race and contain poverty. The medical center they created sought to do more than just provide medical services and jobs to previously excluded Black citizens by attempting to manipulate the perceived backwards sexual culture of poor Black people. It aimed to assist Black male heads of households and every member of their families achieve an individual state of health beyond the absence of disease or illness itself by extending ideas of welfare and well-being culturally associated with the stable employment, health coverage, homeownership, and heteropatriarchal family life of white suburbanites to those living in Black neighborhoods. In so doing, the medical center's proponents, like former CIA Director and chair of the Post-Watts Riots Commission John McCone, hoped its services could help society avoid more punitive and costly responses to poverty like policing.[3]

This book examines the period between King-Drew's origin as an antipoverty program in the late 1960s through its transition into an institution designed to help municipal leaders contain and manage poverty by the mid-1980s. These two decades correspond with a period many scholars refer to as LA's rebirth as a "global city" inclusive and welcoming to racial and sexual minorities of all stripes.[4] White politicians and businessmen had overseen the city's development as an exemplary Western US city for white settlement since the late nineteenth century. But the rise of Los Angeles as a "global city" for multicultural racial and sexual diversity after the 1960s was marked by the joint efforts of white liberal progressives and Black, Spanish-speaking, Asian American, and gay activists to redirect public resources to make the regional economy inclusive for all its citizens. Although leadership certainly became more diverse in composition, the racial and sexual representation of LA's diversity did little to lower rates of poverty and sickness for its queer, trans, and poor people of color.

In the latter half of the twentieth century a series of contradictions defined race and sexuality in American cultural discourse. After World War II, disavowal of formal state-sanctioned racism occurred alongside new economic and diplomatic relations between the United States and newly independent Asian, African, and Latin American nations to remake the contours of everyday public discussions of race in the United States. In the 1950s, ideas of racial liberalism became ascendent as the civil rights movement began to put an end to Jim Crow's legal segregation.[5] By the 1960s and 1970s, these ideas were further elaborated upon to include new ideas of sexual liberalism and cultural nationalism and were bolstered by Great Society initiatives such as Medicare, Medicaid, and antipoverty programs.[6] A greater number of American citizens looked to the election of Black and openly gay officials, integrated neighborhoods, women in corporate leadership, and society's greater tolerance for discourses of Black nationalism, feminism, and gay pride as proof that the nation's diversity was its greatest resource.[7]

Yet, in this era, federal policies tightened access to housing, employment, and healthcare by supporting economic development policies privatizing healthcare, housing, and education. Federal policies further assisted big-city governments and employers with the transition of the nation's postwar economy from a dominant manufacturing base to one centered on financialization and global trade.[8] Although the emergence of this new "global economy" created conditions for inflation and deindustrialization within and beyond the nation's borders, the emergence of a new "service" economy helped augur the inclusion of middle-class racial and sexual elites into "mainstream" society while renewing the criminalization and policing of queer, trans, undocumented, and poor people of color.[9] Rather than attribute the nation's higher rates of unemployment, worklessness, and working poverty to global economic restructuring, white voters and taxpayers interpreted widespread economic crisis as a problem of racialized sexuality. In response they voted for measures to enhance and revitalize existing forms of residential racial segregation, securitize mental health settings, and increase police and prison forces to target undocumented families, women of color on welfare, queer and trans people of color, and so-called absent fathers and wild youth for harassment, caging, and deportation.[10]

Health as Property places the history and development of King-Drew's health system at the crossroads of these economic transitions by exploring the contradictions of liberal democracy, racial capitalism, and sexual liberalism as LA's leaders guided the city's economic development away from a manufacturing economy to a global economy under new racially and sexually liberal discourses of inclusion. These discourses replaced older racist beliefs that Black people were biologically and inherently incapable of being sexually normal and healthy with new developmental discourses focused on reforming the supposedly "backward" spatialized sexuality, reproductive politics, and "culture" of poor, queer, and trans people of color. New scientific discourses of racial and sexual liberalism made it possible for people to think of individuals once thought incapable of self-governance, such as Black and gay people, as suddenly capable of being "normal," healthy, and responsible.

While many white voters by the 1960s accepted these new ideas enough that Black politicians could be elected and Black physicians could be appointed to lead public health programs in Black neighborhoods, Black politicians and physicians confronted the fact that they still needed to service and prioritize the interests of white voters and taxpayers in order to carry out any plan to advance economic development and community self-determination programs in Black neighborhoods. Locked out from accessing credit through traditional banks and businesses, Black leaders and activists turned to the ballot box to access the capital needed to fight poverty and illness. However, like a loan requiring more credit, Black leaders often found they needed more money to fight the scale of poverty illness fostered under racial capitalism than white citizens were willing to part with or give their consent to.

As power brokers betwixt and between LA's Black and white neighborhoods, the city's newly empowered Black political leaders made decisions about the healthcare of people living in Black neighborhoods that were not necessarily aligned with what people living in Black neighborhoods considered good for themselves. Instead, Black community leaders often made decisions based on whether they believed white voters and taxpayers were likely to tolerate those decisions or support them outright. Derrick Bell, the foundational critical race theorist, famously referred to this phenomena by the late 1970s as the "interest convergence dilemma."[11] Tracing the lackluster responses to school desegregation policies in the twenty years after the passage of *Brown v. Board of Education*, Bell posited that Black people's interests in achieving racial equality in a society previously structured by racial inequality would only be accommodated when those interests converged with those of middle- and upper-class white people.

For Bell, ending racism is not just about a "series of quaint customs that can be remedied effectively without altering the status of white people" but also about ending a system that "require[s] the surrender of racism-granted privileges for whites."[12] As his phrasing "racism-granted privileges" denotes, racism is not nor has ever been about whether *all* white people materially hold or retain the privileges afforded to them. Instead, racism is defined by whether white people believe that society reserves those privileges for them as rights over others with darker skin color. According to Bell, it was this "potential sacrifice" of surrendering the literal and figurative properties of citizenship previously reserved for white people under racism, such as decent housing, education, and healthcare, that animated voter and taxpayer defiance to true racial equality after the *Brown* decision.[13]

Rather than being about ending the "immorality of racial inequality," Bell's concept of the interest convergence dilemma reveals that the appearance of racial justice more often than not masks how courts and policy leaders have used discourses of racial liberalism to further advance the interests of white voters and taxpayers.[14] Indeed, Bell argues that the court's rulings during the civil rights movement encouraged "those whites in policymaking positions" to recognize and take advantage of the potential "economic and political advances at home and abroad that would follow abandonment of segregation."[15] As business leaders looked to industrialize the US agrarian South, redevelop abandoned city centers, and invest in new foreign markets in Europe, Asia, Latin America, and Africa, the idea of racial inclusion domestically and diplomatically seemed like a practical way to "secure, advance, or at least not harm societal interests deemed important by middle and upper class whites."[16] In short, for some middle and upper class white people, certain forms of racial liberalism after the 1960s took the place of racism in securing progress and advancement for white communities. That is, racial liberalism functioned to further advance the political and economic interests of those already in power by protecting the property, rights, and safety they enjoyed previously under more racially exclusionary regimes.

The effect of these political and economic relationships made the white taxpayer and the "likely voter" a ghost referent in every aspect of King-Drew's history by positioning its construction and medical services as a line of credit that local Black leaders and their allies accepted as part of a larger political bargain. For Black political leaders and Black physicians from Los Angeles to Washington, DC, the scale and capital of building a Black-led health system was seen as a way to arm Black people with the resources that enabled them to see a future without the imposition of white control over their lives and neighborhoods. The ability to complete this vision, however, required Black political leaders to convince white voters to extend their line of credit to Black economic development programs by supporting referendums favorable to that mission or electing officials who allocated budgets aligned with that goal.

Leaders empowered to oversee King-Drew's operations made calculated decisions on how to discuss the importance of caring for Black citizens who often lived far from many white voters and with whom white voters rarely had daily interactions. King-Drew's academic leaders and board of directors, for instance, hoped to ease growing concern about welfare dependency by designing the center as a new kind of public-private venture that initially would be costly but eventually would be profitable as Black citizens used its services and employment opportunities to lift themselves out of poverty. When eradicating poverty appeared improbable by the early 1970s, Black political leaders sold the costs related to purveying publicly funded hospital, clinic, and housing services as essential in combating homelessness and urban deterioration in white neighborhoods by helping poor people of color to deliberately live in certain neighborhoods and work for lower pay. By the 1980s, Black leaders even began defending King-Drew's importance in contributing new research to emergency medicine through its treatment of gunshot wounds and stabbing victims.

These efforts deepened the asymmetries of power associated with race and sexuality by creating mechanisms for inclusion and progress for some members of historically excluded groups while revitalizing practices of violence and exclusion for those who were already the most vulnerable under prevailing systems of exclusion. King-Drew's services, for instance, provided more opportunities for some people of color to get meaningful employment and healthcare. King-Drew also permitted some physicians of color to overcome structural barriers and gain advanced medical training. It additionally provided some medical academicians with a chance to craft culturally competent medical care.

Yet, King-Drew's overall mission ultimately advanced the public safety and property interests of white citizens who lived far outside its health system boundaries by containing and managing poverty in neighborhoods of color. By no longer seeing poverty as a negative or undesirable trend, the city's and county's investments in managing poverty through expanded hospital, clinic, and emergency room services throughout the 1970s helped city leaders concentrate poverty in neighborhoods just outside of urban revitalization zones. Such investments made LA into a virtual "company town" by encouraging global corporations relocating to its revived downtown to unburden themselves of covering healthcare benefits for the region's lowest paid workers. This taxpayer corporate subsidy drove economic growth by securing cheap workers for a new "global" economy and demarcated a new "thin blue line" for policing based on where LA's private healthcare markets ended and its "medically underserved areas" began. Instead of meeting the health service needs and expectations of the poor, these processes ultimately helped insulate white workers, their neighborhoods, and their private community hospitals from the most volatile effects of global capitalist restructuring by leaving poor people of color exposed to greater rates of violence, sickness, and poverty.

ORGANIZED EMPLOYMENT

Health as Property provides an alternative history from those recently written about the history of urban medical centers in the late twentieth century. Urban historians of healthcare have partly accounted for the revival of city centers since the 1960s by tracing the rise of academic medical centers, an institution emblematic of the shift from the nation's postwar manufacturing economy to one centered on the transaction of personal consumer services in the areas of health, finance, law, education, and real estate. This shift not only changed the nature of work and employment itself but also helped reverse the center of employment away from suburbs back to city centers. Whereas workers once looked forward to stable employment and suburban homeownership after high school by producing tangible goods at a manufacturing plant, workers by the 1980s required a college degree or specialized training to approximate the same level of housing and comfort as pre-1970s factory workers by selling intangible products, such as medical, legal, and financial expertise, that those with accumulated wealth needed.[17]

Academic medical centers buffered the patterns of unemployment and poverty unleashed by this transition by helping regions reabsorb workers laid off or terminated from manufacturing jobs into a new service economy. By linking patient care-focused private health institutions often found in suburbs with the research-focused public health institutions frequently located in city centers, academic medical centers also helped city leaders reverse the flow of capital and people between suburbs and inner cities by giving rise to the modern-day acute care health system. Corporate health systems thus bring the once scattered and loosely connected elements of pre-1960s private physician groups, clinics, laboratories, and X-ray services into greater alignment with the research, teaching, and training objectives associated with academic medicine and teaching hospitals found in urban centers.[18]

The accumulation of all available regional healthcare dollars in the hands of research-focused medical center leaders not only helps account for the economic activity of neighborhoods surrounding regional medical centers but also explains the global reach of some of their increasingly specialized services. Often the largest employer in their respective cities and regions, academic health systems have helped big-city governments avoid bankruptcy by infusing their tax bases with stable well-paid workers once lost to suburbs after World War II and by making city centers attractive for an elite set of financial-sector workers that city leaders regarded as vital for linking their regional economies with the rest of the world. By the 1980s and 1990s, the wealth associated with academic medical centers made it possible for many to advertise themselves as the only places in the world specializing in the treatment of certain rare diseases and illnesses.

The tremendous economic output associated with academic medical centers helps account for why municipal leaders in Los Angeles saw extreme promise in building a Black-led academic medical center as an economic development machine to lift the wages and healthcare standards of workers and physicians living in the city's Black neighborhoods. However, unlike most academic medical centers that continued to prioritize the employment of white workers and professionals, King-Drew's strategy specifically sought to avoid the Black displacement and "slum clearance" that usually follow urban renewal programs centered on the growth of downtown academic medical centers. This book seeks to unpack a central contradiction in the rise of the healthcare industry: Why did the success of economic development programs centered on lifting wages, medical knowledge, and health standards through academic medical centers in city centers not translate to leaders and institutions who were committed to training Black physicians, employing Black workers, and serving Black patients? How, in other words, did efforts to serve the health interests of Black people end up serving the interests of white voters and taxpayers?

Accounting for this contradiction requires calling attention to how society has "organized employment" to benefit certain workers and types of work over others based on race, sexuality, and class. My use of *organized employment* refers to the strategies, tactics, and practices that political actors deploy to order and distribute the basic necessities for reproducing life (such as healthcare, housing, income security, and education) to achieve an idealized arrangement of waged and salaried employment. Paying attention to how certain kinds of work (salaried work, waged work, unpaid housework) are valorized based on workers' race, gender, class, and sexuality not only illuminates how certain types of laborers are considered "fit" for privileged roles in society as leaders or physicians but also highlights how their labor relates to the labor of other workers (both working and not working) in a larger political economy.

Black community leaders and physicians in the 1960s confronted a landscape where Southern congressional leaders and Southern physicians had facilitated the nationalization of Jim Crow through the expansion of the federal government in the mid-twentieth century. Starting in the 1930s, Southern congressional leaders used their power to organize employment through the New Deal and GI Bill to benefit white male breadwinners through federal job programs; generous low-cost loan programs for housing, education, and business ownership; and expanded protections for worker participation in unions.[19] The American Medical Association supported racial segregation in healthcare by opposing federal efforts to mandate desegregation in hospitals receiving federal funds. Although legislatively written without specific mentions of race, these programs almost entirely bypassed Black workers by empowering local actors to apply racially discriminatory practices in implementing federal programs and by making industries with the highest proportion of Black workers—agricultural and domestic services—ineligible for labor protections.

These programs worked in tandem with previous efforts by Southern white physicians to consolidate capital, power, and authority in the hands of white male physicians to corporatize medicine in the form of academic medical centers. Starting with the exclusion of Black physicians from the American Medical Association at the end of Reconstruction, white physician leaders used their power to exclude Black students, medical graduates, and physicians-in-training from achieving each new step that "organized medicine" introduced to authenticate physicians as experts.[20] By the 1960s, health insurance companies helped racialize medical care by regularly denying malpractice insurance to Black physicians. By normalizing and naturalizing income security, health insurance, union membership, and housing as benefits conferred on women by marriage or on children by familial obedience to white male breadwinners, the organization of both employment and medicine since the end of Reconstruction helped consolidate a series of modern amenities offered via the free market, such as housing and healthcare, as properties of whiteness by the 1960s.

Although hopeful, Black political leaders were unsure if the congressional passage of new antipoverty legislation and Medicare and Medicaid proposed by President Lyndon B. Johnson could help break the marginalization of Black workers and physicians given how organized labor and organized medicine continued to prioritize employment and training for white men. In fact, the Watts Uprisings in late 1965 were an opportunity for Black leaders to criticize how the implementation of the federal government's incentive-based antipoverty programs since 1963 had failed both to entice the nation's largest employers to relocate to Black neighborhoods and to inspire union leaders and members to desegregate membership by opening up apprenticeship and training programs for more Black workers. Black physicians, on the other hand, worried new health laws would empower white hospital owners and physicians to tighten their grip on Black patient populations by effectively subsidizing the corporate takeover of Black medical markets that Black physicians saw as properly theirs.

Established at the margins of not only private employment and organized labor but also organized medicine, Black leaders and physicians in Los Angeles helped renew a debate about the relationship between Black freedom and economic dependence that was already nearly a hundred years old. Now famously played out in high schools as a contest between Booker T. Washington and W. E. B. Du Bois, Washington's "cast down your bucket" thesis argued that Black workers laboring under the free wage labor regime of white employers could serve as a foundation for Black people that would eventually lead to the development of Black capital and economic independence through Black entrepreneurship. Skeptical, however, that white employers would ever concede to labor arrangements conducive to the interests of Black workers, Du Bois famously argued in his "talented tenth" thesis that it was necessary to protect the interests of the race by trusting the economic development of Black people to Black professionals and businessmen. White employers allied with Washington, however, rarely supported Black workers' goals to achieve Black freedom and economic independence. At the same time, Black professionals, businessmen, and physicians allied with Du Bois rarely held the capital to successfully dislodge the grip that poverty and predatory white medicine held on Black workers' lives.

Black politicians and physicians renewed this debate by urging local politicians and taxpayers to help them organize employment in favor of Black workers and physicians. By approaching King-Drew as a proposal to organize employment in ways that contested older approaches, *Health as Property* unifies the fields of labor studies and the history of medicine to surface working-class histories and social movements that exceed or cannot be contained by traditional scholarly approaches to "organized labor" and "organized medicine." While scholars in labor history have given us indispensable accounts of how Black worker activism forwarded racial justice aims within "organized labor," their work also points to how Black labor leaders not only blurred the lines between labor and other broader social movements—such as socialism, civil rights, and Black Power movements—but also blurred traditional economic distinctions around "class."[21]

Scholars of the Black middle class note that many Black professionals continued to identify with the Black working class out of what Evelyn Brooks Higginbotham has called the "politics of respectability" and what Michael Dawson has referred to as "linked fate."[22] Since the "social component" and the "economic component" of Black people's lives "were forged during the historical experiences that linked a general subjugation of black life with economic domination by blacks by whites," Dawson argued that Black individuals could not be seen as successful by others without linking it to "group success."[23] As Mary Patillo argues, the service component of Black professionalism also drew upon the practical matter that—in the cases of Black doctors, undertakers, barbers, and insurance and real estate agents—poor and working-class counterparts were their only customers.[24] As "labor leaders" in their own right, many Black professionals took it upon themselves to not only see their plight as tied with the Black working class but also their collective destiny as tied to the legions of the Black unemployed.

The Watts Uprisings opened up an opportunity for Black community leaders to uplift the race because they furnished white establishment politicians and taxpayers in Los Angeles with the urgency and context to impart public money—in the form of a publicly funded Black-led academic medical center and expanded public health budgets—to experiment with federal programs to mount a form of organized employment now better known as "Black capitalism," a term describing consumer and business practices geared to channeling and rechanneling capital toward the development of Black spaces and people.[25] In short, a broad multiracial coalition of actors proposed fixing the problem of capital facing Black physicians and the problem of low purchasing power of Black workers by entrusting public infrastructure and capital to the entrepreneurial vision and leadership of free market–minded Black physician leaders from the National Medical Association.

For many Black physicians, advancing racial inclusion was not just a simple matter of accepting Black people *as is*. Many Black physicians supported new racial scientific theses positing that white supremacy and other structural barriers had stunted the individual sexual development of most poor Black people. In their opinion, the Black community's perceived high rates of "absentee fatherhood," "welfare motherhood," "juvenile delinquency," and homosexual behavior were "arrested" and "suspended" psychological states that illustrated what happened to individual human beings when they were deprived of full inclusion in civilized society. Discourses demonstrating how Black people were as distinctly gendered and sexually complex as heterosexual white men and women were thus not ancillary to ideas about economic development but were central to discussing the modernity of Black communities. They often were understood as both an indicator of Black people's receptiveness to economic development programs and as proof of economic development programs' successes.

In everyday practical terms, Black leaders and physicians operationalized these ideas by using King-Drew as an economic development machine geared toward universalizing employment among Black male breadwinners. King-Drew's designers held an expectation that the conferral of housing, income security, education, and healthcare on women and children through Black male breadwinners would, as it had for white breadwinners in white neighborhoods, incentivize marriage and respectable family life in Black neighborhoods. Planners also hoped that this unique arrangement would keep the dollars earned and spent by Black residents in Black neighborhoods to economically develop them in ways that would eventually match the services seen elsewhere. Although squarely operating in the United States, Black physicians at King-Drew sought to contribute new original knowledge to medicine by experimenting with health distribution models more popularly known as "global health," which sought to develop so-called underdeveloped health markets by balancing public health objectives and acute care services to stimulate free market activity.[26]

THE GREAT LEAP

The Los Angeles that Black leaders and physicians traversed in the 1960s did not have a simple dichotomous racial divide between Black and white residents. Instead, the city developed from the overlapping histories of the conquest of the American Southwest and the nationalization of Jim Crow. Beginning in the late nineteenth century, LA's "Anglo" elites organized employment to settle and build Los Angeles as a destination for white migrants by either attracting or coercively recruiting a diverse mix of ethnic white (such as those of Irish, Italian, and Jewish descent) and Native, African, Mexican, Filipino, Japanese, South Asian, and Chinese American workers to build the region's infrastructure and economy.[27] In the immediate aftermath of World War II, California's residential segregation patterns of dividing neighborhoods between white "Anglo" neighborhoods and nonwhite racially mixed neighborhoods made Los Angeles a popular new destination for Black migrants of the Second Great Migration.[28] The seemingly less strict enforcement of policing by skin color made California a particularly desirable location for Black physicians who saw the conviviality achieved between ethnic whites and people of color as an unprecedented opportunity to treat patients beyond poor Black populations.

However, the GI Bill and massive subsidies for defense industry manufacturers as the United States entered the Cold War dramatically reshaped LA's residential segregation patterns by triggering white flight at the same time that mechanization of agriculture in the US South and programs for Mexican agricultural workers pushed Black and Mexican migrants from their places of origin to California.[29] Alongside the exclusion of homosexuals and those suspected of being homosexual from federal programs, the various migration patterns set off by the war recomposed the landscape of Los Angeles, especially its once "mixed-race" neighborhoods that became more identifiable as three distinct "ghettos": a white ghetto known as a haven for white gays and lesbians west of downtown, a Black ghetto south of downtown, and a Spanish-speaking "barrio" east of downtown.[30] Perceptible to residents of color as an entirely new kind of "suburb" but overlooked by new white migrants as a new kind of "ghetto," however, was a corona of "integrated neighborhoods" that separated the city's new all-white suburbs from the inner city.[31] For anyone walking in a straight line from downtown to one of the city's suburbs, the sensation of postwar sprawl spatially manifested a racial and sexual hierarchy that placed those abandoned most by capital at

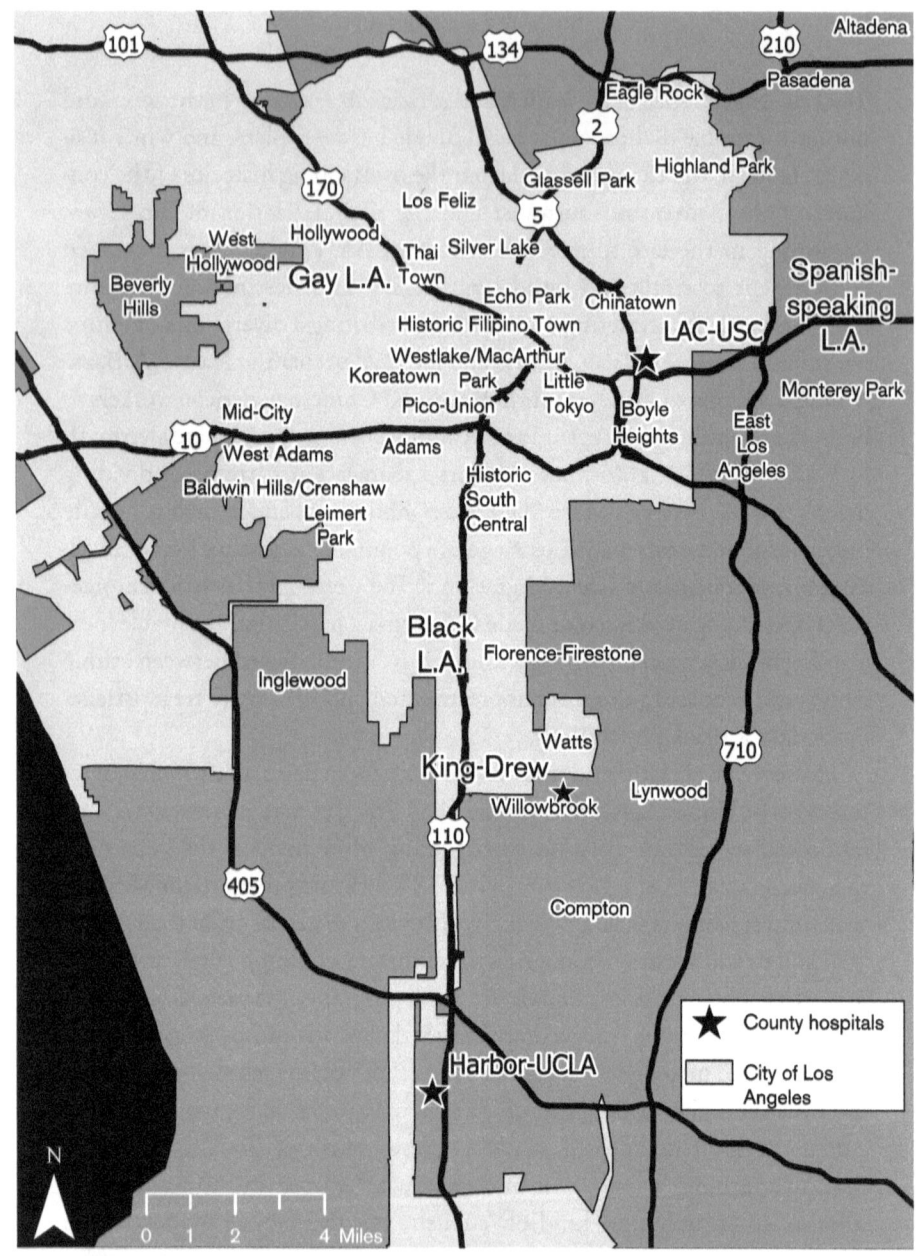

MAP 1. Spatial overview of Los Angeles

The nationalization of Jim Crow through the New Deal along with greater Black, Mexican, and gay migration to Los Angeles dramatically reshaped the city's post–World War II landscape. Shifting migration patterns from the 1930s to the 1960s recomposed the landscape of Los Angeles as its once "mixed-race" neighborhoods became more identifiable as three distinct "ghettos": a white ghetto known as a haven for white gays and lesbians west of downtown, a Black ghetto south of downtown, and a "Spanish-Speaking" "barrio" east of downtown. Map: Tyler Munn. Sources: Oceans (Natural Earth), City of LA Boundary (City of Los Angeles Hub), Neighborhood Boundaries (LA Times).

the city's center and those who most benefited from its development at its outer edges.

The 1965 Watts Uprisings represented a crisis point for the white elites who had ruled over the city's development since the late nineteenth century. The riots not only expressed Black claims for community self-rule and self-determination over their neighborhoods but also helped Chicano, gay, and Asian American activists make similar demands in their own by the early 1970s. As the most tangible product of community aspirations for self-rule, King-Drew's health institutions and programmatic rhetoric quickly served as durable and easily reproducible vehicles for mounting economic development programs as expressions of community "pride" campaigns in identity-based neighborhoods. In 1973, the political coalition built by the flowering of racial and cultural nationalist discourses in the city's Black, Chicano, Asian American, and gay neighborhoods helped lift Tom Bradley into the mayoral office, a feat heralded as a victory for civil rights and multiculturalism given that Bradley served as the first Black mayor of a city with a majority-white electorate.[32]

The revival of Black nationalism and the birth of the Black Power movement, however, made racial and sexual politics in Black Los Angeles as messy as the racial and sexual politics seen in the rest of the city. The sexual politics of King-Drew's economic development program cohered with the ascendence of the Black Panther Party, Ron Karenga's US organization, and the welfare rights and women's liberation movements.[33] The Black Panther Party and welfare rights activists, in particular, offered their own contending visions of organized employment that did not require a male breadwinner or unbridled capitalism to produce progress. As the 1970s wore on, Black activists fighting white supremacy, capitalism, and patriarchy found a terrain where the lines of division had become increasingly unclear. Whereas their targets in the mid-1960s consisted almost exclusively of white men, their conflicts by the early 1970s brought them face to face with Black leaders newly empowered to make decisions around Black health and welfare.

Although the battle for the hearts and minds of the Black masses in Los Angeles was by no means a bloodless affair, the discourses of normality and health offered by King-Drew's Black medical leaders offered everyday Black citizens an alluring and seductive form of politics that felt less confrontational, less violent, and less involved than the pathway offered by the Black Panther Party or welfare rights activists.[34] Like many Black scientists and physicians who used the terms of racial science in hopes of contesting it, King-Drew's Black physicians made arguments promoting traditional gender and sex roles within normative nuclear families to advance Black economic development.[35] In doing so, Black physicians breathed new life into discourses of racial science by propagating their own versions of culture of poverty theory, attributing crime to nonnormative sexual behavior, and treating violence as grounded in pathologies of Black culture rather than as a product of criminogenic conditions. In total, these theories posited a kind of developmental sequence that purportedly accounted for the persistent "under-development" of Black neighborhoods through phantasms of aberrant racialized sexualities, sexual cultures, and allegedly nonnormative sexual practices of women on welfare, absent fathers, promiscuous youth, and queer and trans people of color.

Twentieth-century versions of racial science allowed Black physicians to cultivate trust and intimacy with Black patients where white physicians participating in antipoverty health programs were less successful.[36] Although all physicians involved in antipoverty health programs attempted to use health services to convince Black citizens of the value of desiring work and family life as a key part of achieving individual health, white physicians' ability to inspire Black residents paled in comparison to the credibility of Black physicians and psychiatrists who argued that valuing work and family life were not only important to one's individual health but central to maximizing the health of the entire race. The belief that King-Drew's programs held the promise of unlocking antipoverty program objectives that might actually meet the objectives of getting Black men and women to value work and family helped garner support for its programs well after the initial fervor of support for antipoverty programs waned in the late 1960s.

Black politicians found the racial scientific discourses propagated by ostensibly racially and sexually liberal medical professionals as helpful in contesting anticapitalist visions of Black freedom, gay liberation, and welfare rights that threatened their vision of organized employment. New scientific ideas of racial and sexual normality in urban planning policies empowered local neighborhood leaders to normalize who, by new medical standards, counted as "normal" and police space according to new "community norms." While this helped win greater protection of privacy and property for those living in the city's gay neighborhoods by empowering white gay and lesbian leaders in those neighborhoods to defend themselves, their personhood, and their neighborhoods as "normal," the effect of defining racial normality as heterosexual effectively helped underwrite the policing and exclusion of queer and trans people of color throughout the city's neighborhoods. These processes ultimately re-enlivened the idea that only white people were capable of inhabiting the gender distinctiveness and sexual stability associated with modern sexuality and economic development regardless of whether they lived in gay neighborhoods or in the city's "straight" suburbs.

In general, the idea that nonnormative racialized sexualities, sexual practices, and sexual cultures accounted for Black poverty helped obscure how liberal politicians exploited this rhetoric to hide the deliberate manipulation of poverty to retool the region's economy. As the economic crisis increased in the 1970s, King-Drew's various community health programs helped bring the interests of local neighborhood leaders of color into greater alignment with the interests of global capitalists who saw the city's working poor as an essential workforce to remake Los Angeles into a new center for global finance capital. The rhetoric of Black nationalist clinics and the daily practice of providing health services that citizens were unlikely to find in other cities helped city leaders advertise downtown as a "business friendly" city. Its generous public health, housing, and transportation programs helped employers choose Los Angeles as a place to do business because they could pay workers less than a living wage and not provide private health insurance.

Although promoted by politicians as a solution to high taxes, new welfare reform programs supported by the region's multiracial elite to force poor mothers off welfare and back into working motherhood also did nothing to lower taxes or solve poverty for poor women. Long before Barbara Ehrenreich exposed large corporations like Walmart for employment practices encouraging employees to apply for welfare programs to supplement the company's low wages, the retooling of welfare programs in Los Angeles shows that city and county officials in the early 1970s deliberately engineered the spatial and political relationships that made corporations the true intended beneficiary of the region's welfare programs.[37] Under the banner of celebrating racial and ethnic identity of working-class neighborhoods of color, these programs hid how these initiatives supported global financial firms relocating to downtown. LA's near downtown neighborhoods of color supplied center city employers with cheap, flexible, and plentiful labor to clean and landscape luxury office buildings, hotels, and high-end apartment buildings; cook, serve, and cater food; and entertain, sell goods, and protect white workers returning to live in LA's inner city.

The result of these efforts in the eyes of Black leaders created a city where every neighborhood equally contributed to the health of the city's "global economy" through the interlocking spatial relationships made possible by the arrest and management of poverty in neighborhoods of color. In contrast to when employment opportunities were far from neighborhoods of color, the city's leaders welcomed the return of capital to city centers because they regarded "some work" in a chaotic economy as better than "no work" at all. Rather than regard underdevelopment as the absence of capitalist development, LA's multicultural leaders thus illustrated how capitalist development occurs, as Manning Marable argued, "*not in spite of* the exclusion of Blacks, *but because of* the brutal exploitation of Blacks as workers and consumers."[38]

Despite the fact that King-Drew and Los Angeles's Black neighborhoods served as both keystone and nucleus for the city's thriving regional economy, white voters and taxpayers by the 1980s withdrew their consent to fund public projects premised on racial and sexual inclusion. Instead of supporting the continuation of public funding for social services and employment programs for the poor, white voters responded to appeals by white conservative politicians by criminalizing and deporting Black and Brown citizens they perceived to be burdens on society. Symbolized by the passage of California Proposition 13 in 1978 and the election of President Ronald Reagan in 1980, white citizens reversed course and called in the line of credit that they gave King-Drew's leaders by shrinking the public hospital and clinic services it provided to poor people of color in order to prioritize the emergency medical services they found more compelling and useful for their individual health as they traveled throughout the city. The result diminished the hope that health could be as much a property of Blackness as whiteness.

FOR-PROFIT BIOMEDICINE AND SEXUAL CAPITALISM UNDER RACIAL CAPITALISM

Exploring the interest convergence between racial and sexual elites shows that society's shared belief that biomedical approaches to remedying poor health, illness, and bodily injury produce more favorable outcomes for society than supplying every citizen with decent housing, education, food security, basic healthcare, and income security is a faulty idea. By the 1960s, the premium on solving population health issues through biomedicine ensured that individuals, rather than governments, bore the brunt of responsibility for addressing large-scale public health problems. By the 1980s, this shift resulted in hospitals, pharmaceutical companies, and health insurance corporations holding greater power in determining what counted as a public health crisis and what products were provided to address it.

In many cases, the point of providing biomedical services to poor communities of color also had very little to do with addressing the immediate health needs of the poor and needy. The provision of biomedical services to poor people in the history of King-Drew demonstrates that medical services served, at various points, as a subtext for profitable investment, an excuse to carry out broader real-estate development schemes, or a vehicle to solve larger political and social problems than poor health and illness itself. In the end, white voters decided the meaning of biomedical services in the city's poor neighborhoods by defunding public hospital and clinic services in favor of extending emergency medical services to white suburban taxpayers.

The sum of these processes left sparse medical resources for those who needed them the most while providing a larger and wider complement of expensive, labor-intensive, and around-the-clock biomedical services to those already most able to get access to healthcare. Given the tight relationship between health services and real estate development, the expansion of the health industry after the 1960s also provided jobs and advantages for white people in white-collar and medical service jobs as well as to insurance companies, pharmaceutical manufacturers, investors, and predatory landlords and developers. Together with the rise of policing and prisons, the effect furnished white suburban citizens with a state of wellness that extended beyond the realm of health to include ideas about the protection of one's personal safety, privacy, and property.

All these processes of racial capitalism were sustained by new interpretive frames around the supposedly "backward" spatialized sexuality, reproductive politics, and "culture" of queer, undocumented, and poor people of color living in inner-city neighborhoods. These frames replaced older notions about poor people of color's supposed innate biological inferiority by positing that poor people of color were not able to advance because of their limited individual decision-making skills when it came to their finances, their sexual practices, and their reproductive choices. As founding critical race theorist Kimberlé Crenshaw argues, these ideas were given greater power and efficacy because of, not despite, new discourses of racial and sexual liberalism in law and policy.

In her now famous article "Race, Reform, and Retrenchment," Crenshaw argued that battles over the meaning of racial progress limited the state's remedies around racial justice to ensuring that each individual citizen was guaranteed an "equality of opportunity" when it came to advancing in society. However, racial progress did not include state remedies ensuring that each disadvantaged citizen reached an "equality of outcome."[39] According to Crenshaw, rather than advance racial justice, the result "repackaged racism" by creating the illusion of equal opportunity by failing to address the economic differences created by past discrimination.[40] Theoretically "free" to choose health services but not free to pay for services they could not afford, most working-class Black people learned that racist hospital owners who once turned them away because of their race could now legally turn them away for being poor.

Crenshaw reveals that the explanatory power of culture of poverty theory helped popularize a new belief that poor Black people were no longer victims of racism or sexism but were just victims of their own individual bad choices and negative mindsets. In the context of larger economic restructuring due to capitalist globalization, deindustrialization, and privatization, the state's "remedies" for racism and sexism helped enlarge poverty because it hid how racial capitalism and sexual capitalism continued to distribute fewer and fewer resources to poor people of color with each succeeding generation. The irony of these approaches is that rather than "fix" Black communities of the sexual practices that the state's remedies purported to "cure," the state's remedies for racism and sexism structurally encouraged poor people of color to seek welfare and engage in sexual practices that medical experts and policymakers deemed "dysfunctional" and "deviant."

By the 1980s, politicians and taxpayers responded to the social crises created by economic restructuring and privatization by proposing "solutions" that simply hastened the further privatization of healthcare, housing, and other social welfare provisions. Although historians have rightly associated these trends with the rise of conservatives to political office, many of the policies providing businesses and high-spending consumers with low-cost services and labor were first devised and carried out by leaders in Los Angeles who saw themselves as liberal champions for people of color and the poor. By the 1990s, the narrow pathways taken to advance racial and sexual inclusion in Los Angeles expanded poverty beyond the city by inspiring employers to either seek workers more vulnerable to exploitation, like undocumented immigrants, or relocate to places with more lax labor and environmental laws, like those along the US-Mexico border. Social scientists and labor activists collectively refer to this phenomena as "the race to the bottom" because it encouraged employers to reduce labor and production costs by any means necessary.

My tracing of the persistence of racism, sexism, homophobia, transphobia, and xenophobia after the civil rights, gay rights, and women's liberation movements thus seeks to contribute to larger scholarly investigations of racial capitalism's functions by illuminating the importance of capitalist processes of gender and sexuality in renewing racism after the 1960s. If, as Ruth Wilson Gilmore argues, "capitalism requires inequality and racism enshrines it," then the revival of racial capitalism after the social movements of the 1960s and 1970s shows that its continuation was achieved through the proliferation of other types of inequality to sustain it.[41] In addition to normalizing biomedicine as a response to poor health, this book shows that society's inability to solve its problems also lies in its immersion in notions of gender and sexual normativity that turn difference into domination and exploitation.

Black community leaders invested in using heterosexuality as a norm for racial inclusion and gay and lesbian community leaders invested in using whiteness and gender conformity as norms for sexual inclusion help explain why society's most vulnerable citizens increasingly found little ground for formal economic and social redress by the 1980s. As Crenshaw argued, the manifestations of racial and sexual liberalism in law and social policy were not only inadequate in helping Black women address the racism and sexism facing them but were actually harmful in advancing racial and sexual progress for all people. Using Bell's formulation of interest convergence toward different ends, Crenshaw argued in her article "Demarginalizing the Intersection of Race and Sex" that Black women's interests are only protected when their interests converge with those of Black men or white women under the prevailing belief that Black men's interests represent the racial interests of all Black people and white women's interests represent the gendered interests of all women.[42]

Scholars have responded to these approaches by emphasizing the intersectionality of race and gender with other categories of analysis. According to Crenshaw, the problem with a "single-axis analysis" to issues of race or gender is that it distorts the "multidimensionality of Black women's experiences" but also "imports its own theoretical limitations that undermine efforts to broaden feminist and antiracist analysis."[43] Rather than fight racism and sexism to challenge capitalism, she argued that the state's reliance on limiting remedies to a single axis pitted Black women against both white women and Black men. As she put it, "This adoption of a single-issue framework for discrimination not only marginalizes Black women within the very movements that claim them as part of their constituency but it also makes the elusive goal of ending racism and patriarchy even more difficult to attain."[44]

Rod Ferguson later extended these arguments to address how these processes worked along the lines of sexuality to marginalize queer and trans people in communities of color.[45] Ferguson essentially argues that queer and trans people of color, unlike white gays and lesbians, have been subject to inclusion narratives that have "helped to articulate heteropatrarichy as universal."[46] Under this formulation, queer and trans people of color are protected only when their interests converge with those of straight Black men or white middle-class gender-conforming gays and lesbians under the belief that Black men represent the interests of all Black people and that all white gays and lesbians represent the interests of all homosexual people.

As Patricia Hill Collins has argued, the irony of all of these formulations is that Black men are regularly denied the protection and representation that law and policy's "single axis analysis" is purported to uphold. Citing a rise in police brutality, an increase in arrest and imprisonment, and a resurgence in vigilante violence against Black men, Collins argues that Black men do not just experience violence because they are Black but because their Blackness is produced to expose them to vulnerability and danger in "gender-specific ways."[47] Collins thus argues that discourses of gender and sexuality have continued to steal freedom from all Black people under what she refers to as "new racism."

Rather than suspend the functions of white supremacy, these dizzying mutations of power and representation make sense only when considering how they remain committed to reproducing the functions of white male breadwinning manhood through heteropatriarchy in communities of color and through racism in gay and lesbian neighborhoods. By the 1980s, cultural accounts blaming women of color and queer and trans people of color for slowing social progress made it too easy to ignore how sexual and racial capitalism worked in tandem to expand poverty. As opposed to forging, in the words of Cathy Cohen, "a politics where the non normative and marginal position" of those perceived to be sexually aberrant serves as a "basis for progressive transformative coalition work,"[48] discourses about people's discrete "identities" served to isolate the experiences of Black women, Black queer and trans people, and even heterosexual Black men from each other.

As Crenshaw points out, the single-axis approach to remedying racism and sexism made it increasingly difficult for mainstream (that is, white) feminists and queer activists to understand why women of color feminists and queer activists of color felt the need to defend men of color as much as women and queer and trans people. Crenshaw observed that "although [hetero]patriarchy clearly operates within the Black community ... the racial context" of white supremacy in which Black women and queer and trans people still found themselves made it difficult to develop a political consciousness that "is oppositional to Black men." Such statements mark how many Black feminists and queer and trans activists had less of a problem with men than they had with heteropatriarchy.

Crenshaw was not the only Black feminist struggling to discuss different forms of manhood that did not accept defining racialized manhood in the same exact terms as white patriarchy. Audre Lorde, for instance, understood that discourses of racism and heteropatriarchy used against her as a Black lesbian were intertwined with those facing straight Black men. Lorde argued, for example, against the mainstream appropriation of breadwinner roles in the Black community in her comments about Robert Staples's 1979 article in *The Black Scholar*. She asked, "Why should Black men accept these roles as correct ones?" and referred to hegemonic notions of breadwinning manhood as a "narcotic promise encouraging acceptance of other facets of [Black men's] own oppression."[49] Arguing that racism and patriarchy were systems consented to by not only white men and women but also people of all races and genders, Lorde asserted that it was her wish to "raise a Black man who will not be destroyed by, nor settle for, those corruptions called *power* by the white fathers who mean his destruction as surely as they mean mine."[50]

Lorde's admission that Black people, regardless of their stated gender or sexuality, continued to face oppression illustrates how the supposedly sexually liberal terms of racial liberalism failed to bring forth the fruit of inclusion promised through the politics of respectability. My explorations show that some of the first victims of "culture of poverty" theory were not, in fact, poor Black men or women, but Black male physicians who faithfully reconstructed racial scientific and civilizing arguments about the importance of uplifting the race by policing gender and sexuality in Black communities. These points underline how the categories of Black womanhood, manhood, and queer and trans personhood are all relationally produced in relation to whiteness but also constitute, as Hortense Spillers argues, a Black gender unto their own.[51]

Racial and sexual capitalism prismatically and coconstitutively produced the categories of "absentee fatherhood," "welfare motherhood," "wild youth," and same-sex loving and gender-nonconforming subjects. It is important to attend to this because the so-called remedies devised to manage the economic restructuring of capitalist globalization, deindustrialization, and privatization after the 1960s ensured that these categories of social concern would numerically proliferate as poverty worsened. For employers and high-spending consumers, the social demonization and criminalization of these categories helped underwrite the defunding and policing of poor communities of color that made and make them such a flexible and cheap workforce to exploit. The effect ensured that poor people of color would continue to be seen by white taxpayers and voters as "liabilities" rather than the labor "assets" they actually represent for politicians and employers in a global economy.

As the epilogue shows, LA native Octavia Butler also believed that looking to poor neighborhoods of color in 1980s was important because she felt that the survival mechanisms that poor people of color devised in the face of their abandonment by capital would be important for white suburbanites to learn in order to prepare themselves for the future they were making for themselves. For instance, she intended her novel *Parable of the Sower* to be a cautionary tale about what would happen to suburban homeowners if they continued to vote for laws and referendums that dismantled government programs in favor of biomedical solutions, privatization, and greater policing. Rather than continue to try to "cure" the Black population of female-headed households in pursuit of a mythical family wage unavailable to Black men and a fabled patriarchal domestic sphere at odds with the survival strategies of the community, Butler's approach suggests that we listen to what poor women of color said about solving poor people's actual problems.

HEALTH AS A PROPERTY OF WHITENESS

Health as Property is organized to clarify how histories, structures, and common practices and policies made health into what Cheryl Harris calls a "property of whiteness" throughout the twentieth century. Since "formulations of property" throughout American history "clearly illustrate the extent to which property rights and interests embrace much more than land and personality," Harris argues that just because certain concepts like "whiteness" or "health" are not physical entities, they are not removed from the "realm of property."[52] This book is thus interested in how possessing "health" came to accrue meaning and value as a characteristic of whiteness so desirable and valuable that its attainment became something to ration or bargain with in discussions about gaining access to medicine and health services. To investigate this process, this book relies on archival research in Southern California, Washington, DC, Massachusetts, New York, Connecticut, and Texas to explore the various actors at local, state, and federal levels that federal law legislated as necessary to launch antipoverty programs.

The book moves spatially and chronologically through time over six chapters, starting with a view of Los Angeles from the perspective of doctors and citizens living in the city's postwar Black neighborhoods; then moving "outward" to explore the reproduction of King-Drew's multicultural projects in the city's gay, Filipino, and "Homeless" districts; and ending with a view of the city from the perspective of white suburban residents as they negotiate the meaning of all the expenditures related to public hospital, clinic, and emergency medical care. Readers will notice, however, that detailing a history of King-Drew rarely follows a linear narrative given that multiple storylines unfolded in sometimes contradictory, sometimes complementary trajectories, given the multitude of competing interests associated with the health system and its various constituent institutions. The capillary nature of such a story required a lot of careful decisions on how to tell one coherent story without being too repetitive.

Chapter 1 explores how Black physicians initially responded to their exclusion from corporate medicine and the predatory inclusion of most Black patients as teaching and experimental "clinical material" at the region's white-led teaching hospitals. Black physicians sought to protect the city's poor Black medical markets on the eve of Medicare's and Medicaid's implementation through a "Watts Health District" within which they could build a privately run Black community hospital. Chapter 2 examines how interests in building a community hospital grew to involve more actors than just local Black physicians and explains how plans were expanded to craft the hospital as part of a larger academically oriented health system. With the assistance of national leaders of the African American National Medical Association, the physician leaders of the region's two white-led medical schools (UCLA and USC) and the County of Los Angeles, King-Drew's planners sought to develop the city's poor Black neighborhoods into a thriving private medical market by carefully regulating citizen access to public hospital services through antipoverty health and mental health clinics. Both chapters show the ultimate objective of the academic medical center was to reform the supposedly backward sexuality of poor Black people by employing Black male breadwinners and guiding them to be better caregivers and by retraining the area's Black male physicians to be a new kind of physician specialist—the community medicine physician.

The next two chapters examine the rollout and response by Black residents to the economic development vision offered by Black elites. Chapter 3 reveals the impact of Black nationalist and Black Power narratives on Watts's medical services by tracing the forceful ejection of white physician leaders from an antipoverty clinic owned and led by USC Medical School. USC's clinic leaders sought to use health services as a ploy to convince Black patients to desire work and normative family life as essential features of achieving true health. Although Black physicians shared the same objective, their comparative success in leading poor Black people to desire regular work and normative family life through antipoverty community mental health clinic programs convinced King-Drew's hospital leaders of the need to build all its primary care clinics as Black institutions. Chapter 4, however, shows that such an emphasis on the skin color of physicians obscured the growing frustration and tension that welfare rights organizers and women on welfare had with King-Drew's male-centered health distribution plan. I show that the conflict between the vision of Black physicians to freight economic development and health service distribution on Black men and an alternative vision of Black women on welfare to distribute resources to help all people thrive obfuscated new approaches by Black political leaders to organize employment *through* Black poverty rather than in spite of it.

Although Black political leaders rose to region-wide power partly through the political infrastructure enabled by the reproduction of King-Drew's health programs throughout the city, Black city leaders worked in tandem with county leaders to respond to high rates of worklessness, working poverty, and homelessness related to new global economic restructuring by using the city's and county's public hospital, clinic, and housing services as tools to accelerate the city's transition into a global economy. Unlike overzealous slum-clearance programs that led to rapid population and economic decline in many Midwestern and Rust Belt cities, chapter 5 shows the region's municipal leaders strategically invested in public health infrastructure and policing to achieve two types of economic containment initiatives. First, municipal leaders used public clinic and housing services to supply global financial firms with a cheaper labor force than could be found in other competitive real estate markets; and second, they used strategically placed mental health services to produce a city-ordinance-enforced "homeless" district to furnish global financial firms with real estate elsewhere made "safe" for investment. Guided under the rhetoric and logic of multiculturalism, the city hid the revival of Jim Crow segregation and organized deterioration by celebrating how all the region's neighborhoods—Black, Brown, white, Asian, gay, and even "homeless"—contributed to making Los Angeles the nation's main financial link to the "Pacific Rim."

Although these interdependent relationships between neighborhoods helped prevent population decline and reverse economic deterioration in the city's white neighborhoods, chapter 6 shows that white voters and citizens disagreed with liberal progressive politicians' assertions that the city's new global economy represented progress. Instead of continuing to invest in public hospital and clinic services, white taxpayers shrank public budgets by passing anti-tax measures in the late 1970s and elected political leaders to carry out further cuts to public health and welfare services throughout the 1980s. Despite a deep belief that public hospital and health budgets represented a new form of welfare dependency, however, taxpayers continued to support the enhancement and innovation of King-Drew's publicly funded emergency medical services because citizens saw them as important to saving their lives in a world where gun violence was a more acceptable daily occurrence than universal healthcare or housing.

To make the voices of Black physicians, politicians, and patients central to the history of the healthcare is not simply about representing a "marginalized" group that has been underrepresented in the history of medicine. Instead, it is to demand that we reckon with the freedom dreams, however imperfect, that all Black historical actors in this book sought to make into reality. As my explications above suggest, all the visions offered for freedom—that of Black physicians, of women on welfare, and even of Black politicians—remain unfulfilled and incomplete because of the deep lack of imagination that many white voters and taxpayers exhibited when they entertained the idea of achieving full human equality. The world that Black activists confronted was layered by the overlapping forces of racism, sexism, homophobia, and classism that helped, for better or worse, inform and constitute the various perspectives each Black activist held individually and collectively as they struggled for Black freedom. Their perspectives, in turn, have been elided by conventional accounts of urban history and histories of medicine, and by our scholarly instinct to divide medical history from economic history, and economic history from race and gender and sexuality studies. Rather than present a definitive account of the history of Los Angeles or of King-Drew, my goal is to present a history of medicine and economic development where the achievement of health meant producing more than just the presence of medical services. There are, in what follows, as many histories of roads untaken as there are of roads partially taken; I hope many might see these unexplored paths as more urgent for us today.

ONE

Profiting from Black Sickness

BY MOST MEASURES, Dr. Sol White Jr. had all the education and training needed for a successful private medical practice when he migrated from Nashville to Los Angeles in 1954. White was born in 1931 to a pharmacist and a teacher in Beaumont, Texas; his Black middle-class upbringing gave him opportunities most African Americans could only dream of. With a Fisk University undergraduate degree, a Meharry College medical degree, and a pediatrics residency at the University of Southern California Medical School's training program at Los Angeles County General Hospital, he was an elite amongst racial elites.[1] His education gave him a competitive edge when only 2 percent of all Black citizens held a medical degree and only 2 percent of all Black physicians held a postgraduate medical certificate.

Shortly after completing his residency in 1957, White, with his father's financial backing, sought to capitalize on his good fortune by opening a small private practice in Mid-City, a racially integrated middle-class neighborhood well outside the poor and working-class Black community of Watts. White's decision to practice in Mid-City reflected his belief that his credentials would do more than just give him an advantage over other Black physicians. He believed his training would make his services as desirable as any other well-trained white pediatrician.

His formal education, however, did nothing to prepare him for the realities of Southern California's racist free-market health landscape. In 1960, White decamped from Mid-City to Watts because the area's all-white hospital boards routinely undercut the business of Black physicians by denying them hospital privileges to see and care for patients in acute care settings. He also found practicing in Mid-City difficult because competition for a limited number of middle-class patients in the city's integrated neighborhoods made cultivating a profitable client list complicated for new Black physician migrants.

However, White found practicing in Watts just as financially trying as his time in Mid-City. Although practicing in poor and working-class Black neighborhoods presented him with fewer rivals, he struggled to make a "normal" living because LA's white-led teaching hospitals undermined his business by offering poor patients "free" healthcare in exchange for their willingness to serve as "medical material" for training and experimentation. Locked out of private community hospitals, outcompeted in integrated neighborhoods, and undercut by public hospital care in poor Black neighborhoods, White reportedly took on "10,000 patients" to make in Watts what hospital privileges and fewer clients could produce in middle-class neighborhoods.[2]

White's struggle to doctor while Black demonstrates how by the 1960s Southern California's political economy served Black people's economic interests only when it served the financial interests of white business owners and politicians. It also shows how the region's political economy served Black people's health interests only when their care served the profits, training, and knowledge power of white male physicians. The cumulative effect of offering work, employment, and housing to Black individuals only when it suited employers and politicians created a paradox when it came to Black workers' relationship to healthcare. Unlike white workers, whose employment generally made healthcare accessible to them through their waged labor, Black workers' imposed poverty made them valuable as research and training subjects for white physicians despite their unprofitability.

White's experience in both LA's postwar racially-integrated neighborhoods and working-class Black neighborhoods exposes a core contradiction in prevailing ideas about race and doctoring by the mid-twentieth century. While Black people in Los Angeles were free to choose a Black physician to treat their illnesses and ailments, most with money still felt compelled to see white doctors because of the routine exclusion of Black physicians from hospitals. At the same time, those without money were forced to see a white physician because of the discriminatory staff policies of white-led medical schools and county hospitals. Despite the fact that most citizens believed that it was right and proper for Black physicians to tend to the health needs of their own people, White's struggle shows how Southern California's political economic development effectively made Black people's health an exclusive property of whiteness, excluding most Black physicians from the ability to profit by serving them.

This chapter examines this phenomenon by tracing the development of Southern California's robust public-private health service landscape from LA's refounding as a white-led city after California statehood in 1850 to the 1960s. Despite claims of its naturally healthy landscape, boosters remade the region by repurposing popular Atlantic World racial scientific ideas for the development of the American Southwest that I collectively refer to as *the principle of white male patronage*. Born as a response to calls for slavery's abolition, this principle culturally constructed white men as inherently more capable of healing individuals and governing society than the supposedly less-distinctly gendered and less-sexually evolved complexity of white women, queer people, and people of color. Together with the notion of terra nullius, the city's white employers, politicians, and physicians adapted, applied, and enforced this principle to developing Southern California's political, economic, and medical infrastructure and culture to serve white men and their families above all.[3]

Cultural narratives about white men's supposedly natural fitness to lead and make society civilized, healthy, and thriving was given special meaning by boosters because of the state's early racial and gender imbalances. Southern California remained mostly Mexican and white men outnumbered white women until the 1880s. Developing it thus required boosters to recruit and enlist Native people and Black, Asian, white ethnic, and Spanish-speaking migrants to build their vision of a white ethno-state. Indigenous people and migrant workers of color, however, had their own ideas about the possibilities for advancing their own labor, health, and status in a city filled with different racial and ethnic groups. Despite their exclusion from white society, stories of the different possibilities in the city's multiracial, multiethnic neighborhoods drew increasing numbers of Black migrants to the region after World War II.

The concentration of financial, political, and policing power in the hands of white settlers ensured Black and white migrants arriving in Southern California experienced different cities. Rather than encounter a region designed to promote their wellbeing and health, many poor postwar Black migrants found themselves used and abused by employers, exploited by public hospital physicians for training and research, and hyperpoliced in a small number of overwhelmingly crowded majority-Black neighborhoods. By the mid-1960s, Black residents responded to this treatment in a myriad of ways. Some, like Dr. White, proposed plans to rechannel the business, capital, and energy of Black consumers by using new federal antipoverty and health funding to operate Black-owned businesses, like private hospitals, to develop the

Black community. Others, who took to the streets in August 1965, rebelled in the event known as the Watts Uprisings.

The perceived pragmatism of White's approach helped convince the city's white elites to reconsider demands by Black community leaders. White elites had consistently rejected calls by Black community leaders to enlist their leadership in governing their own neighborhoods, believing that people of color were unfit to lead their own communities. In fact, hospital officials rejected a petition by White to certify a Black hospital in 1964 but later revived it after politicians, health experts, and community activists insisted on revisiting it after the uprisings. While the next chapter explores how these actors used his proposal to plan and build a "Watts Hospital" largely without his input, this chapter explores the intent behind White's proposal to craft a Black health district and build a private hospital within it that he and other Black physicians would own. I contend that by doing so White sought to challenge racism in American medicine by providing Black male physicians the means to lead the community out of poverty while finally profiting from Black sickness.

Serving the financial and professional needs of Black physicians before their poor Black patients may appear antithetical to common ideas about doctoring. Yet a closer inspection of the principle of white male patronage's cultural functions in the history of medicine reveals that profiting from Black sickness and advancing expertise based on exclusionary practices played a central role in developing doctoring as a profession and Southern California as a destination for healthy living. Instead of abolishing all of medicine's exclusionary practices, White sought to contest racism by appropriating Western medicine's culture of entrepreneurship and its discourses of profit, property, and competition to win inclusion for Black male physicians.

Normalizing the idea that Black men, particularly Black male physicians, were fit to lead their own communities toward modernity and health signaled the renewed importance of Black nationalist discourses within a much longer struggle over the terms of racial liberalism. Since the late 1940s and early 1950s, the National Medical Association's (NMA) all-Black and majority-male leadership had begun prioritizing integration of white health institutions like medical schools, hospitals, and military health services over strategies centered on strengthening and building separate Black health institutions. By the mid-1960s, the stubborn unwillingness of white-owned hospitals and medical schools to integrate Black physicians and patients into the fabric of mainstream medicine pushed local NMA leaders like White to advocate a return to Black self-help approaches to healthcare.

For some Black physicians, participating in efforts to wield civil rights legislation towards a budding Black Power movement were also prompted by the threat that some federal programs posed to Black physicians' livelihoods if they fell short in collectively acting on them. The combined use of Medicare, Medicaid, and anti-poverty programs by white hospital owners and doctors threatened to displace Black physicians by transforming Black patients previously considered "valuable but unprofitable" into patient "markets" who were now desirable for their potential profitability. The historical numerical and power imbalance between white and Black physicians threatened to overwhelm Black doctors and exacerbate pre-existing extractive relationships between white physicians and Black patient populations.

Fear of what Black doctors elsewhere in the state referred to as "claim jumpers" and "parasites" led White to lay a claim on Watts in a similar way that prospectors once did in Gold Rush California.[4] He concocted a plan to construct a Black-owned hospital by establishing a new Watts Hospital District that he and other Black physicians could use to regulate competition. His plan offered Black doctors practicing in integrated neighborhoods a chance to unite with those in poor and working-class Black neighborhoods to strengthen a private community hospital whose profits could be reinvested in Black neighborhoods. As White declared, rather than focus on integration, Black leaders needed to embrace "segregation 'for a while' to solve problems in the ghettos."[5] They should approach Black neighborhoods as if they were—as James Baldwin aptly phrased it—"another country," whose people, economy, and health standards could be isolated and sheltered from the very economic and political relations that produced it as poor and "contagious" in the first place.[6]

This proposal to renew capitalism and free market healthcare as an answer to racism is one strand of a larger story increasingly of interest to scholars: how antiracist and anticolonial movements after World War II increasingly relied on similar discourses of development to achieve progress and modernity under the banner of racial nationalism. According to scholars such as María Josefina Saldaña-Portillo and Alyosha Goldstein, urban leaders of color in the United States and "indigenous" leaders in newly independent African, Asian, and Latin American nations mutually inspired each other to think about the future of racial progress within the new pluralist language of state "markets" and national "economies."[7] Despite the wildly different geopolitical contexts facing leaders of color newly empowered to determine the economic direction of their communities and the wide array of political ideologies represented across them, leaders of color willing to speak and act on behalf of their communities all tended to settle on economic development programs relying on the same capitalist mode of development. Instead of breaking with the dominant processes of inequality undergirding colonialism, the renewal of discourses propping up capitalism as a common good by racial elites marshaled old forms of inequality toward new schemes for economic progress under the banner of racial nationalism.

A RIGHT TO PROFIT

A proposal to build a hospital explicitly for Black physicians and Black patients marked a significant shift in strategy and objectives by Black physicians organized in the NMA because it countered the organization's official position since 1945. Vanessa Northington Gamble argues that by the end of World War II the NMA had turned away from "the Black Hospital movement" of the 1920s and 1930s toward integration of white "mainstream" hospitals and medical schools.[8] Since the end of Reconstruction, the movement to build and maintain Black hospitals separate from white hospitals served as the culmination of concerted interracial efforts to help Black physicians and medical school leaders in a period of extreme racial terror and exclusion keep pace with medicine's transformation toward biomedicine and hospital care. The movement aided Black physician efforts to place Black medical graduates from the nation's two Black medical schools—Howard Medical School and Meharry Medical College—at Black-serving institutions.

However, as Karen Kruse Thomas argues, the capital, labor, and cash flow needed to operate hospitals by the 1930s and 1940s caused Southern Black activists to rethink the logic of building separate institutions given the scarcity of capital and low population densities associated with the American South's health markets.[9] Especially as Black hospitals began to falter and close in large numbers after the Great Depression, a new faction of NMA leaders began advocating for the integration of white hospitals and postgraduate medical programs to preserve Black doctoring in an increasingly corporate hospital landscape. These activists worked with lawyers from the National Association for the Advancement of Colored People (NAACP) to desegregate institutions through lawsuits and direct action.[10]

Whereas before World War II NMA activists saw separate Black medical institutions as necessary to ensure opportunities for Black medical graduates and physicians, postwar NMA activists such as Dr. Montague Cobb argued that separate health accommodations simply responded to Black people's desire for equality by serving as a form of "*de luxe* Jim Crow."[11] Cobb's analysis reflected a growing recognition that white-led teaching hospitals were often the only hospitals profitable and large enough to sustain the technology, staff, and expertise to train physician specialists. Such calls to end Jim Crow were also especially poignant after Congress passed the Hill-Burton Hospital Construction Act of 1946, a federal program that sought to solve the high threshold of capital needed to build hospitals in under-resourced areas by subsidizing investors with federal and state money.

To help Black medical graduates keep pace with new medical trends, from 1946 to 1964 the NMA and NAACP focused their efforts on desegregating Hill-Burton-funded hospitals. In 1953, activists successfully desegregated the Veterans' Administration. In 1963, they also won *Simkins v. Cone*, a Supreme Court ruling that extended the US Constitution's equal protection clause to patients seeking care in Hill-Burton-funded private hospitals.[12] In theory, both legal precedents made racial discrimination in hospitals illegal.

Black physicians and their allies, such as the Medical Committee of Human Rights (MCHR), learned quickly how difficult equal protection enforcement would be after witnessing the lengths that hospital owners took to avoid compliance. Southern hospitals actively evaded the law by desegregating wards only during inspection visits and by permanently converting their wards into private rooms requiring higher fees.[13] As the latter suggests, most hospitals avoided compliance by relying on forms of discrimination still protected under the Constitution. In fact, Kevin McQueeney argues that many hospitals instituted policies demanding Black patients prove their ability to pay before receiving medical attention and implemented "delay in treatment" protocols that prioritized serving white patients before serving Black patients.[14] All these policies sustained exclusions once enforceable under Jim Crow by transferring exclusion from "race" to "class," a category still unprotected by the equal protection clause.

The trouble with achieving hospital compliance guided NMA activists to convince President Lyndon B. Johnson to propose congressional legislation expanding poor people's access to hospitals and other health services through new federally funded health insurance programs known as Medicare and Medicaid.[15] Unlike Hill-Burton, which enabled racist hospital owners to enrich themselves and cater to white patient populations without recourse, Medicare's and Medicaid's design encouraged hospital owners and providers to compete for new revenue and profits by reorganizing the culture of their businesses to attract the business of federally eligible patients. For many supporters of integration, such as Cobb, Medicare and Medicaid appeared too lucrative for white hospital owners and medical school leaders to ignore. He believed that Medicare and Medicaid would result in more hospitals integrating their staffs and changing their culture to accommodate Black physicians and patients.

The persistence of racist practices in hospitals and the growing popular attribution of racial progress around Black healthcare to the mostly white membership of the MCHR instead of the NMA, however, led many Black physicians to be skeptical of, if not outright hostile to, the NMA's continued ideological commitment to integration.[16] If anything, new incentives to expand healthcare to poor neighborhoods appeared to inspire white physicians to see profit, value, and meaning where few previously bothered to see it before. Where others saw the end of racism and the beginning of a multiracial integrated society, others saw the unchecked expansion of white medical power over Black communities under the guise of civil rights progress.

Sol White bore witness to these debates after attending the NMA's national conventions in 1963 and 1964 as president-elect and president of the Charles R. Drew Medical Society, the NMA's Southern California chapter. He saw new possibilities where others saw dread. White was inspired by the possible positive effect that new health legislation could have on Black neighborhoods when paired with recently implemented antipoverty program funding. He saw an opportunity to repel encroachment on poor Black medical markets by proposing a plan in 1964 to certify a hospital that he and other Black doctors could operate using a combination of antipoverty, Medicare, and Medicaid funding. He then later amended his proposal to include carving a new Black-led hospital district out of two existing white-led hospital districts to ensure that any future hospital proposal in Watts would have to be approved by him and his other Black physician associates.

By 1966, *Jet* magazine's Simeon Booker sought to help readers understand the dimensions of this shift within the NMA by describing White as an "oddball" among the 135 members of the NMA's Southern California chapter.[17] Booker's coverage reveals that by 1966, White hid his initial time developing middle-class clientele in integrated neighborhoods in order to frame his move to Watts as a choice. According to Booker, "unlike many of his colleagues," White chose to practice in the "virtually all-Negro area of Watts" when most Black medical men "aimed [themselves] toward a more middle-class market—preferably integrated," where wealthy customers owned mansions and had money to spare.[18] Booker contrasted White's dedication to using his middle-class privilege and education to "helping the poor and unemployed in his community" by criticizing Black physicians who were too invested in becoming richer, owning $100,000 homes, and winning "privileges in white hospitals."[19]

Framing White's decision to work in Watts and cater to poor Black patients as a choice rather than a predetermined outcome of racial capitalism helped Booker explain that constructing an explicitly Black hospital and health district did not signal legal segregation's persistence. They symbolized Black people's choice to invest psychologically and materially in the development of their own neighborhoods. While federal legislation gave white physicians the same incentives to migrate and "integrate" medicine in Black neighborhoods, White believed that civil rights law gave him and other Black physicians the means to make claims on Black consumers that were more than the same sort of moral or political claim-making they had used to assert themselves in the past. Leadership of the health district gave him access to the same mechanisms to exclude white physicians from Black neighborhoods that white physicians had used against Black physicians to exclude them from white hospitals.

Booker's 1966 article helped brand White's proposal as a radical departure from the NMA's and NAACP's prevailing emphasis on integration by representing its adherents as ineffective in combating the racism of the white medical establishment and addressing the needs of poor and working-class Black people. However, as the next two sections show, framing White in opposition to other Black physicians and to the white medical establishment hid how White fashioned his proposals by working *within* the common practices, methods, and language of doctoring rather than outside them. His proposals recruited the language of racial difference, capitalism, and heteropatriarchy underlying the principle of white male patronage to counter normative expectations of who counted as a doctor and as a leader by normalizing the idea of Black male leadership over Black health and economic matters as a common-sense approach to eradicating poverty.

THE PRINCIPLE OF WHITE MALE PATRONAGE

Recent scholarship in medical anthropology, ethnic studies, and the history of medicine has demonstrated that the myth of white male superiority is at least as old as the history of the "modern physician" itself. Charles Briggs argues that language around the human body and ideas about health, the work of health, and the work of medicine propagated in the seventeenth century by European and European-descended people began to dominate the language that people all across the globe used to refer to their selves, their bodies, and the health of others.[20] According to Gary Okihiro, the spread of Eurocentric ideas about health served as tools and rationale for the domination of Native peoples and the spread of racial capitalism across the globe.[21]

Historians of medicine have extended these arguments by revealing that the seventeenth century's so-called scientific revolution could not have happened without the expertise of the Indigenous peoples that European and European-descended scientific men encountered during the rise of the slave trade. It is now well known that throughout the more than three hundred years of chattel slavery Atlantic World enslavers and plantation owners largely depended on the talent, expertise, and labor of Black healers—especially Black women healers—to heal themselves, their family members, and other enslaved people. Historians have also traced the origins of early Western scientific knowledge about flora, fauna, and the body to knowledge that Black healing practitioners shared—willingly or coerced—with European and European-descended researchers and physicians.[22] According to Pablo Gomez, rather than existing as "ancillary, adaptive or merely responsive to European institutionalized corporate medical practice," during much of the period of legal slavery "black healing practices and culture" were so "normative and mainstream" that people of all racial backgrounds often did not think twice about seeking care from a Black practitioner.[23]

Normative associations of doctoring with Blackness, however, shifted by the nineteenth century as the violence of slavery's deeper entrenchment made planters more fearful of slave resistance and revolt. Sharla Fett argues planters increasingly directed their anxieties at enslaved healers because of the political and spiritual authority their healing talents gave them in the Black community. She argues planters began relying on paying white physicians for health services because they feared that Black healers exploited their positions to coach enslaved workers to "feign" illness to steal time and labor from planters or used their mobility and leadership across plantation communities to help foment insurrection.[24]

Others, such as Deirdre Cooper Owens, Rana Hogarth, and Christopher Willoughby, argue plantation owners began turning to white physicians because they increasingly offered medical expertise not available from traditional enslaved healers.²⁵ White medical men's newly won reputation as healing experts stemmed from their willingness to exploit slavery's racial hierarchy for medical discovery. White medical men used their access to enslaved people to conduct live human experimentation without consent and created elaborate "body snatching" networks to use enslaved people's human remains for anatomical discovery and training.²⁶ In contrast to an early Atlantic World culture of cross-racial knowledge sharing, by the mid-nineteenth century these medical and scientific exploits provided European and European-descended men with a cache of scientific knowledge and medical techniques that they shared and guarded as their racially-exclusive intellectual property.²⁷

The tight relationship between medical discovery and slavery's economic system highlights how most leading medical men by the mid-nineteenth century either defended the institution of slavery outright or defended the idea of inherent racial difference upon which racial slavery was premised.²⁸ The theory most relevant to the concept of the principle of white male patronage was first popularized by Samuel Cartwright, who argued enslavement and white male control over society were beneficial for human subjects he considered less biologically and intellectually evolved than straight white men. Scholars of medicine have shown that despite being crafted for the political economy of the early nineteenth century, Cartwright's ideas endured for well over a century.²⁹

Cartwright's ideas reinforced a belief that white men's superior intellect and biological fitness endowed them with the power to govern and create order out of chaos. Most famously, he invented the psychiatric disease "drapetomania," or runaway slave disease, a mental illness he argued afflicted Black individuals who attempted to escape the supposedly healing and benevolent authority of white supervisors.³⁰ The invention of such a diagnosis helped underline how many medical men believed white control over Black individuals in the form of enslavement was therapeutic because it allowed the race the benefits of civilization and health they would otherwise not enjoy as supposedly savage people left to their own devices.

Siobhan Somerville argues medicine's racial hierarchy did not just rely on observations about differences between white and Black bodies but also on observed differences between the sexes.³¹ Racial scientists argued that white women were less capable of governing society then white men based on their supposedly less-evolved physiology but also argued they were more evolved than Black women based on the supposedly more "restrained" appearance of white women's genitalia. Similar to drapetomania, racial scientists thus posited that white women were at their healthiest when they served and obeyed white men but went "mad" when they refused their supposedly natural roles as wives and mothers. Both narratives, slavery's racial hierarchy and patriarchy's gender hierarchy, worked together to naturalize white men's leadership as beneficial for all people in society, regardless of their race or gender.

More important, such ideas called upon white men and women, regardless of their rank or class status, to be mindful of the sexual unions they formed with others in order to avoid diluting the white race's supposed intellectually and physically superior racial stock. Based on the matrix of racial science above, unions with people who demonstrated signs of perceived degeneracy either by the color of their skin, by their attraction to individuals of the same sex, or by their perceived gender nonconformity were to be avoided. Although culturally constructed, these ideas reinforced the political economy of slavery by incentivizing white men, women, and children to see their public choices around intimacy and gender expression as part and parcel of possessing whiteness.

These ideas did little to help Black people and antislavery advocates weaken the culture of white male patronage when slavery was abolished at the close of the Civil War. In fact, Black healers were among the first to be targeted for exclusion in a new era of freedom. According to Gretchen Long, the need to address an urgent Black health crisis at the war's end helped expose a health landscape full of traditional Black healers and Black physicians who had trained as enslaved apprentices to white doctors or had received medical degrees from predominantly white medical schools.[32] Rather than treat traditional Black healers as equal to those trained in Western medicine, Union officials helped further marginalize traditional Black healing practices by only reimbursing Black doctors with formal medical degrees.

However, as Douglas Haynes argues, the favored status afforded Black physicians trained similarly to white physicians was extremely short-lived.[33] From the mid-nineteenth century on, white male physicians waged multiple successful campaigns to defer recognition of Black doctors by denying them membership in medical societies, admission to medical schools, and access to hospital training. Haynes argues that physicians used the threat of sectarian divides to preserve the profession as a white and male enterprise by forming the American Medical Association (AMA) in 1847. By 1887, the AMA formalized its anti-Black and sexist policies by reaffirming the right of local chapters to deny applicants membership to the association on the basis of their race and sex.[34]

The exclusion of Black and women physicians from medical society membership paved the way for the AMA to surreptitiously orchestrate the closure of five Black medical schools through proxy control over the Flexner Report.[35] This study raised medical school curriculum standards and medical school costs by elongating matriculation timelines and normalizing hospital internships after receiving a medical degree.[36] By the 1920s, most, if not all, white male physicians had a strong biomedical education, held medical degrees, and had at least some experience applying the biomedical principles they had learned in hospitals as interns and/or residents.

The sum effect of these tactics deferred the legitimacy and authority associated with white male physicians by making becoming a doctor an extremely expensive and time-consuming endeavor for Black students, female students, and their proponents. Higher medical standards attached to training in hospitals required Black students and female students to spend time and money that their families often either did not have or were unwilling to part with.[37] It also required medical school leaders to work with hospitals profitable enough to sustain a training program and willing to take on Black and female doctors. Thus, while Black individuals and women were technically "free" to pursue a medical degree, the AMA's exclusionary tactics ensured that most were not free to profit from the most specialized and exclusive forms of doctoring.

By the 1880s, the principle of white male patronage began to serve as much more than a convenient cultural narrative for racial capitalism. Organized medicine's consolidation of specialized medical expertise in the hands of white male physicians and its support for the belief that white men were "fit" to shoulder the burden of leading and developing society greatly influenced LA's regional development when white physician-businessman Dr. Joseph Pomeroy Widney targeted the city for reinvention as "an Aryan city of the sun" in the 1880s.[38] Widney recruited the racial scientific theories of his physician training to guide the city's physical and economic development. He believed that it was necessary for LA's white civic leaders to address the patterns of overdevelopment and racial miscegenation he feared were leading to white society's degeneration on the East Coast.

He especially saw great urgency for preventing overdevelopment and racial mixture after connecting his encounters with the ruins of a once great "pre-Columbian civilization" to its "lazy" and "dull" Mexican descendants who lived in the American Southwest.[39] By drawing a line from Mexican people's supposed diminished intellect to the ills of crowded racially and ethnically mixed East Coast slums, Widney used the region's pre-1880s architecture and its Mexican inhabitants as living and breathing museum objects to warn white settlers of crowded development and miscegenation. His observations helped lift arguments that industry and eugenics could help guide city leaders to build a model city of "Aryan peoples" that strictly adhered to racial scientific ideas of health and hygiene.

Widney helped build Los Angeles according to the principle of white male patronage by overseeing the construction and funding of the city's railroads, sewage system, street infrastructure, and port. He also contributed to shaping the region's medical standards by founding the Los Angeles County Medical Association in 1871 and the University of Southern California (USC) Medical School in 1885. He also orchestrated the transfer of medical authority over Los Angeles County Hospital's services from the Daughters of Charity, an order of Catholic nuns, to USC Medical School and helped construct a new pavilion-style training hospital in 1878. Widney's belief that racial order and separation were just as important in the work of healing outside the hospital as inside it was reflected in the city's development. Real estate developers marked certain neighborhoods for white settlement while containing the region's multiracial, multiethnic peoples to districts that public health officials often referred to as the "contagious districts."

THE PRINCIPLE OF WHITE MALE PATRONAGE AND ORGANIZED SETTLEMENT

Widney's influence on Los Angeles reveals how racial medicine's biopolitical rhetoric had the power to organize labor and space just as much as it ordered people's individual relationships to healing and hygiene. This narrative power proved especially significant for city boosters and politicians because it gave cultural coherency to a region where white settlers were a numerical minority. Attracting white migrants remained a consistent problem for city leaders because not enough white settlers had arrived to develop it sufficiently as a white ethno-state when the state entered the Union in 1850 and because most migrants arrived single and unattached. In this sense, Widney's wresting control of Los Angeles County Hospital gave city boosters a key institution that culturally narrated the city's future as white while managing the day-to-day material realities of navigating health in a multiracial, multiethnic city.

The Los Angeles County Hospital's change in leadership helped transform it from a custodial institution to a teaching hospital, an institution that many historians of medicine regard as necessary for the birth of modern hospitals in the 1920s.[40] The transformation exposed white settlers encountering hospital care in Los Angeles to the latest advances in medicine regularly used at the East Coast's leading private hospitals. In the eyes of city boosters, providing cutting-edge medical services—normally only available to wealthy paying patients—for free to any white migrant entering the city helped them underwrite their widespread claims that the region's salubrious climate represented a natural destination for health seekers.

In addition to serving the immediate health needs of white migrants, the public hospital also helped city officials culturally maintain segregation by using its public hospital and health services to prevent racial and sexual intermixture between white migrants and the region's racially mixed residents. California's legislators counteracted racial and sexual intermixture by passing the Pauper Act of 1855, which required counties to provide care for indigents.[41] The law targeted single, unattached white men who fell sick migrating alone or ahead of their families from falling into the care of other laymen, women of color, or non-Western medical practitioners. County officials in 1878, then, used the wide latitude given to municipalities by the state to define who counted as "indigent" as a way to serve all white migrants "whether or not they were otherwise receiving public financial assistance."[42]

Legislation privileging white men's health and well-being through public hospital measures was paired with labor policies favoring white workers by subjugating Indigenous workers and workers of color to the lowest-paying, most hazardous, and arduous types of labor. Despite being admitted to the Union as a free state, California's leaders were not shy about adapting the logic of racial domination that had made Atlantic World slavery so profitable. Historians of the North American West argue that California's earliest white settlers directly invested profits derived from enslaved labor to develop the state's early economic infrastructure. They also sought to organize labor in new frontier economies that approximated slavery's profits without reproducing the institution of slavery itself.[43]

This process of using slavery's profits to develop economies elsewhere without enslaved labor illustrates what W. E. B. Du Bois referred to as the reduction of the enslaved worker to "real estate." Du Bois made this comparison in *Black Reconstruction in America* to point out how enslaved labor produced more than just individual profits for plantation owners.[44] It also produced value, meaning, and benefits for a whole host of workers who neither identified as being a part of the slave-owning class nor lived in slave societies. By pointing out that workers in New England and Great Britain benefited directly and indirectly from slavery despite being free, Du Bois sought to show how most citizens came to tolerate or outright support slavery because it made their livelihoods, health, and well-being possible.

White elites' refusal to reproduce chattel slavery in California thus did not represent a rejection of slavery's racial logics but a desire to reproduce its profits using new racialized labor formulations. Michael Magliari, for instance, argues that state legislators instituted a new "species of slavery" by conscripting Native American women and children into peonage systems through vagrancy and indenture laws enacted shortly after statehood.[45] After recruiting laborers from various locations throughout the Pacific Rim and Indian Ocean, California's legislators also passed a myriad of laws designed to prevent workers of color from making unwanted claims to citizenship. Laws governing the immigration of Asian laborers, for instance, limited labor contracts to single men, banned interracial marriage to white women, and forbade the sale of land to nonwhites.[46] Mexican Americans, people of "Mexican-Origin," and "Spanish-speaking" populations, on the other hand, were often offered employment through temporary work programs. In addition to expecting them to return to their places of origin at the end of their work contracts, these programs also exposed workers to deportation, sterilization, birth control, quarantine, and public delousing.[47]

All these practices signal how California's politicians and business leaders crafted policies that prioritized white settlement and business ownership by denying workers of color the right to settle, biologically reproduce, own property, and influence elections. As white migration increased, the occupational and job categories reserved for workers of color increasingly mirrored the same opportunities in agricultural and domestic industries closely associated with Southern Black labor. Indeed, the cumulative effect of California's practices amounted to what Mae Ngai terms "a kind of 'imported colonialism'" by creating "a migratory agricultural proletariat" of Filipinos, Mexicans, Japanese, and Chinese laborers whose labor was central to developing California's infrastructure but whose citizenship status remained "outside the polity."[48]

Despite every attempt to prevent permanent settlement, California's mix of poor and working-class people of color settled in districts that were marked for industrial development by city officials or marked by real estate agents as geographically or demographically undesirable.[49] According to George Sánchez, these neighborhoods consisted of every racial and ethnic group

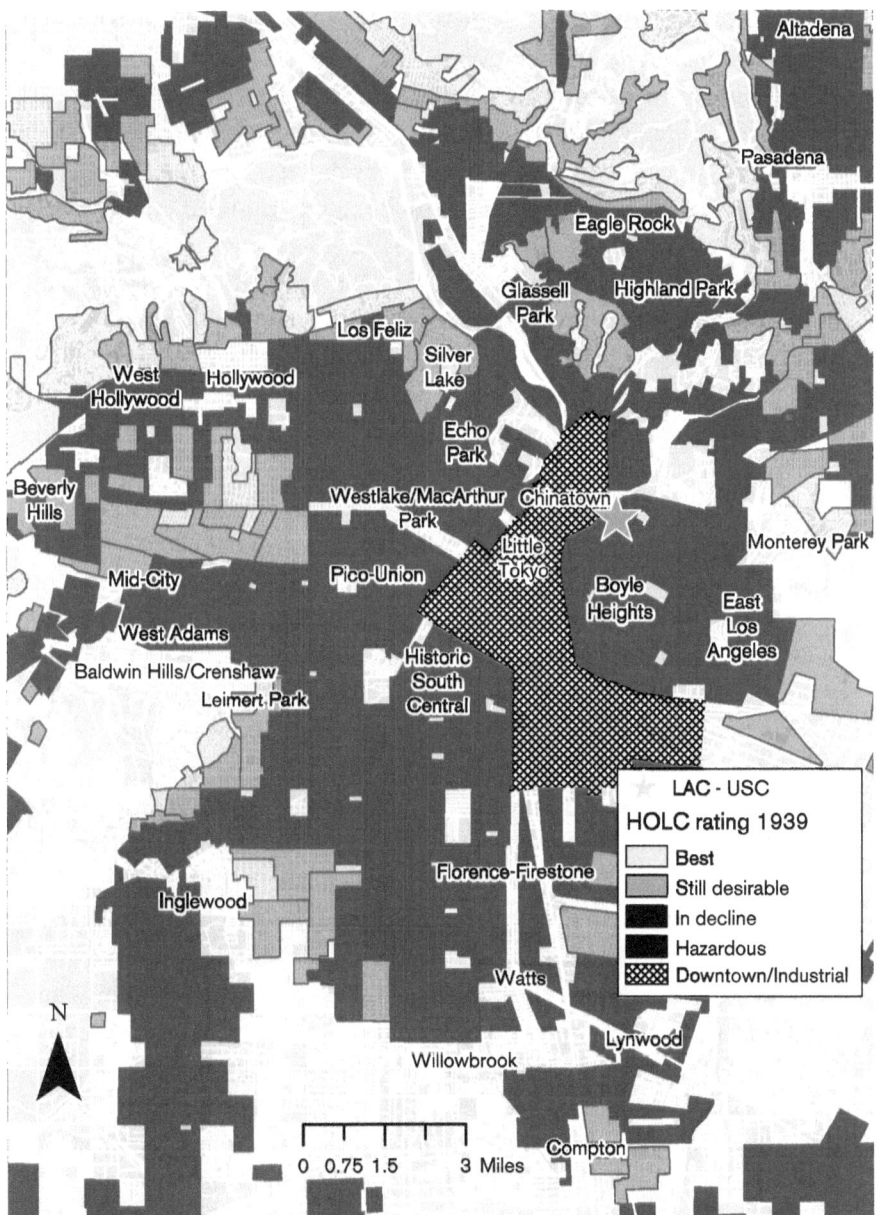

MAP 2. Housing segregation in 1930s Los Angeles

The Home Owner's Loan Corporation institutionalized "residential security maps" to standardize mortgage loan processing by assigning lending risk to borrowers and to real estate based on race. The rating system assigned lower risk to residents and properties in all-white neighborhoods (the lightest shaded districts, like Beverly Hills) and the highest risk to residents and properties in racially heterogeneous neighborhoods (the darkest shaded districts, like Boyle Heights). Many residents of color also continued to live in areas zoned for industrial use (cross-hatched areas, such as Chinatown and Little Tokyo) not residential use. Both the darkest shaded and industrial use districts follow the path of the Los Angeles River. Map: Tyler Munn.

considered by elites to be not white by their standards, such as Mexicans, Mexican Americans, African Americans, Filipino Americans, Chinese Americans, Japanese Americans, and southern and eastern European people not-yet-considered-white, such as Jews, Italian Americans, and Irish Americans.[50] As many historians observe, the districts associated with LA's racially mixed neighborhoods tended to be tightly clustered around overcrowded areas downtown and near the Los Angeles River.

Despite their contributions to building Southern California's infrastructure, city elites routinely attributed the city's prosperity to white business owners and political leaders. According to Bill Deverell, many of the city's earliest white leaders worked to erase the pre-1880s presence of Indigenous and Mexican people by implementing an architectural and cultural program that razed and paved over features strongly associated with the city's Indigenous and Mexican past.[51] More than just the changing of landscapes and narratives, Deverell argues that such programs were also about "race and keeping race in check."[52]

City leaders used bond referendums as way to help educate white voters on the benefits of using public hospital and health projects to attract more white settlement. Voting for referendums thus became an easy way for city leaders to enlist taxpayers in the work of colonization. As the region's white population soared by the 1920s, records show that taxpayers willingly invested and reinvested in the county's public hospital infrastructure to expand, enrich, and enhance its services. Taxpayers, for example, funded Los Angeles County's original hospital in 1878 and reauthorized the construction of a much larger new building in 1930, in the middle of the Great Depression. They also passed referenda to build Olive View Sanitarium in 1920 and Harbor General Hospital in 1946. County leaders often used campaign referendums around hospital expansion as moments to remind citizens of their meaning for the race. A 1930 referendum proposing to build a maternity hospital next to County General, for instance, played on the public's widespread concerns about the region's perceived low white birth rates. According to Natalia Molina, such worry was driven by concerns over the supposedly high birth rates of Japanese Americans and Mexican Americans.[53]

County leaders also used referendums designed to expand services related to contagious diseases as a way to demonstrate how public health services protected white citizens. A 1923 county referendum designed to relieve overcrowded wards in County General, for instance, highlighted the hospital's crucial role in containing contagious disease, a point that resonated with many white citizens because many could not avoid daily interaction with workers of color who traveled to and from white neighborhoods for work.[54] Such messages were also important because it was well known that city officials often bypassed funding programs designed to give the city's racially and ethnically diverse neighborhoods the same basic public health amenities enjoyed by white residents in their neighborhoods.

The idea that public health services earmarked for communities of color served white interests before the health interests of people of color were not lost on white residents. Be it maternity wards or contagious disease wards, many voters, such as Mrs. M. M. James, understood the connection between the hospital's intended purpose and the region's white racial identity by stating that "these bonds must be voted through or we will lose the right to our pride in the 'great white spot.'"[55] Mrs. James's comments reflect how the original vision by the city's white founders to build a landscape centered on the principle of white male patronage had successfully attracted enough white migrants for everyday citizens to claim that it constituted a "great white spot."

By the 1930s, however, the city's status as a white city prompted new debates about the need for well-resourced public hospitals. When County Superintendent John Pomeroy, for instance, proposed a plan to extend the reach of county hospital services to local neighborhoods through county-run neighborhood health centers, citizens led by the county's own volunteer medical staff organized to oppose it. According to Margaret Morden and Richard Bigger, the county's proposed clinics would have consolidated all services related to health and welfare "under one roof," but opponents argued that their formation constituted a "form of state medicine" that would unfairly place county physicians "in direct competition with the private practitioner."[56]

The controversy over public health clinics inspired other physician activists to target the threat that high-quality public hospital services posed to the development of a more robust free market hospital industry. In 1933, Kern County Medical Association leaders won *Goodall v. Brite*, a California Supreme Court decision authored by Judge K. Van Zante forbidding California's public hospitals from treating patients capable of paying for services available in private hospitals.[57] The ruling outlawed the practice of permitting counties to define who counted as an "indigent" by requiring hospitals to screen patients for their ability to pay. County lawyers observing the case noted that the plaintiff's main arguments revolved around a belief that California's public hospitals were "depriv[ing] private hospitals of their normal business" because they offered services "comparable to the Mayo Clinic or the Johns Hopkins Hospital" for free or for a fraction of what private hospitals regularly charged.[58]

The *Goodall* decision helped transition the state's policy of normalizing biomedicine for white migrants through public hospitals towards subsidizing the transition of white consumers to the free market. Lawyers for Los Angeles County observed that Van Zante did not object to county officials using public hospitals that were "equipped, materially and professionally, [with] medical facilities superior to that furnished by standard hospitals" to fulfill their duty to meet the letter of the state's indigent health law. Instead, Van Zante's main objection rested on the ability of "financially able citizens" to use public hospital services, as he put it, for "the preservation of their private resources."[59] The ruling, in effect, argued that paying patients did not have a right to save money when it came to seeking healthcare.

In this regard, *Goodall* marked how California's state-led hospital system was responsible for giving birth to "modern hospitals" in ways that most historians of medicine have previously overlooked or have only associated with private hospitals.[60] Rather than work against the interests of free enterprise medicine, Van Zante clarified the state's role to make certain industries, like healthcare, safer for private investment throughout public entrepreneurship. In quickly applying the most modern biomedical ideas about racial science through large-scale public hospital services, California's health care system also displaced the once common and favorable associations that most citizens had with Black healers and women by creating new associations that associated good healthcare with expensive services rendered by white male doctors in private hospitals.

Ultimately, *Goodall* provided private hospital owners with a protected class of consumers and profits that could be continually used to improve private hospital standards by sheltering them from serving poor patients. In so doing, *Goodall* also left county officials with a new problem: they now had to convince white taxpayers of the value of investing in public hospitals for services they were unlikely to use. They also had to convince the same electorate of white voters to invest their tax dollars into serving and caring for poor patient populations who looked less and less like themselves.

THE PRINCIPLE OF WHITE MALE PATRONAGE AND ORGANIZED EMPLOYMENT

Goodall was much more than just a ruling that helped privatize public hospital and health care. It also served as an opportunity for state leaders to align the state's healthcare policy with the federal government's official response to the threat that rising poverty posed to white families under the Great Depression. By the early 1930s, US congressmen developed a new fear that prolonged bouts of idleness, worklessness, and unemployment were leading to permanent change in the gendered and sexual "character" of white men. Supported by new social science literature on homosexuality and homelessness, they particularly worried about chronically unemployed white men's propensity to explore kinship patterns outside the white heteropatriarchal norm.[61]

Widespread unemployment prompted congressional leaders to be anxious about how quickly poverty and unemployment eroded the power and coherence of the principle of white male patronage under capitalism. Politicians feared that without work, male heads of households lost the proper incentives to provide for their wives and children. With men unwilling or unable to fulfill their role as breadwinners, they feared women would seek life-sustaining arrangements free from the strictures of marriage and patriarchy and that children—disincentivized from seeing respectable marriage and family life as a viable future—would explore kinships outside of traditional marriage to sustain themselves as adults.

The state's responses to public hospital care and white male unemployment in the 1930s, however, advanced the cultural power of the principle of white male patronage to fight the gender and sexual exploration of the Great Depression by expanding its power to everyday white men. State programs rewarding white men and women with material benefits for following the predetermined gender and sexual order of the principle of white male patronage made it difficult for white subjects who might have enjoyed or preferred living outside its strict racial, gender, and sexual arrangements. Especially after the United States's economic success following the Second World War, the policy framework developed by health and labor policy leaders in response to the Great Depression also ensured that white male physicians would benefit from the expansion of capital found in the hands of white male breadwinners.

A closer look at Judge Van Zante's ruling in *Goodall* reveals that his ruling was determined in large part by a concern over the perceived evils that public hospital care posed to white manhood. His ruling affirmed his belief that it was the state's proper role to help "the head of a family" manage his household and that of his community by supporting a free market economy. Van Zante argued that counties fulfilled their duty to promote the community's public health and general welfare by encouraging male breadwinners to part with payment for health services they could afford, thus supporting the business of other male heads of households who cared for their own families on the same terms. Van Zante notably did not argue against public hospital care because he felt that government, particularly in times like the Great Depression, had a duty to help "the honest worker" who would have been able to pay for his own healthcare if it were not for an injury or disease. In this sense, he argued that it was the state's duty to help men *return* to their roles as breadwinners by helping them avoid "indolence and shiftlessness."[62]

Van Zante's use of the phrase "indolence and shiftlessness" pointed to the precise warnings of social scientists and newspaper reporters. White men who had left their marriages and families were increasingly reported to prefer lives without patriarchal expectations that social science experts began to refer to as the "hobo" lifestyle, a euphemism for homosexuality, homelessness, and racial miscegenation among transient men and migrant workers.[63] Similarly, coverage of women bereft of their husbands revealed how women were finding ways to earn money on their own, live on their own terms, and explore their sexuality free of men's expectations.[64] The effect of these processes helped normalize social tolerance for practices and living arrangements like boarding, bachelor dens, intergenerational homes, community parenting, and living next to people of color that were often stigmatized for being nonnormative ways of reproducing society.

While all these practices demonstrated that it was materially possible for men and women to live successfully outside the normative patterns established by racism and patriarchy, legislators responded to the Great Depression's perceived social disorder by passing a series of laws now known collectively as the New Deal. The New Deal and other federal initiatives, such as the Fair Deal and the GI Bill, deliberately organized employment around breadwinning manhood to reaffirm society's commitment to reproducing society through patriarchy and heterosexuality. As opposed to punishing citizens for behavior the state discouraged or condemned, the law worked to reward citizens for behavior it favored.

According to scholars of the "New Deal Order," federal legislation passed between the 1930s and 1950s prioritized employment for adult men through job creation programs that either expanded the government's role as a direct employer or as a contractor subsidizing private companies to work and employ workers on the state's behalf.[65] For some men, the federal government's expansion created new jobs in public works construction, conservation, agriculture, and soldiering in government-run programs like the WPA, CCC, and the US Army. For others, the New Deal expanded employment through government contracts to private companies to build World War II–bound ships, airplanes, and artillery on the state's behalf.

As men returned home from the war, Congress enlarged the scope of benefits available to male heads of households through the New Deal by passing the GI Bill in 1944. The law gave veterans access to low-cost loans to purchase homes, open a business, and receive vocational training or higher education.[66] Together with previous New Deal legislation designed to stabilize employment and employment security by promoting and protecting workers' ability to form unions, the GI Bill helped expand the federal government's strategy to feed, clothe, and house every man, woman, and child through the wages earned by male heads of households by normalizing things previously out of reach for American workers. By the 1960s, the law not only enlarged the number of people who identified as middle class but also made homeownership, college graduation, and health insurance new common features of middle-class lifestyles.[67]

The federal government was careful in designing federal programs to provide male breadwinners with the illusion that their jobs, homes, and educational degrees were the product of their own individual hard work and not government "charity" or welfare.[68] Rather than administer benefits directly to veterans or federal work program participants, the federal government achieved this illusion by entrusting local actors and private agencies to enroll men and implement benefits on the state's behalf. The effect ensured enrollment and eligibility protocols were framed by criteria determined by ideas about race and homosexuality specific to the jurisdictions in which the men lived. The result produced an incredibly uneven landscape of eligibility that often left men of color and white men suspected of homosexuality or caught in a homosexual act ineligible to enroll or receive benefits.[69]

For white citizens, the cumulative effect of these processes assigned real material consequences to certain forms of intimacy that were more or less previously understood by people in abstract racial scientific terms. By the 1960s, the regular exclusion of homosexuals and people of color convinced white individuals that they stood to risk the benefits of an expanded Jim Crow Straight State if they publicly expressed attraction to individuals of color or to individuals of the same sex. The vetting process to produce whiteness and heterosexuality as compulsory for access to the middle class thus helped culturally narrate white flight as a rejection of the racial and sexual heterogeneity that characterized postwar American cities. These ideas, in turn, created a false popular conception that white homeownership conveyed ideas of sexual normalcy and patriarchal benevolence that were not necessarily true in practice.

In fact, as scholars of race and sexuality have argued, the federal government was less successful in achieving the eradication of homosexuality than in creating a white employment culture that valorized and normalized certain forms of manhood that passed as straight. Indeed, Margot Canaday argues that white men who managed to evade detection for homosexuality accessed federal benefits by accepting a "degraded" form of citizenship that required exchanging their true sexual desires for the material and psychological benefits of feeling economically and socially secure.[70] Additionally, policies centered on supposedly protecting and meeting women's and children's needs by encouraging men to serve as their providers and protectors might have inadvertently exposed them to abuse. According to Clayton Howard, the architecture of postwar residential homes and the patriarchal ideas of sexual privacy undergirding them helped hide cases of abuse and neglect at the hands of men in neighborhoods otherwise seen as normal and safe.[71]

Closer and easier access to hospital services for most white citizens by the 1960s largely aided these popular notions because it culturally connected ideas of homeownership to male-centered biomedical care. In addition to the passage of the Hill-Burton Hospital Construction Act as part of the New Deal, California legislators passed the California Local Hospital Districting Law, a law colloquially referred to as the "rural health districting" law because it gave rural citizens the ability to construct their own "privately owned" hospitals. The law permitted voters to partner with neighboring towns to create a "health district" funded by rural citizens to subsidize a hospital corporation to furnish health services on taxpayers' behalf.[72] Although many rural areas utilizing the law remained sparsely populated, the construction of a district hospital often triggered the suburbanization of rural communities. Coachella Valley's Desert Healthcare District, for instance, helped reduce the twenty-five-mile distance to the nearest hospital, while South Bay's Hospital District helped the "Beach cities" of Redondo, Hermosa, and Manhattan Beach to double in total population.[73]

As historians of medicine note, by midcentury the speed and rate of hospital construction and the growth of medical school admissions helped accelerate specialization within hospitals.[74] Unlike previous prevailing standards that held physicians to an expectation of completing at least one year as a hospital intern at a teaching hospital—or, before this, to four years of medical education—the new standard expected physicians to "specialize" in medical fields centered on hospital care. More than just extending medical training through multiyear residencies, specializations increasingly tied the work of physicians to hospitals because most specializations required expensive technology and elaborate labor arrangements that stand-alone doctors' offices could not provide.

By the 1960s, hospital construction and expansion in white neighborhoods in Los Angeles led to concerted efforts by state bureaucrats and hospital owners to slow the rate of construction by requiring hospital owners to obtain a construction certification from an advisory board in order to be eligible for federal hospital funding. Gordon Cumming of the California Bureau of Hospitals declared in 1962 that such measures were needed because he believed that hospital demand in most of Los Angeles had "now largely been met."[75] Such sentiments were shared by James Schooler of the California Hospital Association, who claimed that the new certification was needed to control what he referred to as "overbedding," a phenomenon that produced higher costs by shifting "the cost of maintaining unoccupied beds" to hospitalized patients.[76] The spiraling of business costs prompted the Hospital Association and the Bureau of Hospitals to form a voluntary regulatory body called the California Advisory Hospital Council in 1963.

PREDATORY INCLUSION AND DEBT MANDATES

The California Hospital Association's early 1960s deliberations over how to limit the rate of hospital construction in urban neighborhoods illustrates how most health policy experts assumed that the state's hospital distribution policies had worked as intended. In their opinion, the state's policies had efficiently distributed hospital services according to the invisible hand of the free market to urban and rural citizens.[77] They additionally believed the state's policies provided for the remainder of citizens not covered by private health insurance by relying on taxpayers' continued willingness to fund a robust public hospital system.

White's 1964 proposal for a Watts Hospital, however, forced policy leaders to face the existence of an entire population not served by either public or private hospitals. As this section and the next shows, White's proposals pointed to the growing spatial concentration of poverty in what Arnold Hirsch has termed "the Second Ghetto."[78] The New Deal reorganized LA's racial boundaries as white citizens decamped from older sections to newer suburban developments at the city's edges. Through a combination of civil rights organizing around housing desegregation and white flight, the city's new postwar landscape effectively divided prewar neighborhoods into two zones: a "center city" region of poor and working-class Black, Spanish-speaking, and Asian American neighborhoods and a corona of integrated middle-class neighborhoods.

The reformulation of urban space in Los Angeles shows that the New Deal triggered a different pattern of migration for people of color.[79] Whereas white residents used the New Deal's benefits to move from urban spaces to the suburbs, the New Deal's success in industrializing agricultural crops in the US South prompted the migration of Black citizens to California as displaced workers. Their arrival coincided with greater efforts by California's corporate agricultural firms to recruit workers from Mexico to harvest crops still requiring human labor. Both sets of migrants arrived in LA's overcrowded multiracial, multiethnic neighborhoods just as successful housing desegregation campaigns began to reorganize the city's urban neighborhoods by class. This stratification of neighborhoods by racial composition and class settled the city's poorest Black residents further from a public hospital than other residents of color.

Black residents' spatial isolation from public hospital services also reflected their spatial isolation from the city's major employment centers, given that Black residents were generally unable to access federal housing loans or overcome the outright discriminatory practices of real estate agents and homeowners to purchase homes in suburban neighborhoods. Wesley Brazier of LA's Urban League, for instance, explained to members of the McCone Commission, the official post–Watts Uprisings commission, that a League survey of the region's biggest employers revealed that most had followed the flow of New Deal funding to the city's white suburbs. The result produced an overwhelmingly white workforce.

Brazier was quick to note that employers and union leaders reinforced residential segregation's imposed whiteness by maintaining their own discriminatory hiring employment practices. He pointed out that suburban employers such as Lockheed, McDonnell, and Douglas Aircraft often refused to take federal money designed to diversify their workforces because they considered such programs "socialistic" despite the fact that such firms tended to operate "100%" on federal defense contracts.[80] Brazier also explained that efforts to get union leaders to diversify union halls were just as difficult. Although he acknowledged that leaders in the industrial union movement were more willing to organize low-paid Black workers as part of a larger strategy to organize workers by industry, many higher-paying craft and apprentice-based unions continued to reinforce discriminatory hiring hall practices to exclude Black workers from membership.[81]

Black workers without the resources to travel to and from the city's new employment centers found work where they could. These options included nonwaged work (such as day jobs, temporary work, and contracted work), work outside the informal economy (such as sex work, gambling, and trading in drugs and stolen goods), and work within the formal economy that Brazier described as "the hardest, dirtiest, least desirable work" in labor sectors without union protection.[82] By the 1960s, a growing number of Black workers survived the turbulence an economy pinned to the principle of white male patronage by going in and out of work, sometimes taking on several different kinds of work within the span of a year.

Black workers sometimes tended to describe themselves as "unemployed" because they experienced more bouts of no work than work. Longtime Watts resident Willie Brown, for instance, explained to the McCone Commission that the time, resources, and energy it took to cobble together income in a turbulent work landscape led him to describe himself as "professionally unemployed." Despite the fact that at the time he was driving a thirty-seven-passenger bus bringing domestic workers between Watts and the San Fernando Valley, he explained that for him and others, the effort to get to work was often as taxing as doing the work itself.[83] For example, women picking up day work in the San Fernando Valley as domestics got paid $14 a day; if they took city buses, that cost them $3.06 and took six hours round trip. His bus cost them $2 and took less time.

Black migrants arriving in the city offered testimony that the city felt no different than living in the Jim Crow South. The prevailing opinion that no jobs existed for Black youth that required only a high school diploma prompted a teenager named Winston Slaughter to argue "there wasn't any difference" between his education in Birmingham, Alabama, and Los Angeles.[84] As opposed to investing in jobs and education for Black residents, many respondents observed that the city spent an outsized amount of money on policing Black neighborhoods. Wendell Collins of CORE, for instance, argued that whereas white terrorist groups such as the KKK "augmented" the racist functions of government in the South, the Los Angeles Police Department "almost exclusively" fulfilled this role in the city because there was "no other group to do it."[85]

All these processes produced a different relationship between the public hospital and Black migrants than the one previously established between it and white migrants. As opposed to helping settle migrants and preparing patients for their eventual entrance into free market hospital care, the city's base of majority-white taxpayers reorganized the public hospital's purposes toward training and preparing a new class of hospital-based physicians for employment in private community hospitals in the city's growing white suburbs. Given that efforts to organize employment and labor in Southern California around whiteness had kept Black people at the margins of hospital care since *Goodall*, the effect of these economic processes made being used as medical material by white physicians at the county's training hospitals a compulsory feature of Black healthcare.

By the 1960s, county officials learned to accept the assignment of this function by white taxpayers by carefully monitoring which campaign messages helped them pass public hospital referenda. Taxpayers, for instance, signaled their desire to emphasize physician training over patient experience by passing a referendum in 1960 that voters initially rejected in 1957. Despite similar ballot language, campaigning officials de-emphasized messages around hospital overcrowding in favor of warning citizens about how rejecting county hospital bonds would "seriously handicap the learning of medicine."[86]

The translation of public hospitals' campaign messaging into everyday clinical practice placed the needs of poor Black patients second to the needs of physicians-in-training and medical researchers. According to California Public Health Director Lester Breslow, prioritizing doctor over patient needs helped explain the negative "social attitudes" most medical staff developed toward poor patient populations.[87] It also explained why officials tolerated practices such as long lines, insensitive manners, and short, hurried, and impersonal consultations, which were generally not considered acceptable in private hospital settings.[88]

Despite the well-known abuses associated with public hospital care, California's health policy leaders tended to think of the state's public hospital policies as more racially progressive than those in other states. The fact that Black people were freely admitted into California's public hospitals contrasted with newspaper coverage of the civil rights movement, which emphasized the denial of care to Black Southerners through segregated wards and hospitals. California's Pauper Act entitled citizens to hospital care that was, in the 1930s, considered high quality. Breslow's observations show that by the 1960s, however, that the law and changing market relations functionally entitled poor people of color to the same access to public healthcare as poor white citizens in the 1930s but did not ensure that Black people received the same quality of public healthcare that white citizens had previously enjoyed.

Ultimately, such ideas of racial benevolence hid how Black patient inclusion in California was premised on what Keeanga-Yamahtta Taylor terms "predatory inclusion" because it occluded how public hospital care was transformed by federal legislation to serve the needs of white taxpayers and private hospital owners over the full health needs of poor Black people.[89] As a debt mandate authorizing county officials to take on debt to train and produce physicians, it also shows the lengths that white taxpayers were willing to go to in distributing certain services so long as their interests were served by them.

BACK TO THE FUTURE

The debt mandate animating public hospital care by the 1960s reveals that gaining acceptance into either of the county's two affiliated postgraduate medical school programs served as a ticket to eventually getting a lucrative appointment at one of the area's suburban hospitals. In fact, by 1960, USC's resident physician training programs at Los Angeles County General Hospital (LAC-USC) and the University of California at Los Angeles's postgraduate training programs at Harbor General Hospital (Harbor-UCLA) reportedly accounted for an astonishing three-fourths of all the physicians practicing in LA's private hospital industry.[90] However, until the mid-1950s, both medical schools routinely left the training of Black medical residents to Howard's and Meharry's medical school leaders to coordinate.

This practice of expecting Black medical schools and Black hospitals to graduate and train all of the nation's Black hospital specialists left most Black physician migrants to LA without the necessary social networks to gain hospital privileges. This courtesy enables doctors requiring specialized resources and staff to treat more acute conditions in their patients. To be granted privileges, hospital boards consisting of member physicians vet new candidates based on an existing member's willingness to vouch for the admission of a new member.

Gatekeeping resources based on how familiar a doctor was to a candidate's medical school or how well they personally knew a candidate meant excluding most Black doctors, who arrived in Los Angeles virtually unknown and unseen to the white physicians who had largely been educated and trained in the medical arts in Southern California. They rarely saw a Black doctor or worked next to one as trainees because of the discriminatory policies of the region's two training hospitals. To gain access to hospital privileges, therefore, Black doctors had to rely on the legitimacy and credentialing of their medical degrees and training elsewhere.

Despite all efforts by Black physicians to demonstrate that they were as well trained and educated as white physicians, most found difficulty gaining access to hospitals on their credentials alone. According to Dr. Henry Paul, president of the Drew Medical Society in 1963, hospitals in Los Angeles regularly rejected Black applicants for hospital privileges. Paul intimated that he felt most white physicians feared competing against talented Black doctors. Pointing to Black surgeons in particular, he argued that Black physicians with highly specialized training had a "particularly hard time getting staff appointments" even if they "have been certified as specialists by the American Board of Surgeons."[91]

Being locked out from poor Black patient markets by white-led training hospitals and from private hospitals because of discriminatory hospital privileging practices helps account for why most Black physicians arriving in Los Angeles turned their efforts to targeting middle-class clientele in the city's growing integrated neighborhoods. Cultivating a larger middle-class market for Black physicians pushed many of them to work in deeper coalition with a broader housing desegregation campaign led by an interracial coalition of Black, Asian, and Jewish American civil rights activists. These campaigns relieved overcrowding in the city's prewar "non-white" neighborhoods by leveraging the consumer power of middle-class people of color to desegregate housing by purchasing homes in all-white neighborhoods.

According to Scott Kurashige, civil rights activists crafted this approach to housing discrimination after campaigns designed to convince city officials to invest in "non-white" neighborhoods had failed.[92] The city's lack of investment in basic public health infrastructure such as street lighting, sewage, paved streets, and schools exacerbated the public health crises associated with the city's mixed-race neighborhoods following the increased migration of Black and Mexican people after World War II. As these migrants made certain sections of Los Angeles appear more predominantly Black and Mexican in nature, middle-class residents of color increasingly saw their housing desegregation campaigns as effective tools to both address a crisis of overcrowding in formerly multiracial, multiethnic neighborhoods and preserve the cross-racial business practices and cultural conviviality that characterized their old neighborhoods in newly integrated middle-class neighborhoods.

Longtime Black residents used their testimonies before the McCone Commission as an opportunity to call on officials to recommend riot-prevention measures that helped them preserve and extend the racial and ethnic diversity of the city's prewar "non-white" neighborhoods.[93] Residents like Jean Gregg and John Buggs, for instance, relayed to investigators that they had always lived next door to people of eastern and southern European descent who were not considered white before World War II. They pointed out, however, that like all other residents marked "non-white" by regional standards, they had been unable to purchase homes in middle-class neighborhoods because of racial covenants and racist real estate practices. These practices made Los Angeles's "non-white" prewar neighborhoods "hopelessly heterogeneous" not only in terms of race and ethnicity but also in terms of class.[94]

By the end of World War II, the region's shift from determining citizenship based on race-science ethnological phenotypes toward skin color tested the interracial goodwill of residents who had lived in the city's mixed-raced neighborhoods before the 1940s. Buggs, for instance, explained that neighbors with lighter skin color than him prior to World War II did not have, as he put it, "an opportunity to crystallize attitudes" about his darker skin because residential segregation had made them equal to each other in the eyes of regional elites.[95] By the 1960s, some neighbors had used their newly minted status as white citizens to move out of the city's prewar mixed-race neighborhoods to racially exclusive white suburbs by the 1960s. Others, however, used their money and resources to move with other neighbors of color to preserve the multiracial, multiethnic nature of their old neighborhoods in newly "integrated" neighborhoods.

According to Buggs, the only thing that made these neighborhoods different from the city's prewar racially mixed neighborhoods was their class composition as predominantly middle class. Unlike those who migrated farther out to all-white neighborhoods in the newest suburbs, those who moved with their Black, Asian, and Mexican neighbors to "integrated" neighborhoods near Watts continued to interact with their neighbors of color in ways they had before the war by sharing space, building community, and, more important, doing business with each other.[96] The willingness of middle-class patients in LA's racially mixed neighborhoods to see physicians of a different color, in particular, made California an extremely desirable place for Black physicians.

Black physicians argued, as Dr. Thomas Peyton did in the *Journal of the National Medical Association*, that the openness of patients in Los Angeles contrasted with the closed doors most Black physicians encountered elsewhere. Peyton attributed this to housing desegregation campaigns that not only helped patients open "the door of friendship and opportunity" to Black physicians but also opened the pathway to give them the "merit and recognition" of being doctors that they rarely received elsewhere.[97] The perceived racial tolerance of some California neighborhoods quickly made the state a popular destination for Black physicians by 1960.[98] It was as frequent a landing place as New York and Washington, DC, and more popular than most Southern states, where a majority of Black citizens still resided.

Peyton's comments, however, furnished evidence suggesting that racial tolerance in California had its limits. He warned California could also look like a "gilded mirage" because of the continued discrimination that Black physicians faced in obtaining hospital privileges.[99] Without the ability to access hospitals, Black patients needing more expensive and acute services often left Black physicians to seek the care of a physician with privileges. Peyton observed that hospital discrimination "too often led [the Negro] against himself" because it reduced the practicing capacity of Black specialists to that of general practitioners.[100] The effect, in turn, led to an integrated market saturated by Black physicians who competed for a limited number of generally healthy patients living in integrated neighborhoods.

Peyton's observations were indirectly related to the limits of cultivating middle-class patients that tied Black physician success to housing desegregation. His narrative of "open doors" stood in stark contrast to prevailing mainstream coverage of housing desegregation efforts as signs of "white flight." As Eric Avila has argued, "white flight" often indexed the normative sentiments of white residents who lived in neighborhoods targeted for integration who felt differently than those committed to housing desegregation.[101] In their eyes, the sudden appearance of Black neighbors instilled deep fears about what desegregation did to the equity accumulated in the value of their individual homes. The expansion of banks and residential real estate firms after the New Deal helped enshrine racist financial policies that regularly appraised homes next to or near places where Black people lived as less valuable than those in all-white neighborhoods. The threat of losing capital pushed even the most racially tolerant white neighbors to move to all-white neighborhoods to keep their investments secure.

The overwhelming use of white flight to frame successful desegregation tactics frustrated the efforts of Jean Gregg, a leader involved with Crenshaw Neighbors, a homeowners association for property owners in the newly integrated middle-class neighborhood of Crenshaw. She argued that "white flight" produced a popular amnesia that hid the city's multihued, multi-skin-colored past by pointing out that despite mainstream media's conflation of poverty with Black neighborhoods, "even Watts isn't 100 percent Negro."[102] For her, "white flight" narratives pushed her homeowners association to mount campaigns to keep their neighborhoods middle-class by targeting "young professionals who either don't mind integration or actively support it."[103] By the 1960s, the growing presence of majority-Black middle-class neighborhoods in previously integrated middle-class neighborhoods shows that such efforts were more successful in achieving class exclusion rather than racial integration.

To Buggs, the effect felt like the city was "becoming a much more highly segregated community than it has ever been before."[104] Like Gregg, he felt suburbanization led to "a crystallization of attitudes particularly with respect to the question of where a person would be permitted to live based upon the color of his skin or the language he spoke." Although less willing to join more recent Black migrants who believed that the city felt no different from Birmingham, Buggs admitted that "now," Los Angeles seemed "identical to most of the major metropolitan areas in the North so far as its minority group population concentration is concerned."[105]

These observations mattered to Black physicians because continued integration marked their ability to survive in a medical market where access to practicing in hospitals was not a possibility. Many saw the simple act of having people of different racial backgrounds live next to Black people as linked to their willingness to see Black people as doctors, leaders, and human beings.

By 1964, however, white voters signaled their unwillingness to test this hypothesis by passing Proposition 14, a ballot referendum upholding the right of existing homeowners to discriminate on the basis of race in the selling of their homes.[106] Responding to successful desegregation of neighborhoods west of Downtown and Watts such as Inglewood, Baldwin Hills, and Ladera Heights, the measure effectively helped reestablish a border between

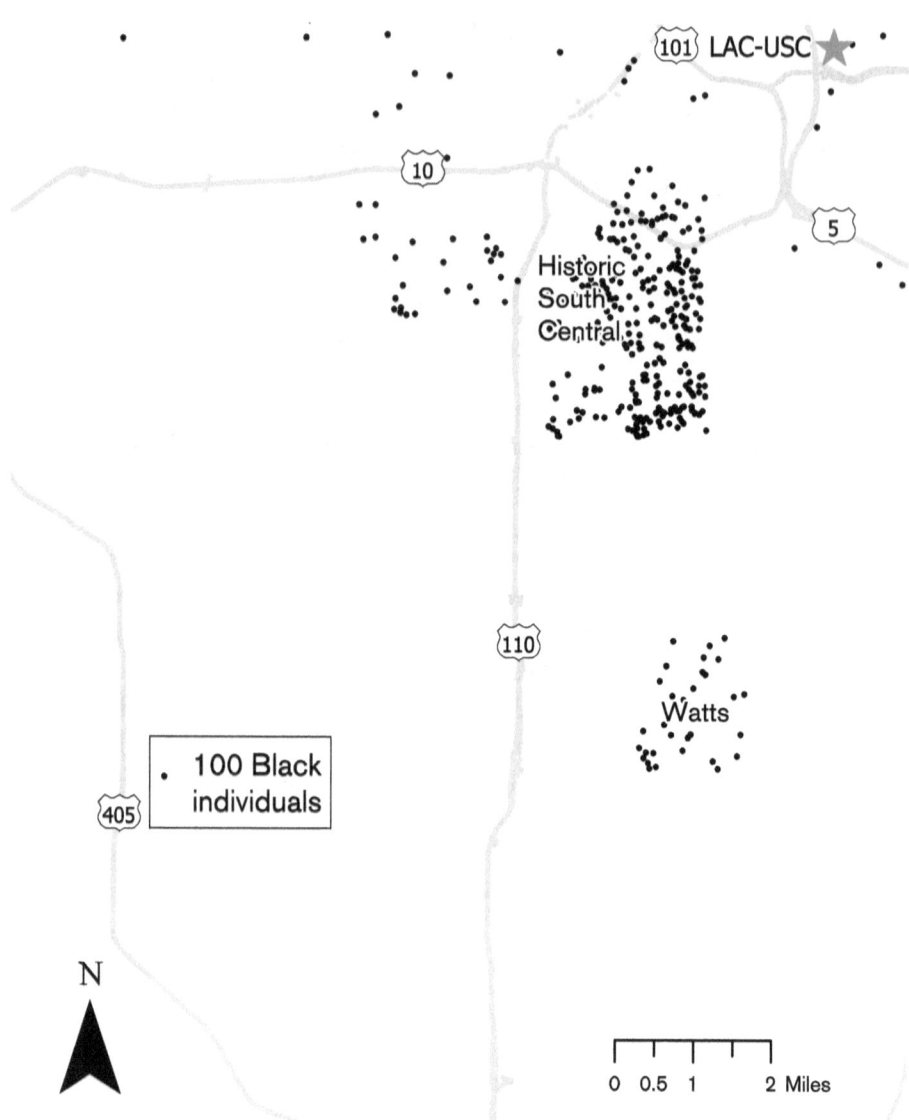

MAP 3. Black Los Angeles, 1930
Los Angeles's Black population in 1930 remained tightly concentrated in multiracial neighborhoods in downtown, along the Central Avenue corridor, and in Watts. Map: Tyler Munn.

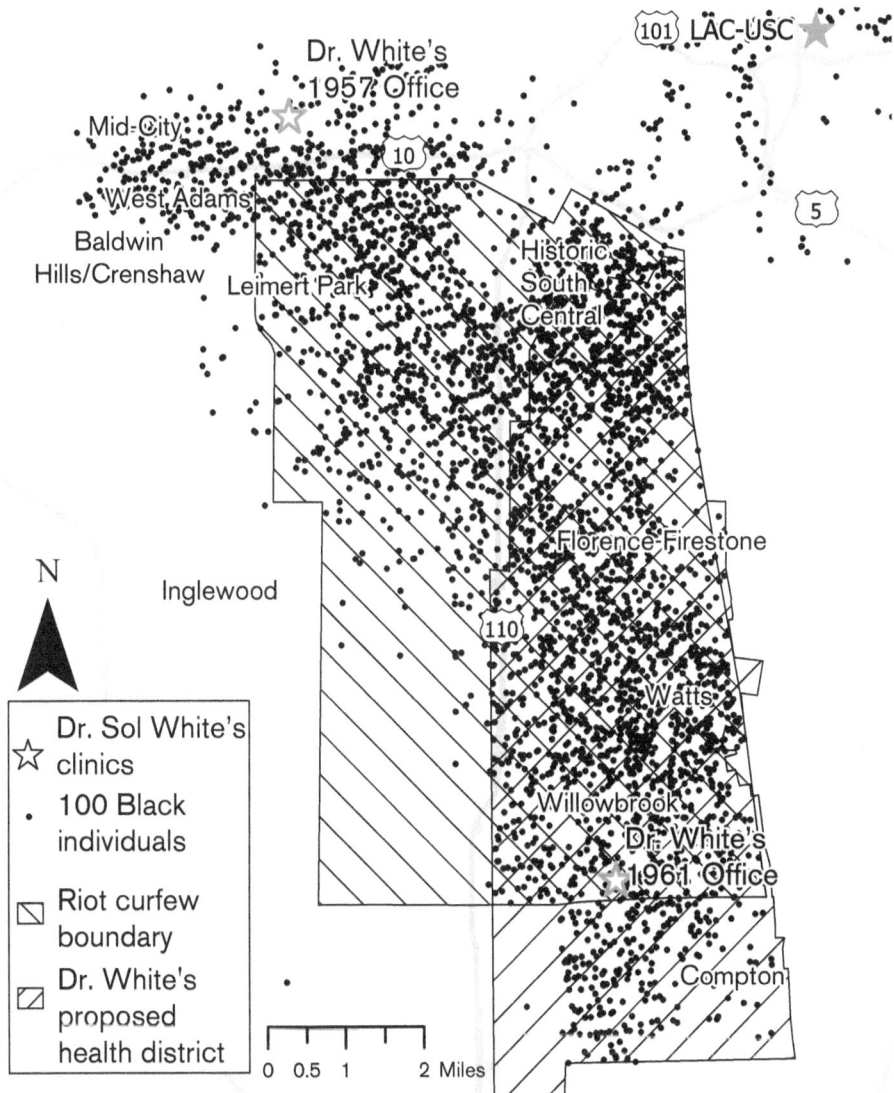

MAP 4. Black Los Angeles, 1960

Los Angeles's Black population ballooned by 1960. In 1965, law enforcement officers imposed a curfew zone to contain rioting in areas understood to be majority-Black neighborhoods. In the same year, Dr. Sol White proposed the creation of a new hospital district tied to the poorest Black census districts. The overlap between the two zones correlates roughly to areas considered by Black residents to be both Black and working class. Areas encircled by at least one zone correlating to areas were considered to be all-Black middle class neighborhoods. Areas outside of either zone were understood as "integrated" middle class neighborhoods. Map: Tyler Munn.

white neighborhoods and neighborhoods of color. Describing it as a "cloud of doom" spreading out "over Watts and the rest of the ghetto," Reverend H. Hartford Brookins interpreted the proposition's success as "further dramatic proof that white Californians do not want to see black Californians in the house next door, in the same neighborhood, in the same schools," and presumably not as their physicians or fellow patients.[107]

TWO VISIONS, ONE HOSPITAL

Proposition 14 likely helped elevate arguments within the Black community for why Black institutions were still needed after the passage of the Civil Rights Act of 1964. Popular discourses around the proposition likely helped account for the appearance of Dr. Sol White's proposal to build a privately owned Black hospital before the California Advisory Hospital Council in June 1964. His first proposal sought to build a hospital on an abandoned twenty-acre petroleum tank farm that could serve the "residents of [Watts's] poverty area" and "attract private patients from the western section of the city."[108]

White's race-neutral phrasing when referencing the integrated neighborhoods west of Watts shows that he believed a Black-owned hospital could equally accommodate the needs of Black physicians committed to integration alongside those, like himself, who had been committed to serving Black patients and developing Black spaces. The hospital that White envisioned would protect Black physicians working in integrated neighborhoods from losing their patients to white physicians when their patients needed more acute care. Although Black-owned, the hospital that White proposed was intended, in theory, to serve all the white, Asian, and Mexican patients that Black physicians had cultivated as their clientele.

The hospital would also address the needs of poor Black patients, who under the auspices of Medicare and Medicaid funding could finally see the Black physicians who had lived and practiced among them for generations. White's hospital would serve as a superior option in terms of not only logistics but also quality because it saved poor patients from having to take the time-consuming journey required to reach LAC-USC or Harbor-UCLA by public bus. He also insisted that the large sums committed to eradicating poverty would also mean Medicare- and Medicaid-eligible patients would eventually transition into paying patients as federal programs achieved their objectives.

White ultimately described the function of the hospital as helping Watts become the "community of tomorrow ... once it has been de-ghettoized and rebuilt."[109] His comments about "de-ghettoization" helped qualify statements he made elsewhere about Black leaders embracing segregation "for awhile." They signal his belief that a Black-owned hospital in Watts might spur integration in poor Black neighborhoods that would make them as middle-class and racially mixed as the surrounding neighborhoods. Such attitudes reflected Buggs's recommendation that post-Uprising measures help "re-create" the multiracial, multiethnic neighborhoods of prewar Los Angeles in Watts by supporting business enterprises that would develop "a real integrated kind of community, rather than the segregated kind of community that we have there now."[110]

However, despite the clear need for a private Black hospital in Los Angeles, the hospital council rejected White's proposal based on the fact that its leaders were engaged in a debate about how to *prevent* more hospital construction in the city. In fact, they argued that White's proposal would have made Watts an overserviced neighborhood based on the measures they used to allocate hospital beds by district and population.[111] Their rejection shows how dividing the state's hospital districts into "metropolitan" and "rural" districts under Hill-Burton made hospital policy leaders unable to see how racialized poverty created barriers to hospital care. It also revealed how unprepared hospital officials were for the implementation of Medicare and Medicaid.

The Uprisings in August 1965 gave White an opportunity to revisit his first proposal by proposing a new hospital plan in December 1965 that included creating an entirely new, separate "Watts Hospital District." White used the meeting as a chance to showcase how a wide cross-section of the community had come together in the wake of the Uprisings to support building a privately owned Black hospital as an answer to Black poverty in the city. White came flanked by Black community leaders and activists representing churches, labor unions, and political offices. Representatives from both the NMA and AMA also showed up to support his application to build a private Black hospital in Watts.

Their supporting testimonies show how Black leaders appropriated mainstream discourses of capitalism and economic development to insist that the expansion of hospital care in Watts be made on the same free market terms as white citizens enjoyed. Ray Parr of the Watts Chamber of Commerce specifically rose to address rumors that the hospital council was considering the possibility of granting certification to the county to build a new public hospital in Watts rather than a privately owned one. He argued against a

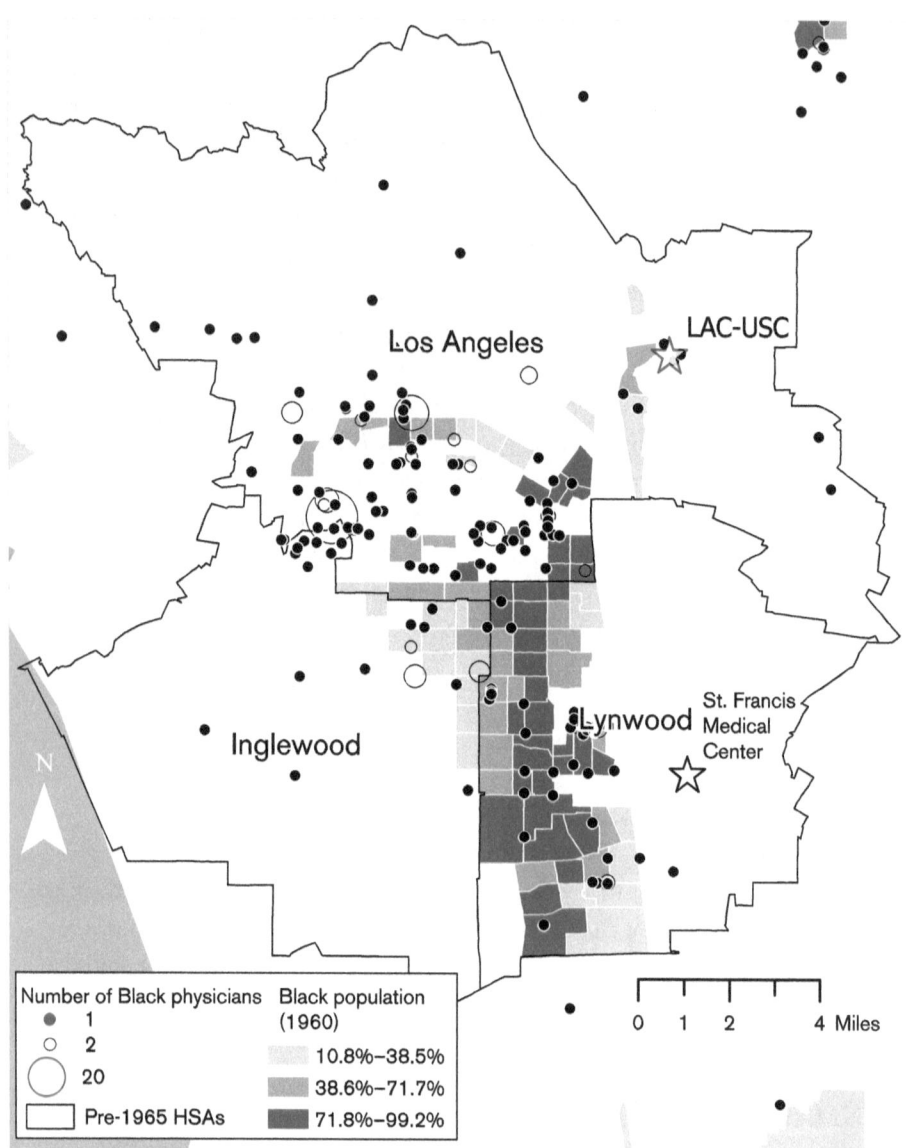

MAP 5. Los Angeles hospital service areas, 1965

Dr. Sol White sought to provide Black physicians working without hospital access in integrated neighborhoods with a hospital centrally located in the most densely populated Black neighborhoods. White hoped the effect would advance the interests of all Black doctors and people by channeling the consumer capital of paying Black working-class patients, Black middle-class patients, and patients willing to see a Black physician towards Black community development. The California Hospital Association, however, rejected his initial proposal after determining that granting his application would exacerbate a perceived crisis of too many hospital beds in the area's existing Lynwood, Inglewood, and Los Angeles Hospital Service Areas. Map: Tyler Munn.

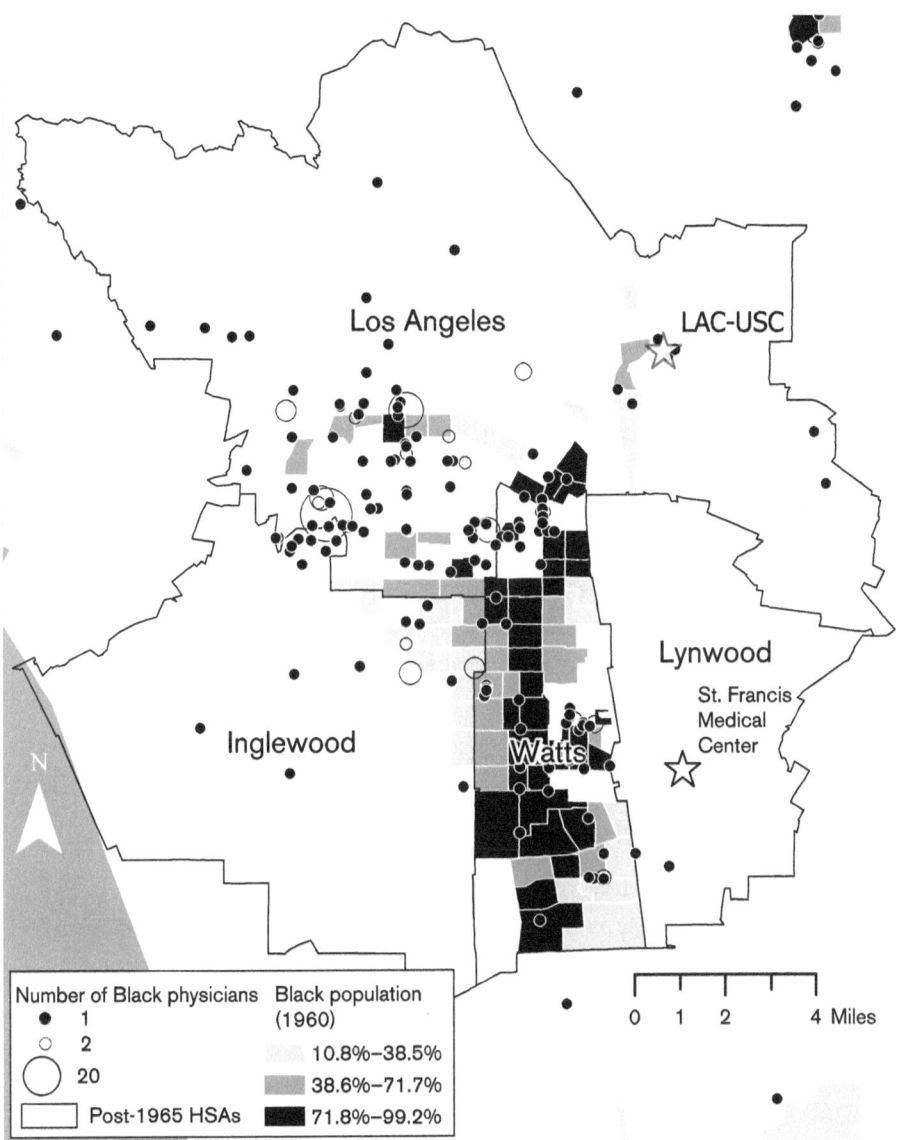

MAP 6. Dr. Sol White's proposed hospital district

After the Watts Uprisings of 1965, Dr. Sol White partnered with the California Hospital Association to investigate the possibility of crafting a new Watts hospital district from existing portions of the Los Angeles and Lynwood hospital districts. Unlike the direction of movement implied by the outmigration of Black physicians from Black neighborhoods seen in maps 4 and 5, White's proposal sought to re-capture the imagination and labor of Black doctors by focusing their attention inwards towards the development of Black neighborhoods. Map: Tyler Munn.

public hospital by insisting that it would place "more people under county welfare" in ways that "just led to more poverty."[112] Dr. Julius Hill of the NMA's Golden State Medical Society agreed. He claimed that the Black community was "sick of the dole and the paternalistic attitude" of the public hospital system's white physicians and social workers and insisted that many likely "would not seek hospitalization at a charity facility" if built.

Hill and others recruited familiar discourses of property and doctoring by speaking about clienteles, services, and constituents as properly belonging to some physicians over others. Whereas white physicians had used such language to exclude Black physicians from treating paying Black populations, Hill used them to claim that paying Black patients were rightfully the property of Black doctors. Hill argued that Black physicians with proper training and education regularly lost the profits they were otherwise entitled to if not for their exclusion from hospitals. As he put it, Black "physicians in the area often lose their patients ... only because adequate private facilities are not available" to them throughout the city. Others, like the Black psychiatrist Dr. Harold Jones, argued that Black physicians were better suited to treat Black patients because being Black gave them a better understanding of poverty. He argued that while medical training in public hospitals might make white physicians "highly qualified" to care for poor patients, the care often given was so demeaning, insensitive, or dehumanizing that it demonstrated a "poor understanding of the people" being treated.

By pointing to the Uprisings as a failure of white leadership, Black community leaders underlined their demands that they be empowered to carry out remediation measures by positioning poor and working-class Black people as properly a constituency for Black physicians to care for and profit from. Black doctors reasoned that making Black doctoring profitable would help Black heads of households be better able to take care of their families through the employment opportunities made possible by Black physicians' entrepreneurship. Hill argued empowering Black leaders with ownership over Black poverty would unburden white taxpayers from supporting increasing welfare rates. He declared that "giving the community the responsibility of supporting its own hospital" would "encourage self-esteem and self-sufficiency in the community."[113] Rev. James Hargett of the Congregational Church of Christian Fellowship made similar statements, saying that granting certification to White would represent efforts to send "the community in a new direction of 'ministering to its own ills and taking care of its own responsibilities.'" As he put it, "The community no longer wants things done for it—it wants to do things for itself."

During the McCone Commission hearings, Wendell Collins offered a more detailed vision of what he thought was possible if more Black leaders were permitted to lead their own communities. Looking to the progress of the Jewish community since World War II as a model for the Black community to emulate, Collins believed that the Black community needed "to do the same things that it seems the Jewish community does, where the big people who develop have a responsibility to putting their time, their efforts, their talents and their money, back into the community so that the Negro community has some community money, some community power."[114] White echoed these sentiments when interviewed by *Jet*: "Who can help these people but their own kin and kind? . . . Who [else] can lead them out of this predicament?'"[115]

Whether Black physicians supported the hospital as an extension of civil rights progress or as part of a renewal of Black nationalist self-help discourses, all efforts to support racial progress required proponents to speak about poor and working-class Black people as an essential component for Black leaders to control. Both visions also posited that poor Black communities were a problem solvable by free market capitalism. Whether owning a Black hospital led to a racially integrated economy or a Black community as economically dynamic as white communities, both visions believed that it was possible to use the scraps of capital distributed under racial capitalism to eventually overcome racism and the economic inequality it produced.

WHO ELSE BUT THEIR OWN KIN AND OWN KIND?

Ultimately, White's proposal to serve the health and economic needs of Black communities by prioritizing the professional and financial needs of physicians like himself reveals how his racial identity as a Black doctor helped illuminate core cultural practices and principles in mainstream medical culture that have often been lauded and commended as favorable attributes in white doctors. For centuries, white physicians celebrated new discoveries and achievements in curing and healing by mobilizing their access to Black populations and Black sickness for profit and gain. However, while these discourses and practices helped authenticate white physicians as bona fide doctors, the same discourses and practices in the hands of Black physicians cast Black doctors as medical interlopers and as threats to white authority and profit.

The Watts Uprisings in Los Angeles temporarily helped unmoor these attitudes. White's proposal to embrace segregation "for awhile" assuaged white people's fear of the threat that the return of rioting and housing desegregation posed to their notions of property and health. On the heels of Proposition 14, his proposal helped encourage some Black community leaders to relent on desegregation campaigns by helping Black physicians turn the community's energies inwards towards developing their own neighborhoods. In so doing, White's proposal offered a vision of developing Black LA under the leadership of Black physicians not unlike the vision offered by Joseph Pomeroy Widney to develop LA as a white city a few generations prior.

More important, White's vision offered a pathway to govern race and health in a manner already valorized as ideal and normative in state and federal law. By putting the financial and professional needs of Black physicians first over the immediate health needs of Black citizens, White's plan reinforced the anti-poverty approach ratified in *Goodall* by ensuring that paying Black patients invested their earnings in the practices of Black physicians who reinvested their profits in the businesses of other Black heads of households. Part of the appeal of White's proposal, then, was its ability to inspire white citizens to support Black nationalism because it offered safety and protection for their neighborhoods through shared ideas of racial fraternity.[116] It offered white citizens a way to imagine that their interests, health, and property would be protected by Black leaders who took their safety and health just as seriously as they took the safety and health of the Black citizens placed under their charge.

White's compelling appropriation of mainstream medical values may have convinced many of Black physicians' cultural fitness to lead community change, but his lack of financial fitness caused many to doubt his ability to lead that change as a hospital owner. Despite Black community activists furnishing what one observer described as a "forceful and sometimes moving account of their community's desire for its own hospital," the hospital council still felt skeptical about granting the certification to White.[117] According to Dr. Milton Roemer, a public health expert from UCLA, hospital council officials later admitted that they felt pressured to reject White's proposal because he "never actually collected any money for his project."[118] According to Roemer, White hoped to eventually gain investors after winning certification from the council.

When asked by the council about hospital financing, White revealed that he had only "been *in contact* with," but had not yet secured financing from, insurance companies, foundations, and other private investors.[119] In fact, by the council's December meeting, White's journey to seek investors had led to three other competing proposals. All three proposals—one supported by the Garland Foundation, another established by a local developer named Arnold Sweeney, and one by a competing group of Black physicians—arose because White had approached them first about investing in his plan.

While the hospital council eventually agreed with Black activists that a Watts hospital was needed, they "expressed skepticism ... over the financial ability of Watts' citizens to support their own hospital," even after taking into consideration new federal funds. They also hinted at the skepticism many had over the qualifications of most Black doctors by raising fears about the "quality of care that patients in the hospital would receive." Eventually, the council members rejected all the proposals for a privately run hospital.

The rejections signaled a more sobering view of Collins's vision to develop Black communities by empowering Black leaders to do what Collins argued Jewish leaders had done in theirs. If the region's political, economic, and medical elites had, since Reconstruction, organized settlement, employment, and medicine to concentrate capital in the hands of white men at a higher rate and larger margin than in the hands of Black men, then the hospital council questioned if it was ever possible for Black leaders to develop hospitals as sophisticated and technologically evolved as those owned by whites. They wondered if a hospital staffed by Black doctors could ever be as good as those staffed entirely by white medical men.

Although Black physician activists did not perceive it at first, the crisis of capital facing Black physicians and Black patients generally helped account for the fourth and most controversial proposal at the hospital council meeting—a proposal submitted on behalf of white Los Angeles County Supervisor Kenneth Hahn by his Black deputy Adam Burton. As the next chapter shows, politicians and health policy bureaucrats in Los Angeles and beyond were inspired to expand White's vision to use the construction of a Watts hospital to solve more problems than just those facing Black physicians locally. Unlike the vision White had to fix a local problem of how to make Black sickness profitable for Black physicians, Hahn and those who rallied around his leadership believed that Watts could help solve a larger crisis of Black male leadership by building an exemplary new medical center and health system designed to eradicate poverty.

TWO

A New Lease on Black Life

IN DECEMBER 1965, white county supervisor Kenneth Hahn made sure his public statements before the California Advisory Hospital Council affirmed his support for calls by local Black community activists to certify construction of a privately funded Black hospital in Watts. He also affirmed the community's demand that whoever won certification also be responsible for regulating the health services in a newly formed health district tied to Los Angeles's densest and poorest Black neighborhoods. These statements demonstrated Hahn's well-known commitment to civil rights progress and Black community self-determination.

However, Hahn's private conversations with staff members, trusted public officials, and health experts reveal that he secretly worried about the financial strength, education, and training of the Black doctors who had come forward hoping to build and lead a privately run Black hospital. The most widely discussed and popular plan was submitted by Dr. Sol White Jr., a Black pediatrician who had assembled a handful of Black physicians organized in the National Medical Association's Drew Medical Society to join his proposal. Many of Hahn's constituents, including Black residents, politicians, and even other Black doctors, were sympathetic to White's vision of helping Black physicians overcome past racial exclusions in medicine but quietly expressed worry that the discrimination they faced in getting training and earning their medical degrees had made them too undertrained and unprepared to lead a community institution as important as a hospital.

The stakes of operating a community hospital in Watts felt even more urgent after the Watts Uprisings. Hahn first became familiar with White's proposal to build a privately run Black hospital after he requested construction certification from the hospital council in 1964 to build a hospital run partly with antipoverty, Medicare, and Medicaid money. Although council members rejected White's original petition under the erroneous belief that poor urban areas like Watts were well served by local hospitals, council members entertained a new proposal by White after the Watts Uprisings in August 1965 called nationwide attention to the problems of economic racism in Los Angeles and other cities.[1]

The uprisings revived White's original proposal and framed it within new federal policy objectives that organized economic development in poor urban neighborhoods around mainstream ideas of breadwinning manhood. Although later more popularly associated with Undersecretary of Labor Daniel Patrick Moynihan's "culture of poverty theory," the policy objective of targeting the perceived backward spatialized sexuality, reproductive politics, and "culture" of poor urban people of color for reform manifested after the uprisings in the McCone Report. Authored by former Central Intelligence Agency (CIA) Director John McCone, it issued an official recommendation that a "comprehensively-equipped hospital" be built in the area. As we saw in chapter 1, by the time the hospital council convened to revisit White's proposal in December 1965, McCone's recommendation had inspired multiple proposals, including one from Hahn to build the proposed hospital as a new public hospital.[2]

Discussion of an antipoverty-funded hospital and health district prompted politicians and health policy leaders to build more health institutions than just a hospital. Funding a health district through federal antipoverty programs inspired them to imagine building an entirely new *health system* linking community clinics, community mental health services, and emergency medical services to a hospital attached to a new medical school. Discussions around a "Watts Hospital" morphed into a project briefly known as the "Los Angeles County Southeast General Hospital" until it was renamed the Martin Luther King, Jr. General Hospital and Charles R. Drew Postgraduate Medical School (King-Drew) in 1968. When it opened in 1972, King-Drew Medical Center served as the crown jewel of a much larger health system.

The next chapter explores how King-Drew's acute care hospital and medical school provided coherency and purpose to a whole host of smaller and less expensive antipoverty projects built ahead of the hospital's opening—such as USC's Multipurpose Neighborhood Health Center and Central City Community Mental Health Center. These institutions gave poor people access to low-cost preventative health services. The effectiveness of these services, however, still required antipoverty advocates to address how to provide poor people with access to more expensive and labor-intensive services without enlarging the burden on white taxpayers. As construction of King-Drew's acute care medical campus drew nearer to completion, conversations about how to acculturate poor people to modern biomedical services without encouraging them to be dependent on state assistance programs increasingly transformed concerns about Black people's bodily health into concerns about their mental health and consumer subjectivity.

This chapter reveals that King-Drew's health system created a shared space of contested meanings for a wide cross section of political and medical leaders who came to support its construction as an antipoverty machine. For liberal progressive politicians yearning for lasting political change such as Hahn, Councilman Tom Bradley, and Congressman Augustus Hawkins, King-Drew provided a political vehicle outside the reach and control of white conservative "Dixiecrat" mayor Sam Yorty. It served as an example of how activists in neighborhoods of color, gay districts, and poor communities could build economic development schemes to counter white supremacy using ideas of community self-determination, political power, and identity. For medical leaders of all races, the health system's ability to control and regulate costs and the flow of patients to and from clinics and hospitals provided them with the means to help themselves overcome the greatest obstacle confronting healthcare's expansion at midcentury. By creating a new type of physician specialist called a "Community Physician," medical leaders believed that it was possible to turn poor patients into paying patients. This, in turn, would transform risky healthcare markets into new consumer markets for profit.

Finding Black medical leaders capable of managing a much larger and complex health system than the one originally imagined caused politicians and regional health policy leaders to target poor Black physicians and their patients as two kinds of citizen-subjects in need of reform.[3] Building the hospital and health system they imagined also required them to find more capital than was available through Medicare and Medicaid alone. The raised stakes of such an endeavor made politicians and health policy leaders fearful that the training and standards once tolerated under Jim Crow made Black doctors, their past training, and their past education too outdated and inadequate to make medicine in Black communities modern following the Civil Rights Act. They also feared that the imposed poverty Black physicians experienced also made them more eager to get rich from new federal programs than to help uplift the poor.

To protect their interests as well as those of white taxpayers, politicians and health policy leaders conspired to raise the capital needed to build a new health system with the help of local Black physicians in 1966. By the end of the decade, however, politicians and regional health policy leaders had laid a pathway leading to the appointment of elite Black physicians hand-selected from the NMA's national headquarters to carry out what all proponents referred to as King-Drew's "Master Plan." In theory, the master plan guided and coordinated the participation of any health provider, public or private, willing to serve Black patients in the context of antipoverty objectives. Formed over several years under the auspices of Dr. Mitchell Spellman, Drew Medical School's dean, and Dr. M. Alfred Haynes, Drew Medical School's chair of community medicine, the master plan aimed to lead the community out of poverty by creating a class of Black physicians fit to lead the way.

An examination of King-Drew's master plan reveals how racial elites devised a scheme to prevent the return of crisis through what Neil Smith refers to as a "spatial fix."[4] Smith argues that events like the Watts Uprisings are products of uneven development that require "some sort of spatial solution, a 'spatial fix'" that attempts to "resolve or otherwise displace [uneven development's] inherent contradictions."[5] In the case of a "Watts Hospital," LA's municipal and medical leaders sought to stave off another uprising by organizing employment around healthcare to challenge the abandonment of inner-city neighborhoods of color since World War II.

The McCone Report ensured that King-Drew's master plan did more than just employ Black people. It also sought to fix space by "fixing" what Hortense Spillers calls Black gender.[6] According to Spillers, Black gender names all the sexual manifestations that proponents of the culture of poverty theory argued prevented Black individuals from economically advancing. In the case of the Watts Uprisings, politicians and health policy experts blamed white supremacy for preventing Black families from taking their "normal" shape as heterosexual patriarchal nuclear family units by portraying Jim Crow as primarily an injury to Black men. Politicians and health policy leaders believed that the lack of proper incentives around breadwinning manhood under Jim Crow accounted for what by the 1960s was perceived as the Black community's high number of homosexuals and "heterosexuals on the outside of heteronormativity," such as so-called absentee fathers, women on welfare, and delinquent and sexually promiscuous youth.[7]

Proponents of culture of poverty theory saw their approach as a more benevolent alternative to older racist narratives portraying Black men as biologically and intellectually incapable of self-governance because it sought to marshal the federal government's resources to rehabilitate their manhood. The theory, however, helped obscure the processes of racial and sexual capitalism that accounted for poverty in poor neighborhoods of color. It hid how absentee fatherhood, welfare motherhood, youth delinquency, and homosexuality were also features endemic to many spaces and places that society represented as white, middle class, and straight. Rather than make poor people of color criminally and sexually "deviant," their reliance on the leadership of strong women, the presence of men who continued to love kin despite their empty pockets, and alternative kinship patterns (inclusive of intergenerational, same-age, same-sex, and gender-diverse living situations) all represent how humans organize themselves to survive in neighborhoods abandoned by capital.

And yet, as Cheryl Hicks has argued, Black people's appropriations of mainstream discourses of respectable marriage and family and active defense of normative expectations of gender and sexual roles have rarely won Black people the same protection and privacy as their white counterparts.[8] Although Hicks explores these dimensions among poor and working-class Black migrants in New York City in the 1920s, this chapter extends her analysis to "poor" Black physicians working in poor and working-class Black neighborhoods like Watts. As Black middle-class professionals working in poor urban neighborhoods, Black physicians were perhaps the most representative embodiment of what Evelyn Brooks Higginbotham calls the "politics of respectability."[9] They willingly appropriated white society's norms of medical education, physician training, and sexual respectability as part of a larger strategy to make themselves "fit" to both doctor and lead the race. However, King-Drew's master plan shows that most Black physicians by the 1960s, except for a select few, were generally not considered fit for anything but medical reform.

The idea that Black physicians and male heads of households fell short of normative expectations about fitness to lead and care for families—regardless of how well-educated, distinctly gendered, and distinctly middle class they were—exposes a ruse at the center of racial and sexual liberalism's discourses of inclusion. If a plan for inclusion based on being highly educated and sexually respectable requires those who have arguably been most committed to those values to still be subjects of reform, we should ask who is benefiting from these discourses. If poor Black communities in the 1960s and white communities during the Great Depression all demonstrated that it was possible to live and care for each other despite a lack of capital, then what could societies look like if those arrangements were given as much social and state investment as breadwinning manhood?

FIT TO BE PHYSICIANS?

That most Black physicians supposedly failed to match the fitness of most white male physicians in the 1960s was not for Black physicians' lack of trying. Through the formation of the NMA, the National Hospital Association, and the *Journal of the National Medical Association*, Black physicians did everything in their power to ensure that medical school curriculum, training standards, and continuing education in Black medical schools, hospitals, and private practices matched those expected in white medical institutions. By the 1960s, the combination of the AMA's efforts to exclude Black physicians from medicine and Jim Crow's hold on Black labor since the end of Reconstruction forced Black physicians to make difficult decisions about their own physician identities vis-à-vis both other physicians and their own communities.

As historians of Black doctoring argue, Black physicians debated the meaning and significance of pursuing expensive forms of biomedical education and training because such pursuits often placed their skills at odds with the economic and material realities of the majority of Black individuals. Scholars have, for instance, argued that many Black physicians took umbrage at Abraham Flexner's recommendation in 1910 that Black physicians "humbly" forgo careers in biomedicine by serving "their people" as "sanitarians" after completing medical school.[10] Flexner's comments suggest that he, like many other white medical leaders, believed that Black medical students "were considered 'colored' doctors working towards a predetermined future that was worlds apart from the white medical mainstream."[11] His comments thus also underlined a belief that Black medical graduates should avoid directly competing with white physicians by limiting their practices to public health jobs paid by the state.

Lynn Miller and Richard Weiss, however, argue that Flexner felt safe to make his recommendations based on the public statements of Meharry and Howard University's own leaders, who regularly stressed the nation's need for Black physicians to provide "instruction for the people in hygiene and sanitation" and the need for the Black masses "to adopt proper sanitary regulations."[12]

They contend too that such calls by Black medical school leaders were also likely made to win the support of liberal white philanthropists who stood willing to help fund instruction of biomedicine in Black institutions. By the 1920s and 1930s, Thomas Ward argues that white philanthropists' relationships with Black medical school leaders were reproduced between Black hospital leaders to help Black medical graduates get the training needed to keep pace with white physicians.[13]

Vanessa Northington Gamble argues that these philanthropic relationships not only helped Black hospitals survive but allowed them to meet standards set by national accrediting boards. She contends, however, that "such support was not without consequences" because it "frequently enabled white philanthropists, not the Black community, to determine the policies of Black hospitals."[14] By the 1960s, the dilemma facing Black physicians was exacerbated by the proliferation of hospital specializations and sub-specializations requiring Black physicians to train in academic medical institutions with departments catering mostly to paying white patients in the suburbs.

Before his appointment as King-Drew's chair of community medicine, M. Alfred Haynes explained the dilemma facing Black physicians by the late 1960s as a choice between pathways disproving two widespread beliefs: that Black doctors were incapable of being highly talented and competent physicians, or that Black people were inherently incapable of personal hygiene and being healthy. The first required Black physicians to practice in research settings often far from neighborhoods of color, while the latter required Black physicians to give up fame and notoriety by toiling in marginalized neighborhoods. Haynes understood this as an impossible choice.

He argued that Black doctors made themselves vulnerable to attack no matter what choice they made to challenge racism. According to Haynes, a Black doctor who "establishes practice in the suburbs" to show how competent he is exposes himself to attack because the Black community will wonder why he lacks "social consciousness" since he works so far away from Black neighborhoods, while his "white colleagues will wonder why so few Black physicians practice in the ghetto."[15] On the other hand, "if he practices in the ghetto, they will assume he is incompetent, for why would a dedicated, competent physician practice in the ghetto?" This no-win, false choice for Black physicians illuminates how capitalism and white supremacy worked in tandem to alienate Black physicians' own sense of self by pitting their professional pursuits against that of their communities.

Black physicians who could not keep up with the education, training, and practice of their white counterparts compensated by keeping up with what they believed it culturally signified to be a doctor by midcentury. By the 1960s, Black physicians organized in the NMA did everything they could to demonstrate their readiness for inclusion in the AMA by adhering to all the AMA's principles except for its stance on racial exclusion. During the twentieth century, this readiness increasingly called upon Black doctors to follow their white counterparts' strict adherence to gendered ideas about medicine's division of labor.

This shift reflected a different approach to doctoring than when the NMA was founded in 1895. Likely influenced by the AMA's concurrent exclusion of women, the NMA's founding documents show that the organization supported the medical education of women by stating that it was inclusive of both "men and *women* of African descent." This decision reflected the fact that the world's most prominent women's medical college, the Woman's Medical College of Pennsylvania, had readily accepted and trained Black women medical students since its inception in 1850. By 1925, the college was responsible for graduating eighteen Black women physicians.[16]

However, the activities of local NMA chapters show that Black physicians had begun to subjugate the role of women in the organization, reducing them from doctors to wives, by establishing Woman's Auxiliary units in 1936. This followed on the heels of the AMA's founding of a Woman's Auxiliary for white women in 1924 and mirrored the AMA's convention of referring to the club as an organization for "physician's wives." According to Kelly O' Donnell, these organizations enlisted physicians' wives into providing local chapters and the individual practices of their physician husbands with unpaid administrative and logistical labor under the concept of "medical marriages."[17]

Out of all the tactics deployed to assert Black male physicians' legitimacy, the work of Black physicians' wives appeared to be crucial. Through the publication *The Mouthpiece*, Black physicians' wives instructed each other on rearing children, keeping house, and helping their husbands carry out the NMA's policy decisions.[18] They were also frequently responsible for setting up spaces for doctors to meet for their continuing education workshops, holding scholarship drives for Black students, and carrying out elaborate galas and awards dinners for Black doctors to culturally authenticate themselves as middle class.

Black physicians' wives were also more willing to be explicit about medicine's unspoken gendered divisions of labor. Mrs. Marcus Tucker of Los Angeles, president of the NMA's Woman's Auxiliary in 1965, for instance, lamented the lack of "a satisfactory reservoir of college students to channel into medical careers" given that "Negro women outnumber Negro men in college by a ratio of 2 to 1."[19] For her, the idea that colleges were too full of Black women not bound for medical careers required Black physicians' wives to do their part in encouraging Black men to become doctors by raising money for scholarships and holding social events to help medical students and graduates matriculate through school. She argued that it was a physician's wife's calling to meet the challenge of recruitment because they, "more than any group, other than the doctors themselves," were able to speak "with authority . . . on a medical career."

These efforts show that most Black physicians did not consider gender norms and patriarchy as ancillary to the work of doctoring. In fact, in the absence of having the social connections and capital to back up their medical education and training with specialist certifications and high-end suburban practices, many Black physicians relied on the social policing of gender norms as an easily accessible way to authenticate status as a physician. For many, the idea that Black physicians were men and that they were married to women was such an ingrained concept that it often did not need comment or explanation.

FIT TO BE MEN?

The testimonies of Black politicians, community leaders, and activists in the wake of the Watts Uprisings show that the use of patriarchy's discourses to make arguments around racial equality was not just limited to Black physicians. Between the August uprisings and the hospital council's December meeting, the community's attention turned to the McCone Commission's recommendations. This sequence of events implicitly sent a message to any party hoping to gain approval for hospital construction that proposals aligned with McCone's recommendations would ultimately win.

Appointed by Democratic California Governor Edmund "Pat" Brown shortly after the uprisings, John McCone was charged with conducting a full investigation of the causes and reporting on ways to remediate and prevent future rioting. McCone and his team compiled evidence from a series of hearings and investigations that he gathered from September to November 1965 into a volume ominously titled *Violence in the City—An End or a Beginning?* Rather than design entirely new programs to address poverty, McCone issued policy advice to municipal leaders with large poor urban constituencies on how to marshal new antipoverty programming and previously existing poverty-oriented programs into a more coherent economic development strategy.

This pragmatic approach to craft responses from existing policies and programs extended the logic of congressional responses to white poverty during the Great Depression to solve Black poverty in the 1960s. Similar to the political rhetoric of the 1930s, McCone argued that intergenerational poverty flourished in Black communities because society had failed to incentivize its male breadwinners to maintain marriage and family as foundational institutions. He argued that permitting Black male breadwinners to be chronically out of work not only produced "hopelessness and permanent dependence" in Black neighborhoods but also produced "damaging side effect[s]," such as laziness, sexual promiscuity, and social delinquency, in Black women and children.[20] Rather than attribute poverty to the economic inequality required by capitalism, McCone's solution sought to save Black people from what he imagined as a crisis of "no work" through a plan centered on getting men in Black communities back to work.

The similarities between McCone's recommendations and Daniel Patrick Moynihan's culture of poverty theory caused many to believe that McCone was pressured by President Johnson or Moynihan to issue policies favorable to federal policy positions. McCone insisted, however, that he conducted his investigations "independently of Washington DC."[21] A closer inspection of McCone's hearing transcripts shows he was influenced indirectly to support federal initiatives by local Black political leaders who were already familiar with the policy underlying Moynihan's thesis. By the 1960s, most local Black political leaders would have been familiar with and supportive of similar social science narratives popularized among Black leaders, including work by Oscar Lewis, Gunnar Myrdal, Robert E. Park, Emory Bogardus, St. Clair Drake, Horace Clayton, E. Franklin Frazier, and W. E. B. Du Bois.[22]

Local Black political leaders organized their testimonies in hopes that McCone's recommendations could, in tandem with new federal policy recommendations, help them neutralize the threat that Mayor Sam Yorty's leadership over the city's antipoverty programs posed to progress in communities of color. Mike Davis argues that Yorty, elected in 1961, famously "threw his weight behind the police and the growing white resistance to civil rights demands" by supporting laws like the passage of Proposition 14, a referendum repealing a prior housing desegregation law.[23] Yorty's white supremacist approach to policing and housing manifested in tactics that either stalled antipoverty programming or directed funding to ineffective leaders and programs.

According to Charles Schultze of the Federal Budget Bureau, Yorty's approach to maintaining white supremacy had national reach because he also fought for mayoral oversight of federal antipoverty funds as president of the US Conference of Mayors. Yorty knew that antipoverty funds had the potential for leaders of color to create "a competing political organization in their own backyards," and he set up bureaucratic mechanisms to help city leaders with large Black and Brown urban populations to delay antipoverty funds and evade demands made by civil rights activists to challenge economic racism.[24] His national leadership exemplified how cities defied federal law and deferred civil rights action through administrative means.

Growing recognition of LA's importance as a new front for national civil rights battles helps explain why federal authorities provided an advanced copy of Moynihan's report to local activists to use as a guideline in crafting their own comments before the McCone Commission. They hoped making recommendations aligned with Moynihan's culture of poverty theory would assist civil rights activists in other majority-Black cities, like New York and Atlanta, pressure their own local governments to follow federal policy recommendations. They also believed McCone's recommendations could assist other neighborhoods in LA, like the city's Mexican and Asian American neighborhoods, to implement programs aligned with culture of poverty theory in their locations. Ultimately, they optimistically dreamed that McCone's well-known reputation as a conservative Republican could help activists present culture of poverty theory as a bipartisan solution to racial progress in cities led by Republicans, not Democrats.

The testimonies of Black politicians before the McCone Commission reveal their belief that white leadership, supervision, and proxy control over antipoverty programs had indirectly contributed to the uprisings by perpetuating the status quo. According to Rev. H. Hartford Brookins of the First African Methodist Episcopal Church, Yorty's antipoverty programs were led by Black operatives who were "selected for the Negro community by the white power structure."[25] Their appointments led Councilman Tom Bradley to described Yorty's antipoverty programs as "temporary 'make work' projects" that did little to improve Black workers' chances for gainful and meaningful employment.[26] The fruitlessness of Yorty's antipoverty programs was apparent to James Baldwin, who toured a boys' correctional program, which tasked them with "mak[ing] wooden frames for hassocks."[27] Baldwin argued that the whole thing was clearly "nonsense" to everyone—including him, participants, teachers, and even the school's principal—who knew its objectives did nothing to help Black youth develop a "useful" trade.

Such arguments allowed local Black leaders to make claims about what their leadership could do to prevent future uprisings if they were empowered to independently carry out their own antipoverty agendas. Their claims centered on addressing the injury to Black men and Black families inflicted by Jim Crow, particularly in the wake of its nationalization through the New Deal. Brookins summarized the problem by arguing that white employers' unwillingness to hire Black men combined with Black women's access to welfare programs disincentivized Black men from stepping into their roles as male heads of household. As he described it, in such a situation, "there was nothing for [Black men] to do but get out and get from [marriage], because his wife was better off through the welfare programs and agencies of this country with him not being present than they were with him being present."[28]

Black politicians argued that growing Black poverty since the New Deal demonstrated a radically different outcome than the prosperity associated with white neighborhoods. Assemblyman Mervyn Dymally reminded McCone that the "fundamentals" of marriage and family were "challenged" during the Great Depression but that the perceived problems of independent women and homosexual unions were, as he put it, "taken apart, seam by seam, and reconstructed" with the New Deal.[29] Congressman Augustus Hawkins's comments thus used Dymally's comments to portray antipoverty programs as an effort to reorganize economic development in Black neighborhoods along the same lines as the New Deal. As such, he argued antipoverty programming potentially could give Black communities what he believed they had always wanted, which was for "the family union to be recognized in its proper role with reverence for our women and respect for the manhood of the house."[30] To do that, it was necessary for white leaders to work with trusted Black leaders to govern Black neighborhoods.

Discussion over "trusted Black leaders" was a ploy by many elected Black officials to encourage McCone to make recommendations in their favor. They sought to steer resources and political favor toward themselves and away from Black leaders they found divisive and extreme. These included Yorty's

"Uncle Tom" appointees and the growing presence of Black nationalists, who (Brookins argued) had a proclivity to "counsel separation, nationalism, and the utter hopelessness of a future of isolation for Negroes in a totally Negro world."[31] Brookins argued that standing aside and letting either camp grow in power would only lead to another uprising.

The point of giving this topographical lesson on local politics was to strengthen efforts to preserve and grow an "integrated" multiracial, multiethnic city that many felt was being overshadowed by rioting and segregation. John Buggs of the Los Angeles County Human Rights Commission, for instance, reminded McCone that Black residents living in middle-class neighborhoods did not riot because they were less willing to burn property that they themselves owned.[32] He called upon McCone to "use whatever influence is possible with all of the agencies responsible" to encourage more business ownership and activity in Watts so that "we can begin to develop in the area a real integrated kind of community [like those in middle-class neighborhoods outside Watts], rather than the segregated kind of community that we have there now."

These messages resonated with McCone because his tenure as CIA director had informed him of the dangers of reproducing older forms of colonialism in the US's economic and diplomatic relations with newly independent nations abroad. He understood that the profile of leaders who came to power after gaining independence from their colonial possessors was crucial in determining their nation's willingness to work with American diplomats, businessmen, and military officials after achieving independence.[33] McCone also knew that American diplomats, businessmen, and military officials regarded leaders who appeared to be hand-selected by former colonial powers to be just as difficult to access economically because of the continued political instability in nations rejecting capitalism and democracy as methods to develop their economies.

Hawkins built on such statements by reminding McCone that threats to American democracy and capitalism were also present in American cities. The multiple political divisions within the Black community proved that "more than a local issue or civil rights" was at stake in McCone's recommendations, because how local governments addressed the Watts Uprisings and how the federal government dealt with emerging and undeveloped nations were one and the same. He contended that successful outcomes in Watts could inspire global citizens "yearning for self-government, freedom, security, and human dignity" in "troubled spots" around the world to know that progress and modernity was possible under a shared banner of democratic capitalism.[34]

All these arguments by Black political leaders convinced McCone that the primary target audience for his report was neither white political leaders nor Black Americans but white taxpayers, whom he believed ultimately held the power and resources to end violence in inner cities through the ballot box. His report strove to convince white taxpayers that it was necessary to expand state support for education and training programs for young Black adolescents so that "in the long run" they could compete for better-paying jobs as adults. "In the short run," he argued that white taxpayers needed to support welfare programs, Medicare, and Medicaid programs because they were necessary to "create an initiative and an incentive on the part of the recipients to become independent of state assistance."[35] Both approaches, in theory, would eventually work together to reduce not only white voters' tax burdens but also the threat of violence to their health and their property.

McCone issued his report as a sort of cautionary tale. He warned that if Black leaders were not empowered to take leadership of their families and their communities, Black citizens "would become more and more estranged and the risk of violence would increase." In the absence of a new direction, he prophesied that "the cost of police protection would increase, and yet would never be adequate"; "unemployment would climb; welfare costs would move apace" in ways that would only give "preachers of division and demagoguery . . . a matchless opportunity to tear our nation asunder."[36]

McCone felt that action preventing the disaster he predicted was so urgent that he issued recommendations in his final report to bypass Yorty's municipal oversight of antipoverty programs. He highlighted that programs focused on health would make the county, not city, responsible for administering health-related antipoverty federal funds. Among his recommendations, McCone attested that "immediate and favorable consideration . . . be given to a new, comprehensively-equipped hospital" in Watts.[37] He also stressed that a "broadly-based committee" consisting of citizens and representatives of the area, the Los Angeles County Department of Charities, and representatives of the region's medical associations and medical schools should be appointed to craft it.

FIT TO BE LEADERS?

McCone's recommendation for a comprehensively equipped hospital in Watts was an early indicator of how politicians and health experts had begun to take White's hospital and health district plan more seriously since the uprisings. Recommending, however, that it be built with the oversight of a broadly based committee consisting of agencies and institutions well known for excluding Black physicians indicated that politicians and health experts did not take White as seriously as they did his plan. In theory, the support that local politicians and their allies had thrown behind White's plan should have made his proposal the strongest out of the five plans submitted.

The events surrounding the hospital council's December proceedings, however, suggest that the stakes of who should lead such a hospital had been raised by talk about its possible non-medical uses. Discussion about the hospital's use as an antipoverty machine elevated expectations about the proposed hospital's purposes and the quality of healthcare found within in it. If it was to be both a hospital and an antipoverty tactic, this required its leaders to simultaneously be medical experts, businessmen, and social workers who were savvy enough to inspire poor patients to consume more medical services without encouraging more dependency on state assistance programs.

By the council's meeting, Hahn had done enough reconnaissance to be concerned about White's motivations, qualifications, and financial acumen. Deputies working on his behalf had informed him that White and his associates did not have enough capital on hand to win certification. Other informants also indicated that the hospital council was wary about granting certification to any Black physician group based on the McCone Commission's own investigations into the care standards observed in Black neighborhoods. It did not help that many Black leaders, including Black politicians, physicians, and activists, also provided Hahn with anecdotal evidence corroborating the claims that White and his associates were not fit to lead the hospital they proposed to own.

One of Hahn's deputies, Harry Marlow, for instance, uncovered information casting suspicion on White's motivations for building the hospital. White's journey to secure capital had led him to Arnold Sweeney, a Black consultant for several East Coast philanthropic funds. Sweeney's interactions with White convinced him that White seemed more interested in profits than in serving the poor. As Sweeney explained, White erroneously believed he could attract investors by winning certification before showing independent proof of funds. White also believed that it was possible after opening the hospital to run it, if need be, entirely on Medicare and Medicaid funds.

The sum of these revelations gave Sweeney the impression that White sought to profit handsomely from the venture but wanted others to shoulder the financial risk. As Sweeney phrased it, White and his associates "want[ed] everything handed to them, a hospital in which they would work and which they would eventually take over" but that "no one," including White, was "ready to put up any single dollar in assistance for it."[38] Sweeney's frustrations led him to cast aspersions on White and his associates by stating that this "is no society of doctors. They are [just] Negro doctors... practicing in the area."[39]

Black politicians who had shown up to publicly side with White, such as Congressman Hawkins, quietly shared frustrations over Black physicians' claims to a commitment to serving the Black community. After word reached the leadership of the Drew Medical Society that USC was contemplating opening an antipoverty clinic in Watts, Hawkins shared with USC's leadership that none of the Black physicians who rushed to meet with him in his office in Watts appeared to have lost sleep like him.[40] His observations underlined the fact that most Black physicians never thought about living or practicing in Watts until Medicare's and Medicaid's implementation in late 1965.

Black residents echoed these sentiments with their own observations. Some activists, like Jim Bates, noted that most Black physicians in the area "maintained practices outside of [Watts] altogether," while others directly questioned the sudden interest of Black doctors to serve the community. One anonymous leaflet circulated among residents claimed that most people living in Watts could not name even one—yet alone two or three—Black physicians working in the area.[41]

While Black physicians were less willing to be as publicly critical about their colleagues than local politicians and residents, they did quietly critique White and his associates through their actions. Some Black physicians, such as Dr. Julius Hill, for instance, indirectly criticized the training and care standards of White and his associates by forming a separate medical society. In 1962, Hill and others started the Golden State Medical Society as a venue for Black physicians to reaffirm the NMA's commitment to biomedical innovation, racial integration, and high educational and training standards.[42] Although open to all doctors, the society in practice served as a means for Black physician specialists to exclude general practitioners already organized in the Drew Medical Society. By 1965, the existence of competing societies effectively served as the loudest form of criticism of Drew Medical Society's standards.[43]

The most consequential and widely circulated evidence casting doubt on local Black physicians' readiness to lead a new hospital came from the California Advisory Hospital Council's own investigation of White's proposed Watts Health District and from the McCone Commission's report on health conditions in Watts. White's proposal carved out a new hospital district from the region's poorest Black neighborhoods that would provide a pathway for him and other Black physicians to build a two-hundred-bed independent hospital. All in all, White's proposed district encompassed a twenty-square-mile area of approximately 344,000 residents (a population roughly equal to that of the nation's fiftieth-largest city).[44] Bordered by Jefferson, Artesia, Alameda, and Broadway Boulevards, the proposed district encompassed the county's lowest-income Black census tracts.

The council's report provided a clinical overview of the proposed health district. The report gave credibility to White's claims about the need for a hospital in Watts but eroded the qualifications of anyone currently working in the area to lead it. The report revealed that out of forty-two hospitals within and near Watts, only four institutions, with a total of 180 hospital beds, existed inside the boundaries of the proposed district. A closer examination of their average occupancies demonstrated that all four institutions struggled to achieve bed occupancies over 60 percent. The difficulty in filling beds helped account for the startling discovery that all institutions in Watts failed to win accreditation under new Medicare and Medicaid standards. The council's report thus shored up White's claim that a hospital was needed in the area but painted Black providers as generally unable to manage the business and health standards needed to run one successfully.

The McCone Commission's report on healthcare was more aggressive in passing judgment on local Black physicians and the institutions they had built. Authored by a committee of white medical experts led by Dr. Milton Roemer, a public health professor from UCLA, the health report described physicians who lacked training beyond a hospital internship, who negligently allowed their specialist certifications to lapse, and whose waiting rooms were always overcrowded.[45] The report compiled other findings from relevant health regulatory agencies to argue that the area's physicians and administrators failed to maintain basic standards of order and cleanliness by quoting evidence of mice droppings in patient care areas, confirmation of failed health inspections, instances of understaffing, proof of improper medical waste disposal, and observations of broken medical equipment.

The sum of these reports portrayed Black physicians and medical staff working in Black neighborhoods as unqualified and unfit to care for patients. Both reports did so by pointing to the seemingly poor business practices of these health institutions. By using health standards in white neighborhoods as standards for what constituted good care in Black neighborhoods, their

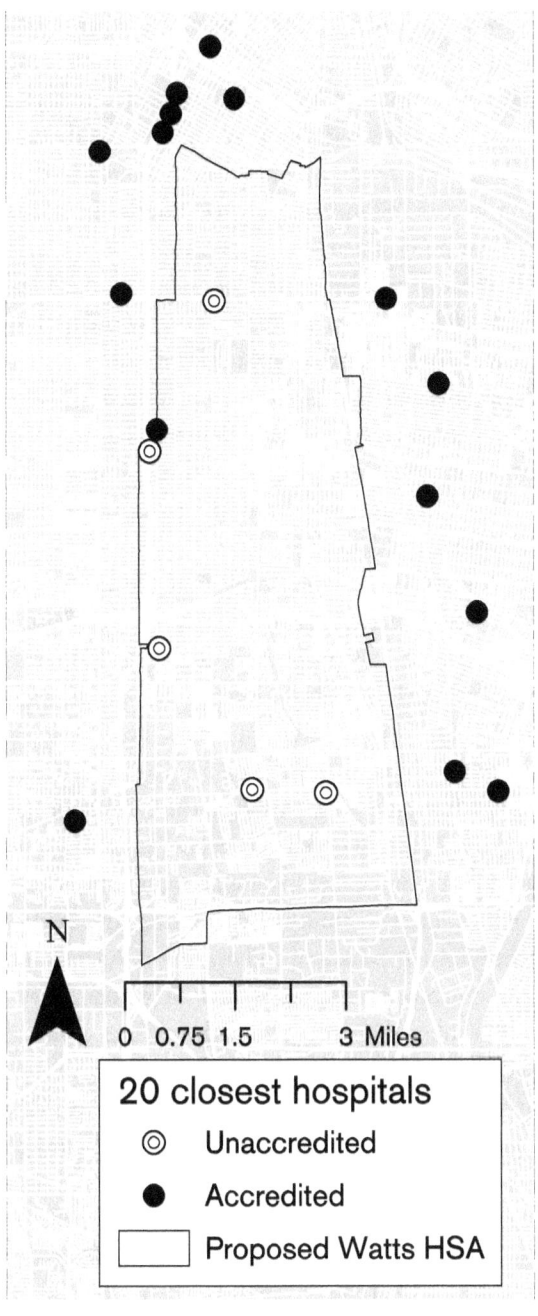

MAP 7. Hospitals in and near to Watts

All four of the hospitals inside White's proposed hospital district faced closure at the end of 1965. None of the service area's hospitals met new federal care standards for Medicare and Medicaid. Map: Tyler Munn.

reports elided the different ways that Black physicians and medical staff, regardless of being there by choice or circumstance, attempted to provide the best care they could under dire economic circumstances. Rather than argue that their investigations found proof of what providers did to provide care when confronted with poverty, these reports helped health policy leaders portray the health providers who worked in poor neighborhoods of color as equally in need of reform as their poor patients.

As the next section shows, these determinations, alongside the anecdotal findings of local citizens, helped white physician leaders portray themselves as agents more ready and able to help Black communities improve health standards than the Black physicians who had historically practiced in them. The facts gathered in the discovery process of vetting White's plan inspired them and Hahn to imagine what their own hospitals and medical schools could do with Medicare, Medicaid, and antipoverty funding to advance their own interests in poor neighborhoods of color.

Hahn's and health policy leaders' immediate problem at the December hospital council meeting was that they had no legitimate way to enter Watts's health market without the participation of Black physicians. In 1963, Congress authorized federal funding for a whole host of antipoverty programs through what bureaucrats termed the "citizen participation" mandate, a requirement tasking federally funded agencies with recruiting the poor into the planning and implementation of poverty alleviation programs. Be it the County of Los Angeles or some private investor, Hahn believed that whoever built a new "Watts Hospital" would need help from Black physicians and community members in order to win certification, win antipoverty funding, and be successful in recruiting poor people into its planning and operation. As it stood, White had brought a convincing array of Black politicians, clergymen, physicians, and local residents who spoke adamantly about their belief that the proposed "Watts Hospital" should be a private, not public, hospital.

Hoping to thread an impossible needle, Hahn brokered an offer to those present at the meeting, stipulating that the Los Angeles County Board of Supervisors would authorize the construction of a badly needed hospital in Watts if privately raised funds could not be secured to build a free market "community hospital" by the council's next meeting in February 1966. In the interim, Hahn requested that the hospital council approve the health district boundaries as outlined by White. In so doing, the authorization of a "Watts Hospital District" would begin a process to prime Black neighborhoods in Los Angeles for the same political and economic interventions being designed for developing economies in the colonial and former colonial possessions of European empires.

According to Timothy Mitchell, the technology of visualizing poverty as a discrete and manipulable object by spatializing its dimensions on a map was the product of the "development of the economy as a discursive object" between economists and state technocrats between the 1930s and 1950s.[46] Plotting the Watts Hospital District as distinct from other districts provided health experts with a geospatial representation of hospital markets "in which the world was pictured in the form of separate nation-states, with each state marking the boundary of a distinct economy" and "provided a new, everyday political language in which [a Black neighborhood] could speak of itself and imagine its existence as something natural, spatially bounded, and subject to political management."[47]

Creating a health district without naming its leadership was a tactic that helped Hahn, Black politicians, and mainstream health policy leaders focus community attention away from the demands of local Black physicians and toward discussions about the low number of providers and perceived low standards of healthcare in the neighborhood. More important, establishing the district diverted attention from more troubling questions about the political and economic relationships that helped constitute Watts as a space lacking capital and resources that were available in other neighborhoods. Instead of addressing the processes of racial capitalism that enmeshed Watts's health with the rest of the city, the formation of a district simply asked residents who had the capital and know-how to fix its problems.

RULE OF EXPERTS

Hahn's request to delay deliberations on who should lead efforts to address the health problems in Watts hid how Black politicians sought to buy more time to convince residents and other Black physicians to support a plan to build what Hahn later referred to as a "county community hospital," a term suggesting the possibilities for new public-private partnerships in healthcare after Medicare and Medicaid. As this section reveals, the hospital council's investigation of White's original proposal and the McCone Commission's exploration of health services in Watts encouraged regional health policy leaders like California Director of Public Health Dr. Lester Breslow, USC Medical School's Dean Dr. Roger Egeberg, and UCLA Medical School's

Dean Dr. Sherman Mellinkoff to analyze how antipoverty, Medicare, and Medicaid funds could transform and extend their efforts to advance biomedical research and innovation. Like Black politicians who could not help but be inspired to see a way to advance their own political goals, these health leaders could not help but see a vehicle to advance new medical knowledge.

The health reports by the council and commission served as an occasion for a wide swath of health policy leaders to investigate White's claims more seriously. White's proposal rested on his belief that Medicare and Medicaid laws now gave Black patients formerly reliant on public healthcare a "choice" of where to apply their benefits. Under the stipulations passed by Congress, Medicare- and Medicaid-eligible patients could consume healthcare in private hospitals so long as those institutions voluntarily enrolled in each program and met the standards for providers set by the Joint Commission on Accreditation of Hospitals (JCAH) and the Centers for Medicare and Medicaid. The law thus gave patients the freedom to choose their own healthcare by denying them the freedom to choose healthcare the federal government deemed substandard.

White also sought certification of a new hospital district because it would give him and his associates a monopoly on Black patients. Under the established protocols of hospital construction governance, hospitals in a given district were given the power to approve or reject any new health service application. White hoped that being the first owner to operate a hospital in a newly established "Black" hospital district would give him and his associates the power to control who practiced in Watts because he and his associates would have the power to control who received construction grants.

For Dr. Lester Breslow, the problem posed by White's proposal was not that it was too narrowly focused on organizing profit for Black physicians but that it overlooked the potential benefits a Black-led teaching hospital could provide for revitalizing biomedical research at a crucial juncture in the history of medicine. After extensive medical advances to counter contagious disease and to advance biomedical research, the nation stood poised by the mid-1960s to mount research on a suite of diseases, such as heart disease, cancer, and stroke, that required physicians to establish long-term study relationships with their patients. This intimacy required medical school leaders to consider how they could get patients to willingly choose care at their research hospitals rather than at a proprietary hospital. Medical schools thus had to consider the potential threat that Medicare and Medicaid posed to undermining their ability to continue medical research using Black patients.

Instead of lamenting the end of public hospitals as people knew them or celebrating the potential growth of private hospital power, Breslow welcomed the potential market turbulence of Medicare and Medicaid because it would force teaching hospitals to compete with private hospitals for the same patients by humanizing healthcare.[48] In late 1965, Congress more or less incentivized teaching hospitals to experiment with improving patient care standards by passing the Heart Disease, Cancer, and Stroke Act, a piece of legislation later programmatically known as Regional Medical Programs (RMPs). Congress passed the law with the explicit intent of reducing death rates related to the three biggest causes of morbidity in the United States, but the act has since been understood by historians of medicine as being responsible for defining the basic elements of what constitutes an academic medical center.[49]

Unlike Medicare and Medicaid, RMP funds were selectively given to an extremely small set of teaching hospitals based on their top status within a particular regional market. To receive RMP status, teaching hospitals were required to demonstrate their ability to serve a large racially and socioeconomically diverse patient population. They also had to demonstrate that they could sustain consistent long-term relationships with patients across all socioeconomic classes to mount effective research on heart disease, cancer, and stroke.

The combination of these factors made White's original plan extremely attractive to county hospital administrators and regional medical school leaders because involvement in Watts strengthened their own ability to compete for federal research dollars. By late 1965, the medical school deans of USC and UCLA, Roger Egeberg and Sherman Mellinkoff, each expressed willingness to support Black physicians in developing a medical school of their own. Egeberg even went so far as to integrate the operation of a federal antipoverty health clinic that he and his medical school staff had won grant money for toward the development of King-Drew's health system.

Their involvement effectively helped broker a peace between them and the Drew Medical Society by committing resources to help the society build and open a medical school named after Charles R. Drew in exchange for their willingness to allow the hospital to be built as a new county hospital. By 1969, this commitment was made real by an agreement struck between the two deans to pledge portions of their RMP funding to recruit the Drew Medical School's inaugural faculty. As their public correspondence shows, both leaders invested in King-Drew's academic arm to help bolster its status as a regional leader not only on how to administer healthcare in LA's poorest neighborhoods but also on how it could serve as a "prototype for other American ghetto communities" to follow.[50]

These agreements helped Hahn and the county's hospital leaders broker a peace deal with Drew Medical Society's leaders by encouraging them to think of their potential leadership of a new medical school as de facto ownership of a new county hospital. The idea of a privately owned medical school leading a hospital paid for by taxpayers was not such a difficult concept to sell given that both USC's and UCLA's teaching and research facilities were effectively all paid for by taxpayers through county referendums and military funding. Such relationships affirmed a common practice of using taxpayer-paid resources to lubricate free market medicine.

The difference that made county leaders eager to enter into a new relationship with Black physicians was the fact that Medicare and Medicaid helped the county supervisors imagine a new role for its county hospitals. Although Medicare and Medicaid did not release them from treating indigent patients under California's Pauper Act of 1855, the supervisors signaled hope that new federal programs might one day make them profitable by changing the names of their institutions from county hospitals to general hospitals. The name change signaled to residents that public hospitals could now accept paying patients and potentially generate revenue for the county's coffers.[51]

The idea that a public hospital could be entrusted to Black physicians to be run like a private hospital and that an antipoverty clinic owned by USC could work in concert with a medical center owned ostensibly by another competing medical school illustrated early on how people understood King-Drew's master plan would work. The point of the master plan was not to dominate or monopolize healthcare in Watts but to coordinate the health resources in the community to maximize the health standards of Black residents and assist in developing job opportunities to elevate their income-earning potential. Rather than an aloof and detached medical center, King-Drew was intended to anchor, regulate, and direct the traffic of capital and patients across a wider health system that included physician groups, primary care clinics, and community health clinics owned by various public and private agencies.

According to Harvard's Dr. Alonzo Yerby, a Black professor of public health brought in to develop King-Drew's master plan as a consultant, the objective of coordinating services across agencies run by different proprietors—like USC, UCLA, the county, and private doctors—within a single health system was to make healthcare services desirable and attractive enough for poor Black patients to eventually want to pay for them on their own.[52] Yerby believed that federal health programs would "fail to satisfy the health needs of the poor until services [were] arranged more for the convenience of the patient than for doctors and hospitals." Without this, he believed that "the lack of coordination which exists in most communities between private doctors, public programs, clinics, hospitals and the larger number of public and private agencies concerned with health care for the poor" would not inspire poor patients to seek healthcare on their own enough to return to use services, let alone pay for it themselves.

In the eyes of leading health experts and medical school leaders, the true question of how to solve the health crisis in Watts was not how big and well-equipped the medical center needed to be but how small and how basic enough it could be to stimulate job growth and economic activity to attract more investment in the neighborhood, either by others or by Black people themselves. The true aim of King-Drew's master plan was thus not to build a health system that allowed Black physicians to monopolize control of health services in Watts but to make Black people's lives appear healthy and normal enough for others to invest in the area. It was thus important for the master plan to address both the general lack of consumer power in Black neighborhoods and the lack of hospital training and experience of the physicians practicing there.

By late January 1966, successful discussions to get White and other Drew Medical Society members to agree to build their proposed hospital as a public hospital were aided by a concerted campaign by Black political leaders to get residents to rally around the same idea. Over two months, Rev. Roy L. Thompson of the South Central Area Welfare Planning Council, John Manning of the Watts Labor Community Action Committee, Shirley Spencer Taylor of the United Neighborhood Organizations of Watts, and Dr. J. Alfred Cannon of People in Community Action all organized meetings and sent letters attesting to their members' desire for a public hospital.[53] The combination of these two campaigns resulted in the hospital council granting certification to the County of Los Angeles at its February 1966 meeting.

For Hahn, the excitement that health and medical school leaders exhibited in having a stake in elevating the status of the Watts Hospital project to that of a full-fledged academic medical center presented a challenge because no one at the time, including the County of Los Angeles, had the capital or the taxpayer authorization to build it. By March 1966, the Watts Hospital Committee, which included members from the Drew Medical Society, the Watts community, the County Hospital system, and the medical school leadership of USC and UCLA, all looked toward passing a June 1966 referendum called Proposition A, a bond measure put before county voters to build a new public hospital in Watts. In so doing, the referendum put the McCone Commission's theory of social change and racial progress to a vote by the county's majority-white electorate.

UNDERWRITING BLACK HEALTH

Proposition A made McCone's recommendations real for white taxpayers because it, unlike congressionally approved antipoverty programs, directly asked them to debate the merits of culture of poverty theory by placing an exact dollar amount on the price of public safety after the Watts Uprisings. The ballot measure called for raising $12.3 million for a 438-bed hospital to be built in the southeast portion of Los Angeles County, consisting of "hospital buildings for medical care and treatment of children and adults, surgeries, laboratories, post-graduate medical training and other related facilities."[54] Voters rejected the ballot measure by a slim margin.

The rejection placed the Los Angeles County Board of Supervisors in an awkward political position. By late 1965, the board began committing resources to transform the purpose of its existing public hospitals to be aligned with the purposes of its new Black-led public hospital. The excitement of using health services to develop the poor and working-class neighborhoods of East Los Angeles and the South Bay surrounding LAC-USC and Harbor-UCLA pushed the supervisors to go against a trend among other county boards to close rather than save their public hospitals.

Elinor Blake and Thomas Bodenheimer argue that most county officials in California shuttered their public hospitals because they initially and falsely believed that Medicare and Medicaid would sufficiently incentivize private providers to take over the state's historic responsibility of caring for the poor. By 1975, eight counties had closed their public hospitals and an additional five had transferred their care responsibilities to for-profit hospital operators.[55] Merced, Mendocino, and Trinity Counties, for instance, all transferred management for medically indigent care to National Medical Enterprises, a predecessor company to Tenet Healthcare. Whereas sixty-six public hospitals were spread out over forty-nine of California's fifty-eight counties in 1966, less than half of California's counties operated a public hospital by 1985.[56]

LA's supervisors, however, joined the leadership of other counties, such as San Francisco, Santa Clara, and Oakland, who kept their public hospitals open to take advantage of the growing economic potential associated with academic medical centers. Others, such as Orange, San Diego, and Sacramento Counties, joined this trend by transferring authority of their county hospitals to the University of California, transforming each facility into a teaching hospital connected to newly established medical schools. All these measures demonstrate that King-Drew's identity as a publicly financed hospital run by a privately run medical school was not new or novel except for the fact that it was designed to be led by Black physicians.

Public debate about Proposition A shows that white voters used the McCone report to interpret the proposed hospital within McCone's proposed framework of considering federal antipoverty programs as important elements in protecting white people's public safety and property. Some voters, like Tony Cimurusti, an editor for Monrovia's *Daily News Post* and a former Watts resident, used McCone's frame to urge voters to remember the existence of the "many fine Afro-American persons who own property in Southwest LA and who have seen their property values shattered by the riot and the resulting damage, physical and to the reputation of their area."[57] He argued that authorizing the hospital was essential to helping "these people" fight poverty, sickness, and violence in their own neighborhoods in ways that simultaneously protected the public safety and property interests of white voters. As he put it, "It is for these people that a hospital should—and must—be constructed in the Negro section of Los Angeles."

Others, however, interpreted McCone's recommendations as a way for Black people to hold white voters hostage in order extract modern amenities that many believed Black people neither earned nor deserved. Signaled by "Don't Reward Rioting" bumper stickers distributed by a local white citizens' council, a growing amount of voices began interpreting Proposition A as "racial blackmail," a phrase expressing how some white voters believed that McCone's predictions of a more violent, disorderly, and tax-burdened city seemed designed to extort money from white taxpayers for people and neighborhoods they considered inherently violent and permanently dependent on welfare.[58]

While McCone's framing ultimately did not convince enough voters to pass the referendum with the needed two-thirds majority to authorize the hospital's construction, the supervisors' actions show that his framing did convince them to fund it regardless of the referendum's outcome. Preparations to announce funding of the proposed hospital in advance of the election outcome included compiling a list of past projects rejected by voters but built with county funds. A list showing that county leaders had authorized the construction of two juvenile hall centers, a men's jail, and a superior court house suggests that the supervisors all prepared statements defending the allocation of hospital funds for public safety purposes.[59]

Hahn's public statements show that he ultimately decided to use arguments suggesting that the nearly-two thirds majority vote served as a "mandate" to authorize the construction, but the decision to use alternative funding arrangements pushed the supervisors to enter into riskier financial arrangements. By the end of 1966, Hahn and the other supervisors worked alongside Hawkins, Dymally, and Bradley to broker a deal allowing Mayor Yorty to build a proposed new convention center downtown in exchange for his support in building a hospital in Watts. In 1967, the city and county finalized deals to support both projects by entering into a Joint Partnership Agreement. According to Destin Jenkins, such agreements bypassed public bond referendums by creating "special districts" that raised capital through bondholder agreements with higher interest rates and shorter loan servicing periods.[60] Politicians often defended such projects by limiting their use to so-called revenue-generating projects, such as toll bridges, parking garages, and stadiums, that "paid for themselves" through user-generated fees.

The less favorable financial terms of the proposed hospital made securing competent medical center leaders an increasingly significant objective. The higher financial risk associated with it compelled the Watts Hospital Committee convened by the McCone Commission to underwrite the new risks associated with operating an antipoverty hospital by enlarging their search for medical school leaders beyond Los Angeles. The results of their search reveal that Jim Crow medicine had produced an extremely small elite set of Black physician leaders concentrated in Washington, DC.

Unlike other urban areas with high concentrations of Black physicians by the 1960s, like New York, Los Angeles, and San Francisco, the District of Columbia's metropolitan region was the only city with a Black-led medical school and training hospital. The tight spatial relationship between Freedman's Hospital and a Black population large and wealthy enough to sustain training programs for Black specialists and subspecialists allowed Howard University to develop a small community of successful Black medical academicians. By the 1960s, Howard University's leaders also had invested enough in the building of specialist programs, which they did earlier and more consistently than their Meharry counterparts, to boast several highly trained subspecialists on its faculty roster.

The city also played an important role in guiding medical policy by serving as the national headquarters for the NMA. Likely in response to the competition facing Black physicians in light of key federal legislation such as the Civil Rights Act, antipoverty programs, Medicare, and Medicaid, the NMA appointed Dr. Mitchell Spellman of Howard University's Medical School and Dr. M. Alfred Haynes of Johns Hopkins University's Medical School to serve as leaders of the NMA Foundation. Created in 1968, the nonprofit was meant to be a policy clearinghouse allowing the NMA to better understand how federal funds could be used to aid the free market development of Black medicine.

The foundation played a significant role in rebranding the NMA's purpose after the Civil Rights Act ended the legal exclusion of Black physicians from the AMA. Haynes used his research skills to highlight the significant racial imbalance and poor spatial distribution of Black physicians as context to call upon white physicians to assist Black physicians with recruiting and training more Black physicians.[61] More important, he used his role as a spokesman for the NMA to call upon white physicians at the AMA's national convention in 1969 to join them "in removing barriers between government medicine and private medicine; in once and for all abolishing charity medicine; in bringing the poor into the mainstream of American medicine; and in helping every American, black or white, rich or poor, to enjoy the benefits of adequate health care."[62]

The foundation allowed the NMA to highlight the accomplishments of Black physicians who had been handpicked by white philanthropic organizations for training and leadership opportunities usually foreclosed to most Black physicians. In fact, Spellman was the product of a practice developed by Howard University's Numa P. Adams to train faculty members for new academic departments by working with leading white faculty members at predominantly white teaching hospitals whose Black graduates would take positions at Howard upon completion of their postgraduate programs.[63] In the 1950s, Howard University doctors Joseph Johnson and Paul Cornely worked with Dr. Owen Wagensteen of the University of Minnesota to train Spellman as a thoracic surgeon.[64]

Philanthropic foundations solidified these arrangements by providing Black trainees with material aid while serving as an intern, resident, or fellow.

In Spellman's case, Johnson's and Cornely's assurance of a faculty position helped persuade grant officers at the Commonwealth Foundation and John and Mary Markle Foundation to underwrite his training at the University of Minnesota with scholarships and fellowships. Unlike most Black physicians, who often needed to work during medical school and skipped postgraduate medical school to pay back debt and earn income, Mitchell's financial aid package permitted him to conduct research and publish in medical journals, secure an academic appointment at Howard University, and win awards as a member of the American College of Surgeons.

As Spellman's eventual appointment as the inaugural dean of the Charles R. Drew Postgraduate Medical School demonstrates, an elite Black medical graduate pipeline created by Black medical leaders and their allies did more than just help Howard University's Medical School keep pace with white medical standards. It also served as a vetting process that helped white medical school leaders, such as those at USC and UCLA, authenticate which Black candidates in their hiring pool fit the standards of training believed appropriate to lead a medical school of their caliber. Under the leadership of Dr. Sherman Mellinkoff and Dr. Roger Egeberg, the Watts Hospital Committee recruited Dr. Mitchell Spellman to serve as both dean and medical director of the Charles R. Drew Medical School and King General Hospital in early 1969.

Spellman's selection signaled several important things. First, even though local Drew Medical Society representatives and local Black community representatives sat on the Watts Hospital Committee, their presence was outnumbered by USC's and UCLA's representatives. It was also likely unbalanced due to USC's and UCLA's financial commitment to fund the Drew Medical School's faculty recruitment effort through their RMP funds. Second, Spellman's recruitment indexed a future-oriented desire to invest in Black physicians whose profiles looked more like his curriculum vitae and less like those already practicing in Watts. In so doing, Spellman's appointment sent a message that a physician's familiarity with extremely expensive and labor-intensive biomedical care was ultimately more important than their demonstrated commitment to working in poor neighborhoods of color.

Ultimately, Spellman's arrival in 1969 literally and figuratively represented the culmination of a four-year process to secure a vision to advance racial progress on terms that balanced Black people's desires for health and income with the wishes of white voters to preserve their personal safety and property from future violence. It did this by giving Black politicians a leader they could trust to help them build more political power in challenging the region's white power structure. It also gave county officials and regional medical school leaders the assurance that their investments would eventually turn a profit or produce value through the achievement of successful economic development schemes or by the attainment of new medical research knowledge. For local Black leaders, however, Spellman's arrival marked their transformation from being community leaders to being subjects for reform.

ORGANIZING KINSHIP THROUGH MEDICAL PATRIARCHY

Spellman's actions after arriving in 1969 show that he understood his first task as translating all the discussions that had culminated in his hire into a coherent operational program. To make explicit what had been implicit, Spellman won a grant from the John and Mary Markle Foundation to conduct a series of conferences to develop King-Drew's master plan. In addition to all the constituents already involved with the hospital planning process, the conference series brought together leading health experts in urban and rural healthcare, including Dr. Alonzo Yerby, chair of Health Services Administration at Harvard, and Dr. M. Alfred Haynes of the NMA Foundation.

The Markle conference series also resulted in Haynes's hire as the Drew School's inaugural chair of the Department of Community Medicine, a job that entrusted him to author the master plan. Using the guidelines established by his own hire and Haynes's hire, Spellman proceeded to appoint physicians to fill the chairs of seven basic academic departments, all determined by RMP funding as necessary to conduct research and training around heart disease, cancer, and stroke. The appointments mostly drew Black physicians who had training and service experience in predominantly white medical schools, and only one physician, Dr. J. Alfred Cannon, held a Drew Medical Society membership prior to his appointment.

As we have seen, the challenge for Spellman and Haynes went beyond carrying out an antipoverty program that serviced the wishes of Black politicians, health policy leaders, and local residents. They were also faced with the challenge of addressing the *local* health concerns of Black citizens by using the basic infrastructure provided to them by the federal government to research and treat diseases such as heart disease, cancer, and stroke that were

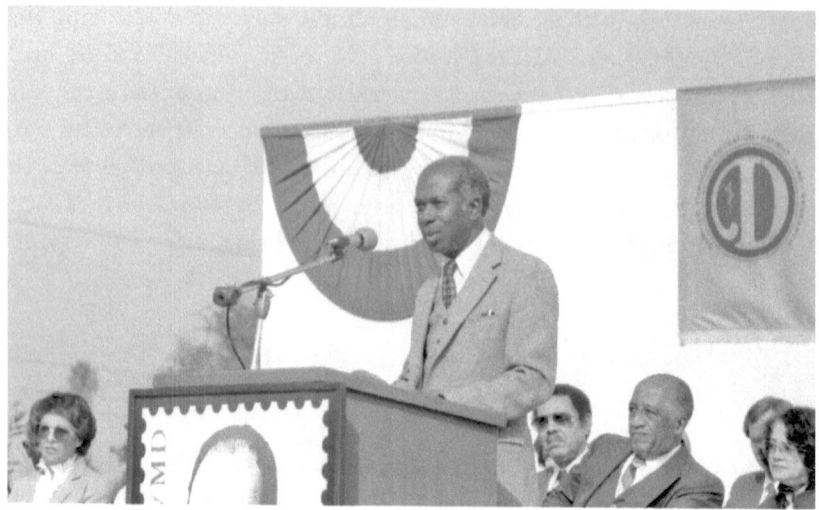

FIGURE 1. Dr. M. Alfred Haynes, 1982

Dr. M. Alfred Haynes's extensive research in global and community health eventually led to his appointment as Drew Medical School's dean in 1979. Source: Guy Crowder Collection, Courtesy of the Tom and Ethel Bradley Center at California State University at Northridge.

predetermined by others to be of *national* importance. Long ignored by mainstream health institutions, both Spellman and Haynes accepted the exclusion of local Black physicians from leadership as part of the terms of leading an institution of unprecedented scale and importance.

Dubbed variously the "Drew School's master plan" or the "Department of Community Medicine's master plan," King-Drew's master plan prioritized the protection of taxpayer interests by using its hospital services to introduce Black residents to high-quality modern hospital care. Rather than build a medical center outfitted with every modern health amenity available, Spellman and Haynes avoided launching services considered too expensive or sophisticated for underdeveloped health markets like Watts. Instead, they developed mechanisms to engage community members in the collective pursuit of developing the neighborhood's economy to better target health issues like maternal and infant mortality, tuberculosis, venereal disease, and "mental retardation" long considered by Black medical leaders to be Black health issues.[65]

Rather than ratify the idea that such a thing as a "Black disease" existed, Spellman and Haynes sought to show that higher incomes and access to biomedical resources in Black neighborhoods made sickness less a property of

Blackness than of poverty. For them, it was more important for residents to see health services in Watts not as the product of white benevolence or welfare but as a product of their own collective labor in developing services they figuratively "owned" as a community. In their vision, it was less important to "match" services found in white neighborhoods and more important to develop services sensitive to the neighborhood's existing resources.

The medical center's truer purpose was thus not per se to provide greater access to healthcare but to serve as an employer and generator of new opportunities for Black men, particularly Black physicians and other new high-paying allied health workers such as physician assistants, radiology technicians, and paramedics. Haynes described the school's Allied Health Sciences Center as being primarily responsible for training residents to take "tasks now performed by physicians [that] could be appropriately delegated to other categories of health personnel."[66] To showcase the medical center's intended purpose to shore up the authority of Black men as heads of households, the center's first program centered on retraining "discharged military medical corpsman" from the Vietnam War "to become extensions of the physicians" through a physician assistants program more popularly known as Medex.[67]

In theory, as incomes rose through the proliferation of antipoverty training programs, Haynes hoped that King-Drew's system could mirror the coordinated care approach of Kaiser Permanente, a private healthcare system that was emerging as a leading advocate for health maintenance organizations. The health district was key to making this vision of tracking improved health outcomes at a population level because it allowed health experts to imagine that the health of district residents could be cordoned off and manipulated as if it were a fully independent "market" or "nation" to develop. The health district concept allowed public health experts to approach Watts as a giant petri dish and made it possible to make claims about the efficacy of public health campaigns through the district's surveillance functions.

Haynes's research was crucial to leading this endeavor because his extensive experience working in communities in the United States and abroad that were widely considered undeveloped, underdeveloped, or deteriorating made him an expert in a growing field known as community and social medicine. Prior to his appointment, Haynes had served as a medical officer on a Cheyenne reservation for the United States Public Health Service; an assistant professor of preventative medicine, epidemiology, and community medicine at the University of Vermont; a USAID-funded visiting professor at Trivandrum Medical College in India; and an associate professor in the

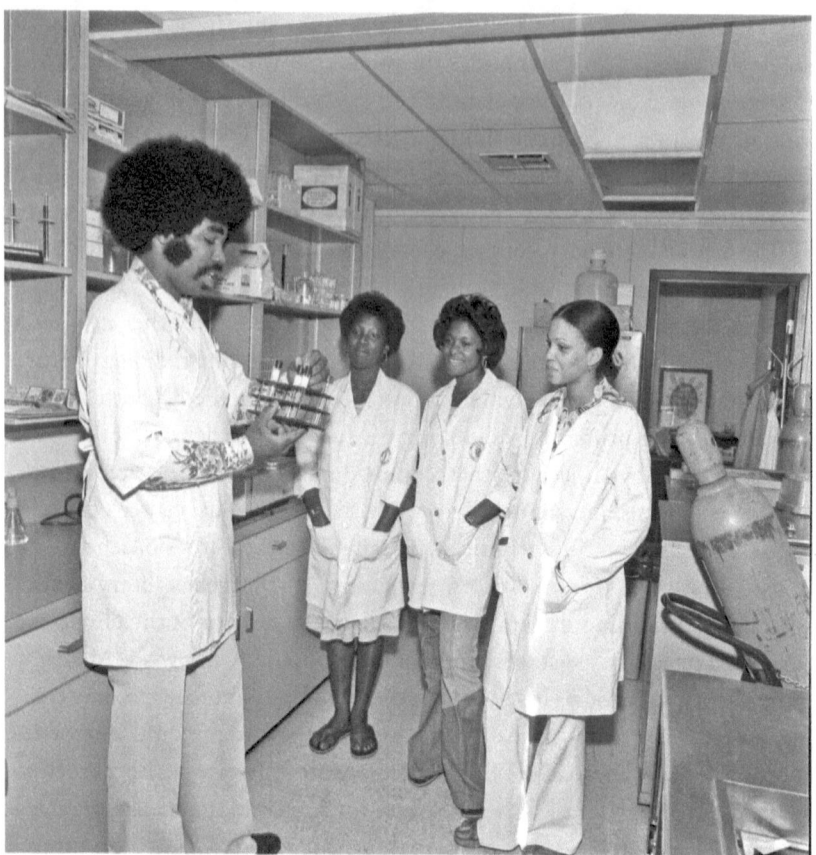

FIGURE 2. Training at Drew Medical School, 1976
Drew Medical School's Allied Health Sciences Center sought to help Black workers compete for a growing amount of jobs in healthcare. Source: Guy Crowder Collection, Courtesy of the Tom and Ethel Bradley Center at California State University at Northridge.

Department of International Health at Johns Hopkins School of Hygiene and Public Health.[68]

Haynes's experience working in poor health markets helped him introduce the concept of community health centers to regulate the flow of poor patients to expensive taxpayer-paid services in the hospital. Instead of being granted immediate access to the hospital, patients would be instructed to obtain a referral by first seeing a physician assigned to them in a low-cost clinic situated closer to their home. Haynes's design also proposed limiting hospital access only to citizens living in the hospital's health district and proposed restricting access to "emergency waiting room" services to nights and weekends.

Similar to Kaiser Permanente, Haynes proposed assigning every family in the health district to a new kind of specialist, a community medicine physician, whose role was to guide male heads of households on how best to manage the sickness and health of their families by referring them either to the hospital for specialist care or to an in-house team of public health nurses, medical social workers, and patient education experts for preventative care. The point of these arrangements was to transform poor citizens into ideal citizen-consumers capable of utilizing healthcare services equitably and responsibly on their own.

Haynes believed that the calmer and less expensive health setting of a neighborhood clinic offered physicians the ability to develop intimacy with Black families that would allow them to prescribe therapies based on the personal financial and social details of each individual in a household. Haynes developed the idea based on his experience as director of the Family Care Unit at the University of Vermont's Department of Preventative Medicine. In that post he piloted a teaching program pairing medical students with one hundred local medically indigent families selected to participate based on their ability to expose students to a "wide range of medical and social diagnoses and [provide] a fair representation of each age group, from infancy to old age."[69]

Haynes designed the program to develop "an appreciation of the influence of environmental factors on health" in order to apply it to "the study and management of a family."[70] Such approaches were intended to help physicians see how environmental factors such as unclean, unventilated homes, stressful work environments, and internal family tension contributed to the causes that brought patients to seek interventions in acute care hospital settings in the first place. They also sought to help physicians see themselves as teachers who could intimately shape the community's heads of households into independent, self-sustaining, and responsible health and financial decisionmakers.

Implicit in such approaches was the expectation that community physicians be familiar with the medical resources available immediately and nearby to cure or heal. Haynes thus expected community physicians to be knowledgeable about all the resources available to them to treat patients with primary care medicine but also be knowledgeable about specialist resources and technology available at the hospital. In this way, Haynes argued that community medicine doctors elevated "the role of the traditional family physician" by having "modern facilities at his disposal in order that he may provide a higher quality of medical care in a shorter period of time."[71]

Haynes's emphasis on families as society's most basic administrative unit suggests that he expected male heads of households and their families to bear the brunt of responsibility for addressing bodily harms and injuries caused by structural inequality. It made sickness and injuries stemming from lack of safe housing; the common presence of toxic hazards in Black neighborhoods; or Black workers' frequent exposure to occupational hazards and unsafe working conditions into problems for male heads of households to solve, primarily through biomedical means. By extension, it also made any socially organized answer to these issues a problem for a medical firm to solve.

In Haynes's opinion, the result of these relationships replaced older biological ideas of "Black diseases" with new socially constructed ideas of Black community health "solutions." In this regard, Haynes expected community physicians to help Black heads of households solve the health issues of family members by being familiar enough with local community institutions and agencies to have them contribute to the matrix of health decision-making.[72] He, for instance, encouraged physicians to get to know the neighborhood's public school teachers, social workers, and police officers as part of basic physician knowledge. The total effect sought to transform the relationship between patient and physician into a power dynamic more akin to a student and teacher. As Haynes put it, the real measure of success for community physicians was not measured by the number and volume of a physician's billable procedures but "by the degree of active participation of his patients in their adventure of healthful living rather than their otherwise passive acceptance of medical care."[73]

The aim of these relationships hid a higher purpose in helping community physicians gather the data and statistics required to chart a health economic development program relevant to local conditions. Noting that "communities have their own goals and priorities," Haynes offered the issue of high maternal mortality rates as a prime example of a health issue long considered abated in mainstream medicine through technological advances but that continued to need solutions in Black community contexts.[74] Implicitly, Haynes's observations about mainstream approaches to maternal mortality posited that differently situated communities could produce similar health outcomes using different approaches sensitive to the financial means and social and political capacity of their neighborhoods.

Thus, in addition to serving as a conduit for physicians to triage care in a calmer and less expensive health setting than the hospital, data gleaned from community clinics was also intended to provide community physicians with insight on how to conserve and direct scarce healthcare resources toward the community's most pressing healthcare problems through the clinic's surveillance functions. Haynes argued that clinic data allowed for "a continuous analysis of the health problems of the community," which would allow community physicians to "facilitate the coordination of existing resources for care within the area with the aim of providing those services which can best meet the needs of the community and diminish or eliminate existing problems."[75] In Haynes's opinion, organizing community members along these lines gave poor citizens a sense of pride and ownership through having "a piece of the action" and sharing "the real power of decision making."[76]

Despite all of its grand and elaborate vision, the plan put forth by King-Drew's leaders conveniently did not engage residents in transforming society's overall distribution of capital and resources. It simply asked communities of color to collectively reorganize the substantially scant capital and resources distributed to them under prevailing processes of racial capitalism in the belief that the community's collective sense of self-esteem, pride, and sense of ownership would produce more favorable outcomes than providing high-quality, high-cost healthcare outright. In this way, King-Drew's master plan revealed how elite Black physician leaders shared a belief with mainstream white society that newly accessible hospital services in urban poor neighborhoods would foster welfare dependency if such services did not stabilize the employment of the male breadwinner as the most efficient way to distribute society's most basic life necessities. Thus, instead of using Medicare and Medicaid to make healthcare more universal and democratic, King-Drew's designers worked to make public healthcare more exclusive by making access to hospitals contingent on clinics designed to heighten surveillance of and data collection from the area's poorest residents.

THE FINAL INSULT

Ultimately, King-Drew's master plan symbolized the renewal of constrained freedom for Black medical schools and hospitals in an era normally understood as legal end of Jim Crow. Framed as assistance to help Black physicians achieve greater autonomy and control over medical research and practice, King-Drew's master plan repackaged the problematic relationships between Black hospitals and white philanthropic funders of an earlier era with an even larger set of stakeholders. The sum total of these relationships expanded the number of obligations, financial or otherwise, faced by King-Drew's leaders. In addition to servicing the interests of white philanthropies like the Commonwealth and Markle Foundations, the corporate scale of a Black-led medical center sent King-Drew's leaders deeper into debt and obligation to taxpayers and a slew of other stakeholders.

These stakeholders were often motivated to invest in King-Drew for reasons other than serving poor Black patients. For political leaders such as Hahn, Bradley, and Hawkins, King-Drew served as a political vehicle to build a base of power that could eventually challenge the region's white power structure. For County administrators, it offered a possible plan to reduce welfare rates and generate public revenue. Lastly, it offered white medical school leaders an opportunity to maintain access to research and training opportunities in Black neighborhoods without the troublesome direct colonial relationships of a previous era. Be it paying back capital or servicing a social obligation, each partner in King-Drew's establishment exacted demands that were mostly at odds with the wishes of most poor Black patients.

Outwardly, the establishment of King-Drew served as an occasion to celebrate the community's new "opportunity" to improve health and become independent by entrusting Black physicians with large sums of taxpayer money. Hahn and Los Angeles County officials proudly lauded King-Drew's leaders for their innovative and cost-conscious approach to healthcare. They referred to the medical center as the county's first "county-community hospital," a designation noting the hospital's status as a private hospital with public financing, and described its master plan as a potential template for transforming its two existing public hospitals into county-community hospitals. The projection of such optimism demonstrated how the politicians and health and policy leaders who came to support Dr. White's original plan were pleased with the plan's outcomes.

However, not everyone involved in creating King-Drew's master plan was as content as the politicians, health policy leaders, and King-Drew's elite medical school leaders. Instead of local Black doctors being freely admitted into the hospital with physician privileges as originally intended, both Spellman and Haynes signaled that King-Drew's system would remain closed unless these doctors agreed to a series of reforms subjecting them to further training, assessment, and certification before they would be allowed to treat their own patients in the hospital.

The goal of these requirements appeared to be for Black physicians who had been practicing in the community for decades to earn specialization as "community physicians." Indeed, in many cases, local Black physicians were required to not only participate in learning sessions alongside new medical graduates being trained as community physicians but also help teach their future competitors the art of providing humane care in poor patient settings. For physicians already seriously overburdened with large patient volumes, these requirements appeared to be unrealistic and unnecessarily patronizing. The suggestion that those with day-to-day experience working as community physicians get retrained alongside new physicians also struck many Black doctors as insulting and demoralizing.

Rather than shore up the stability of Black breadwinning manhood, then, the development of King-Drew's master plan reveals the inherent instability of gender categories and Blackness. Arguably, the fact that most Black male physicians could not be seen to occupy a strong enough position of authority and expertise to guide Black families out of poverty destabilized the very premise underlying the medical center's plan. That is, despite often exemplifying the shared gendered and sexual politics of mainstream society, King-Drew's leaders could not help but see local Black physicians as subjects to reform or exclude. Such deferral of fitness to lead in people thoroughly groomed by vocation and culture to govern over matters of community health and wealth underlined the difficulty of stabilizing a community through the rhetoric of gender and sexuality.

THREE

The Psychological Wages of Blackness

IN 1967, *LOS ANGELES TIMES* reporter Jack Jones gave readers a sense of how federal, state, and local funds were not just building another teaching hospital in South Los Angeles but creating an entirely new health system with various public and private agencies.[1] As Jones explained, South Los Angeles's Black residents were beginning to know and understand the purpose of their new health system through two antipoverty-funded clinics built ahead of the hospital's opening. He noted, for instance, the presence of the South-Central Multi-Purpose Health Service Center (the "Watts Clinic"), a primary care clinic funded by the Office of Equal Opportunity (OEO) and owned by USC, and Central City Community Mental Health Center (Central City CMHC), a community mental health clinic funded under the auspices of the National Institutes of Mental Health (NIMH) and led by Dr. J. Alfred Cannon, a Black psychiatrist from UCLA. As Jones's article detailed, however, the community's opinion on each clinic diverged greatly based on the racial background of their respective leaders.

Local Black doctors and community members discussed their apprehension over the new Watts Clinic by describing USC to Jones as a "white-oriented school." According to Dr. Walter Tucker, a Black dentist practicing in Watts, the term "white-oriented" expressed the community's shared "feeling" that "once again the white community was imposing its own solutions on the Negro area." Black residents cited the fact that USC's majority-white trustees and doctors still ultimately owned and governed the clinic as reason to continue to regard USC as a colonial employer, neighbor, and healthcare provider because of its long history of abusing Black workers, displacing Black residents, and using Black patients for medical experimentation and training. Black physicians, in particular, saw USC as an intruder hell bent on

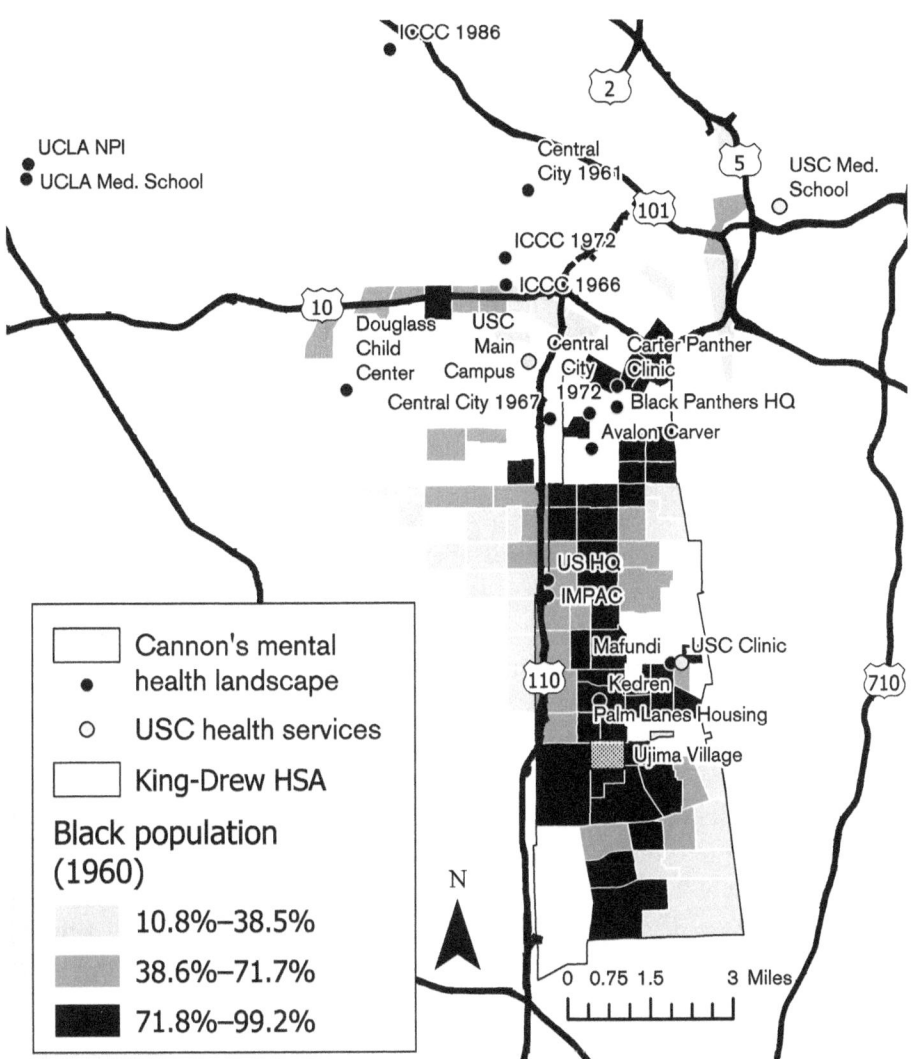

MAP 8. Constructing Black mental wellness in LA

USC's white clinic leaders and Central City's Black clinicians sought to fight poverty and racism in an era with active debates about the meaning of Black freedom, health, and mental wellness. Map: Tyler Munn.

"stifl[ing] the Negro practitioner" by outcompeting them in a corporate bid to force them "to take jobs under them." Such arrangements seemingly did not allow Black individuals to stand on their own two feet—as patients, doctors, or community leaders.

In contrast, Jones's article offered a glowing description of the Central City CMHC, a former donation-based mental health clinic recently expanded and moved to a larger location closer to Watts through an infusion of new federal and state funding. The article portrayed Central City as more successful in responding to the needs of poor and working-class Black people because its founder and director, Dr. Cannon, a neuropsychiatrist, held lived experience as a Black man. Cannon boasted of the center's success in growing clientele by emphasizing "short-term therapy," maintaining an open-door policy "to never turn anyone down" or "have a waiting list," and by characterizing the center as a place to dispense "help" and "advice" rather than "diagnosis" or "treatment." Cannon's supposedly race-sensitive sensibilities permitted Central City to reach populations usually fearful and suspicious of accessing mental health services because of psychiatry's long history of unfairly diagnosing and incarcerating Black individuals as "mad" or "insane."

Jones's narrative frames eventually accounted for each clinic's divergent fate within King-Drew's health system by 1970. By 1969, discourses describing the Watts Clinic as failing because it reproduced Jim Crow's racial hierarchies convinced King-Drew's leaders to distance themselves from USC's clinic and hire Cannon in 1970 as the health system's first Chair of the Department of Psychiatry. By the close of the decade, racial conflict caused King-Drew's leaders to cease plans to integrate USC's clinic into its health system over fears that local Black physicians would refuse participation in the hospital's entire network because of it. The desire to build primary care clinics led and directed entirely by Black physicians eventually set King-Drew on a path to open its entire master plan to scrutiny by federal and private funders (see chapter 4).

A narrative emphasis on the melanin of USC's and Central City's leaders, however, obscures how physician leaders at both of LA's experimental clinics shared the same assumptions about poverty and mobilized the same methods, practices, and approaches to acculturate formerly excluded patient populations into mainstream medicine. The similarities between the approaches, however, have been muted—in some ways by design. By the early 1970s, Black physicians were increasingly recruited into the profession in the belief that their past experiences were essential to shaping more humane and culturally competent approaches to healthcare in the wake of new federal health programs.

Historians have also rightly narrated the history of community clinics as separate from community mental health clinics because their functional relationships each explain their distinct purposes within a larger health service referral system.[2] Primary care clinics, for instance, regulate costs and services around bodily health normally associated with acute care hospitals, whereas community mental health clinics helped professionals control involuntary commitment rates associated with state hospitals. Keeping their histories separate, however, hides how community clinics of both types saw it as their unique historical responsibility to inculcate patients with a sense of financial and sexual responsibility that few mainstream physicians saw as necessary for their own patient populations.

Their collective work in the 1960s and 1970s sought to produce ideal citizen-consumers who extend what Nayan Shah refers to as ideal citizen-subjects.[3] Rather than exclude subjects from citizenship solely on the basis of their gender, race, nationality, or economic standing, Shah argues that increasingly over the twentieth century the "objective of liberal governance" aimed "to cultivate citizen-subjects who can govern themselves" by "granting authority to professionals who are licensed and empowered by the state to create norms of individual conduct, make judgements, and administer policies."[4] As professionals "licensed and empowered by the state," clinicians extended public health's early twentieth-century concern over personal hygiene to the realm of consumer responsibility through the expansion of third-party taxpayer-paid health insurance programs such as Medicare and Medicaid.[5] Whereas professionals once relied on relatively low-budget public health approaches centered on personal hygiene to maximize population health, such as universal handwashing and latrine use, clinicians after 1965 increasingly saw it as their responsibility to teach the poor how to manage different health options while being, in their opinion, mindful of the wishes of white taxpayers footing the bill.

Thus, rather than solely focus on the skin color of King-Drew's health clinic leadership, this chapter traces how leaders at Los Angeles's antipoverty clinics sought to produce ideal citizen-consumers who shared the medical belief that breadwinning manhood's supposed culturally evolved kinship patterns of gendered distinctiveness and sexual complexity were necessary prerequisites for individuals to possess "good health" and the capacity for "economic rationality." Through the associative properties of how medical authorities defined health in relation to gendered labor participation, antipoverty clinicians offered poor citizens the ability to psychologically inhabit "normality" and "health"—two related states of being that they believed proved more seductive and durable than economic security itself. More important, poor people of color, in particular, had long been denied them on the basis of race and class alone. Whether the clinic was led by a white or a Black clinician, King-Drew's antipoverty clinics encouraged the poor to see work and respectable marriage and family as practices that made them healthy and normal citizens regardless of their skin color or class.

The state's involvement in regulating and orchestrating the seemingly private economic and sexual behavior of poor individuals and their families reveals a central contradiction in histories of racial and sexual liberalism. It demonstrates that schemes designed to eventually grant poor people of color the freedom to exercise independent economic and health decision-making required the state to expand its reach into the private lives of poor households. Although middle-class consumers freely engaged in the sexual and economic behaviors targeted for reform in poor communities without impunity, poor individuals were expected to follow middle-class prescriptions of how to "properly" consume healthcare in ways often at odds with the daily realities of poverty.

LA's antipoverty clinic leaders not only confronted the daily realities of poverty facing poor patients but also faced a Black political landscape where Black people thought divergently about what constituted "good health" based on ongoing debates within the Black community about the relationships between race, poverty, and illness. In fact, many antipoverty recipients sought to test the limits of federal programming guidelines to advance ideas about Black freedom and community autonomy using "bottom-up" approaches to organizing not tied to the "top-down" programmatic visions of antipoverty "experts."[6] Community activists such as Caffie Greene, Ivory Perry, Bobby Seale, and Huey Newton all famously used federal funds to train organizers for social movement work and for other purposes that caused grant authorities to tighten funding criteria to achieve outcomes closer to the vision of antipoverty programming experts.[7]

USC's and Central City's leaders additionally confronted a healthcare landscape reshaped by a larger consumer and patient rights movement increasingly suspicious about whether physicians, psychiatrists, hospitals, and state hospitals could truly hold the best health interests of patients in an unregulated health market. Nancy Tomes argues that the aspiration to establish a "medical democracy opened up opportunities for groups outside the new middle classes ... to lodge their own complaints about the inequities of the health care system."[8] As the civil rights movement transformed into the Black Power movement and amid the rise of patient and consumer rights, clinicians found themselves deeply invested in testing which methods and narratives of racial citizenship best produced the subject that most closely resembled their idea of an ideal citizen-consumer.

THE PROBLEM OF DESIRING INDIVIDUALS

Designers of antipoverty legislation sought to expand democratic practices, processes, and institutions while preventing the misuse of funds through what federal authorities referred to as the "citizen participation" mandate, which required that all beneficiaries of federal money recruit the poor into the design and implementation of all antipoverty programs. While the law appeared benevolent in its commitment to inclusion of once-excluded populations in matters of shared governance, historians of antipoverty programming argue that the mandate's true intent sought to acculturate the way the poor thought of and saw poverty to the same ways that economists thought of and understood it.[9] That is, rather than see poverty as a natural product of capitalist inequality, antipoverty programming's bureaucratic designers sought to teach the poor to think of their poverty as a problem created by past practices of social isolation and poor individual choices.[10]

According to Alyosha Goldstein, antipoverty programming's objectives were inspired by Milton Friedman's theory of human capital, "which defined individuals as rational, self-interested, profit-maximizing agents who operated along the same principles as capital itself."[11] In theory, antipoverty programs provided the poor with all the starting elements—such as capital and consumer education—necessary for rational economic actors to "increase future returns, including economic mobility and improved aggregate productivity" without the state's assistance. Although the theory was originally designed in the 1930s to inspire economists to imagine ways to maximize productivity at a macroeconomic level, by the 1960s it also enabled an entire suite of actors concerned with the economy to name certain actors and their individual practices and behaviors as "irrational" within human capital theory's idealized economy.

As opposed to viewing the end of legal Jim Crow and the implementation of Medicare and Medicaid as bad for capital, antipoverty's architects saw the mainstream civil rights movement's emphasis on capitalism and democratic participation as rhetorical mechanisms capable of unleashing the market potential of Black consumers in markets formerly "isolated" from the mainstream economy. In other words, antipoverty's policy designers saw the Civil Rights Act as legally opening up the opportunity for Black people to have and hold jobs, homes, and services from which they were previously barred, regardless of how real the access to those jobs, homes, and services was. According to legal scholars such as Kimberlé Crenshaw, a shortcoming of this approach is that it focused on remedying racism by addressing the capital and capacity of Black individuals rather than on addressing the exclusionary practices and policies designed to keep Black people from jobs, housing, healthcare, transportation, and education in the first place.

Crenshaw argues that rather than view the state's true responsibility as supplying a "guarantee" that every citizen achieve a similar economic outcome, the state mobilized antipoverty programs to ensure that every citizen was afforded the same "opportunity" to obtain a well-paying job, own a home, and have access to comprehensive healthcare on the same "terms" as white citizens before the civil rights movement. According to Crenshaw, this shift from targeting employers, real estate agents, hospital owners, and educators and toward targeting individuals not only made anti-discrimination discourse "fundamentally ambiguous" but also accommodated "conservative as well as liberal views of race and equality."[12] Although this policy design theoretically treats all individuals "equally," it exacerbates existing inequality by treating differently-situated individuals similarly, shifting the burden of responsibility of addressing inequality from those in power to individuals who must prove discrimination on extremely narrow terms.

The problem, then, as most antipoverty bureaucrats saw it, was not how to empower the poor to determine a completely new future for themselves through antipoverty programming's shared governance and funding, but how to help the poor help themselves to the future that others had designed for them. At first, as the formation of King-Drew's master plan demonstrated, antipoverty program planners found it acceptable for educated middle-class Black community members to serve as representatives of the poor because the terms *Black* and *poor* were culturally understood to mean the same thing. Black politicians, medical professionals, and middle-class homeowners, however, tended to share the same view of Black poverty as antipoverty's architects because they shared educational backgrounds and class interests with antipoverty experts, rather than with most working-class and poor Black people.

When, for instance, white county supervisor Kenneth Hahn announced plans in July 1966 to demolish a thirty-acre, 470-unit public housing complex called Palm Lanes to construct King-Drew's acute care hospital tower, he strove to make sure in official press releases that the public knew it was not a unilateral decision by county officials but one supported by the Willowbrook Plaza Home Owners Improvement Club, a homeowners association formed by Ruby Daniels and Wilhelmina Shamberger.[13] As Black homeowners who lived near Palm Lanes, Daniels and Shamberger worked at the end of 1965 to gather other property owners into town halls held in their living rooms to "listen to complaints and suggestions on how to improve the Watts-Willowbrook area."[14] They had heard about the county's interest in finding a suitable location for the new hospital and saw the potential of a "center of pride and medical service" near their homes as a boon to local real estate values and agreed with Hahn that Palm Lanes was steadily becoming a "potential slum." Although they later admitted many Palm Lanes residents were friends, they "organized a survey and got the votes to replace the project with the hospital."[15]

While striving to show how Daniels and Shamberger acted as "rational" economic actors, Hahn's press release also highlighted the problem of "irrational" economic actors, who antipoverty programs by the late 1960s were increasingly more interested in targeting for economic reform. In contrast to his praise of the members of the Willowbrook Plaza homeowners association, Hahn registered dismay upon discovering that "some of [the Palm Lane residents] had Federal, State, and County jobs and could afford to buy their own home and pay taxes like every other property owner."[16] In highlighting the presence of residents who refused to live independently of state assistance yet appeared to have every opportunity to do so, Hahn sought to draw public attention to a form of independent thinking that was no longer tolerable under the state's expansion of healthcare and housing programs—namely, citizens who consumed state benefits in ways that countered new ideas of appropriate use.

As historians of medicine and psychiatry have shown, however, ideas of "appropriate use" in medicine were in flux given the rise of a consumer and patient's rights movement and two interrelated community health and community mental health movements. Each of these overlapping movements sought to diminish the unquestioned authority of the physician over people's bodies and minds alongside the two preeminent sites of their expertise: the acute care hospital and the psychiatric state hospital. Despite the growing association of American medicine with technology and medical discovery, by midcentury many white middle-class insured patients increasingly questioned how their own deference to medical authority and compulsory ignorance of the business of healthcare had contributed to its stunning costs. Patients increasingly viewed news coverage of unnecessary surgeries, hospital overbedding, inflated pricing, and service duplication as evidence that physicians and hospital owners were more than happy to profit from people's need to feel normal and healthy.[17]

Although rising healthcare costs were the direct result of the unscrupulous profit-driven business practices of hospital owners and physicians, the patient and consumer rights movement increasingly moved to check the power of big business by turning to the deferential patient-consumer as the "problem" to solve. As Nancy Tomes argues, rather than strongarm hospitals and physicians into making healthcare more patient-centered, efficient, and affordable, patient rights advocates increasingly framed change around the production of an empowered, well-educated patient consumer, whose eventual ubiquity would, in theory, entice hospitals and physicians to make healthcare more welcoming and "consumer-friendly."[18] Although "once derided as a threat to the 'American way' of medicine," Tomes argues, "discriminating patients became [free market medicine's] salvation: by conscious choosing and wise consumption, [well-educated patients] could redirect American medicine toward higher standards, in both therapeutic and economic realms."[19]

The crisis of physician authority, however, was not just relegated to American hospitals. As Gerald Grob argues, another patient's rights movement challenged the centrality of psychiatry and psychiatric state hospitals within the realm of mental health.[20] By the 1960s, a growing number of patient advocates began to contest psychiatry's claims that involuntary commitment and isolation from society constituted the best care for those diagnosed as mentally ill. In particular, patient rights advocates and psychiatrists involved in a community mental health movement increasingly questioned mainstream psychiatry's continuing commitments to racial scientific ideas that deemed women, homosexuals, and people of color automatically more prone to mental illness.[21] Citing the promise of new alternative treatment models and new approaches based on psychoanalysis, many psychiatrists, patients, and politicians were increasingly convinced of the viability of diverting patients bound for state hospitals toward a new community mental health infrastructure and releasing those involuntarily committed from state hospitals through deinstitutionalization.

State and county mental health officials were eager to support the objectives of deinstitutionalization because they saw it as releasing the proper responsibility of overseeing mental health to the free market and feared the future fiscal impact of a state hospital and prison system overburdened and overcrowded by the increased migration of Black and Spanish-speaking residents to California since World War II. Indeed, to stem the explosive growth of California's state hospital system, which reached 37,211 residents in 1955, state officials began to coordinate the work of the Department of Mental Hygiene and the Bureau of Social Work to detect and divert presumed mentally ill "at-risk" populations from state hospitals toward community treatment and welfare services that paid greater attention to improving socio-environmental factors such as better schools, education, and general standards of living.[22] California then passed its first deinstitutionalization law, the Short-Doyle Act, in 1957 to balance services between state hospitals and those in community settings by enticing county, municipal, and private operators through subsidies to build mental health services in the community.

As the next two sections show, community clinics not only manifested the desire of patients, politicians, and physicians to decenter the power of physicians and hospitals but also carried the hopes of patient rights activists and physicians critical of established medicine to produce a more equitable health landscape through more informed and more assertive consumers. As a patient population formerly excluded from healthcare and newly minted as "consumers" through state subsidies, physicians and politicians ironically could not help but see Black neighborhoods as laboratories to test out new mechanisms to produce in Black patients what unregulated free market healthcare had previously failed to produce in white middle-class insured patients. That is, as the crisis of hospital costs detailed above suggests, most hospital owners and physicians not only tolerated but encouraged consumer habits in insured patient populations that many health experts feared normalizing in new Medicare and Medicaid-eligible consumers. Namely, they feared poor Black people would also utilize health services with the same unregulated frequency, rate, and haphazard gusto that most white insured patients had previously demonstrated in their pursuit of feeling healthy and normal.

THE MIND, THROUGH THE BODY

The overlapping objectives of antipoverty, community health, and community mental health advocates within a broader patient rights movement demonstrates how new 1960s healthcare benefits strove to do more than just expand the number of consumers within free market medicine. Policymakers built an architecture of programs and laws seeking to produce something more difficult and elusive for bureaucrats to achieve by pinning the maximization of the nation's economy and overall health to an independent self-governing individual who consumed healthcare resources responsibly. Rather than exclusively reform the bodily health of antipoverty programming participants, this dimension of state objectives prioritized the subjectivity of poor people as the state's true target of reform.

Historians of the community health movement, however, have generally underanalyzed the psychological and subject-forming objectives of early neighborhood health clinics in order to privilege how they expanded health access to low-income neighborhoods of color and challenged the primacy of expensive hospital care. Despite the community health movement's heterogeneous origins, scholars also have often uplifted the work of Dr. H. Jack Geiger in order to highlight the movement's origin as coextensive with the civil rights movement.[23] As a member of the Medical Committee for Human Rights (MCHR), the so-called medical arm of the civil rights movement, Geiger pushed the organization's mostly white middle-class base of medical volunteers to move beyond their focus on narrowly tending to the health needs of civil rights workers to fighting segregation by operating free clinics in Mississippi's poor Black communities.

As a physician who shared in the patient rights movement's growing criticism of medical authority and corporate profitability, Geiger's leadership also brought the civil rights movement into greater alignment with the burgeoning field of social and community medicine. At the time, the field was primarily led by left- and liberal-leaning medical professionals concerned with mitigating the effects of free market healthcare. Geiger saw the civil rights movement as an opportunity to transplant the work he was exposed to as a Rockefeller grantee at Sidney and Emily Kark's Pholela Community Health Centre in South Africa to the United States. The Pholela clinic used health services to engage Black South Africans in a larger community development scheme. By the end of 1965, Geiger helped MCHR activists in Mississippi use health services to advance the civil rights movement and convinced OEO officials to fund seven antipoverty clinics across the nation, including USC's Watts Clinic, to use health services as part of the federal government's War on Poverty.

In contrast to Black residents' views of USC's leadership as "conservative" and relatively mainstream, USC's leaders—Dr. Roger Egeberg, Dr. Elsie Giorgi, and Dr. Robert Tranquada—tended to share Geiger's criticisms of mainstream medicine. As dean of USC's Medical School, Egeberg famously advocated for a comprehensive health plan for all Californians and criticized the AMA's opposition to Medicare and Medicaid.[24] In the aftermath of the Watts Uprisings, Egeberg appointed two white liberal progressive physicians, Giorgi and Tranquada, to direct the clinic and oversee its progress. Giorgi had experience screening children in Watts as a Head Start health volunteer and ran Cedars-Sinai Medical Center's community clinic and home care program.[25] In 1966, Egeberg appointed Tranquada as USC's inaugural chair of community medicine and public health.

Opened in September 1967 to much fanfare by Sargent Shriver, director of the OEO, USC's $2.4 million, 53,500-square-foot clinic was built on land leased to the university for $1 by the Los Angeles City Housing Commission. In keeping with King-Drew's general plan for community clinics, USC's Watts Clinic was designed as the future hospital's "new front door" by serving as the primary point of health service for the clinic's surrounding patients. With three separate wings splayed out from a "central core" of supporting pharmaceutical, X-ray, clinical laboratory, and data-processing services, Giorgi explained that the clinic's architecture reduced costly duplication of health services and got "rid of fragmentations" by giving poor Black residents a "one stop neighborhood health center ... designed to provide all medical, dental and all health services (except hospitalization) for [the] whole family."[26]

Although its services were nominally free, OEO officials strove to clarify that all clinic health services were contingently offered on the premise that the poor would reform their own opinions about poverty and themselves. As an OEO brochure explained, federally funded clinics endeavored to do more than to just reduce "the incidence of disease and disability—important though that is."[27] Their true purpose was to, as the brochure put it, help the "neighborhood" see itself as "a source of physical and social contamination" that was "costly and menacing in both physical and political terms" for "the broader community of which the neighborhood is a part." Rather than place blame on society for their ill health and living conditions, the brochure sought to help the "neighborhood" see itself, through its "improved physical health" and "social self-sufficiency," as having the means to overcome social exclusion by helping itself "earn acceptance for itself and its residents."

The phrase "earn acceptance" reveals how clinic leaders interpreted the Black Freedom movement as not a plea for Black self-determination but as a plea for Black citizens to enjoy, as consumers, all the same benefits, services, and treatment conferred on insured white patients. Such a frame accounts for why Giorgi and Tranquada worked diligently to reeducate the poor through the architecture of the clinic itself. As Tranquada explained, the clinic's design attempted to "organize medical care" in ways mirroring healthcare practices among insured patients by ensuring "every patient saw the same doctor on each visit."[28] Tranquada understood such a change constituted a "drastic departure" from the "emergency-type medical care that people who are unable to afford care have traditionally received" but firmly believed that poor patients would gladly trade the hasty, impersonal, and brusque healthcare interactions of pre-1970s emergency room care for the supposedly more relaxed, intimate, and humane care associated with family physicians.

The idea of assigning each poor family to a family physician with immediate in-house access to other specialists and services was more than a ploy to give poor Black people a consumer experience befitting an insured white patient. It was also the primary means, as USC's grant application phrased it, "of interrupting the cycle of poverty" that tied "illness" and "under-education and unemployability" together.[29] Through the "exchanges of confidence" made possible by the clinic's pairing of a family physician with poor patients, Tranquada claimed that it was possible for clinicians to get to the problems "which seemingly have nothing to do with health" such as "worry over money problems or worry about a son who has gotten into trouble [that] can cause or aggravate medical problems."[30] Once identified, the clinician could refer the patient to a team of psychiatrists, psychologists, social workers, and neighborhood health agents to "change situations which cause problems in their day-to-day living" or to a health education team "to help individuals and groups prevent and control health problems" through a range of available self-help literature.[31]

In this regard, USC's OEO application did not define good health as the absence of disease, illness, or even poverty itself but as the psychological presence of a striving subject intelligent enough to improve their individual capacity "to function responsibly on their own behalf."[32] USC leaders explained their hope to achieve this by recruiting the discursive "total health" framework of Dr. Julius Richmond. As Head Start's director, Richmond argued that racism had "so chronically debilitated and demoralized [poor Black people] biologically and/or psycho-socially" by depriving them of all the elements thought needed for "total health" that they were, by the 1960s and 1970s, "powerless to improve their health or socio-economic condition without assistance or leadership" of antipoverty agencies.[33] According to Mical Raz, Richmond's "total health" theory defined good health as an equilibrium that tied it, for better or worse, to the presence of many internal factors, such as life within an emotionally healthy family, biology, and genetics, to external factors, such as good housing, schools, employment, nuclear families, and nutritional food, all considered abundant in white neighborhoods but lacking in poor Black neighborhoods.[34]

The challenge for antipoverty officials like Giorgi and Tranquada, then, was creating desiring subjects who wanted good housing, schools, employment, nuclear families, and nutritional food on the supposedly same free market terms as white people. In this regard, the entire architecture of antipoverty programming demonstrates how planners thoughtfully created all the mechanisms they believed necessary to conjure this subject while knowing that they ultimately held little to no control over how actual participants would use the clinic's services. In this regard, Giorgi and Tranquada were extremely optimistic. In their own proposal, they stated: "It can be very safely assumed that this type of participation will produce eventual self-esteem and self-sufficiency, by overcoming the powerlessness of the poor, and allowing them a greater control over their own lives and welfare."[35]

However, as Merlin Chowkwanyun has argued, Watts residents had their own ideas about how well the center served the interests of Black people.[36] Some residents responded positively to the new clinic. Mrs. Dolores Morado, for instance, echoed the sentiments of many Black residents, in rural and urban parts of the nation, who celebrated the arrival of once scant and far-off medical services to their neighborhoods through federal programs. She told reporters she welcomed USC's clinic because it was "close to her home and she no longer had to go to the County-USC Medical Center for emergency treatment for her children."[37] Comments like Morado's underlined how many Black citizens were eager to access any form of healthcare, regardless of a physician's skin color, because costs, distance, and concerns about quality made healthcare a luxury many poor people could not afford.

Others used the center's hiring practices as a barometer for how well it served the community. Some, like Mrs. Birdell Moore, claimed that the clinic appeared to hire more community people "on this project than any other, excluding Operation Head Start," while others, like Mrs. Ruth Robinson, argued the center was not "employing enough people from the community."[38] Statements like Robinson's highlighted the absence of Black leaders at the top of the center's organizational chain of command, which Mrs. Alma Wood put in more blunt and aspirational terms: "I hope there will be a day when we take over." Indeed, the center's greatest criticism came from Black community physicians who argued that the center overlooked their expertise and actively undermined their ability to practice. Despite serving as an advisory board member for the clinic, Dr. Charles Hall, for instance, argued that the clinic had caused a loss in his practice in the month since it opened in September 1967.

These public comments were surface indications of much deeper conflicts over how the center shared power with community members. For instance, despite all its best-laid plans, Tranquada admitted that criticism, funding cutbacks, and high-volume caseloads had "forced" the center "to rely on emergency-room type care—the very thing it was trying to replace with a family-centered program weighted heavily with preventative medicine."[39] More important, conflicts with the clinic's community board, patients, and Black physician leaders precluded any progress on the clinic's hidden objective of intervening on the psychological dimensions of poverty in the community. As an unsigned letter written to Black congressman Augustus Hawkins in October 1968 detailed, "The primary emphasis, has been and still is, medical and dental care, rather than on *total health care* and use of the health center as a tool of *social intervention*" (emphasis mine).[40]

Since such criticisms increasingly focused on the white racial character of USC's leadership, Giorgi and Tranquada felt pressed to relinquish control of the clinic to Black physicians. From late 1967 into early 1968, USC initiated steps to assuage community tension by hiring Dr. Sol White as a co-medical director. As White was the physician who had devised the whole scheme to create a Black health district and hospital (see chapter 1), the move sought to strengthen relations between USC's white leadership and local Black physicians and provide White a position befitting his contribution.

However, as Chowkwanyun argues, Giorgi found White was too willing to politically conspire against her and the center's leadership and was, as she put it, more "motivated towards self rather than the task."[41] White leaked confidential information from the center's leadership to community members, unilaterally made contractual agreements on behalf of the clinic that personally benefited him, and disrespected the clinic's organizational model and chain of command. The combination of these factors led to his dismissal just one month after being hired.

The fallout of the ordeal led Giorgi and Tranquada to elevate Dr. Clifton Drummett, a Black dentist, to the role of associate director and caused them to lean more heavily on the leadership of Dr. Charles Thomas, a Black psychologist appointed as the center's director of education and training.[42] By late 1969, USC had also appointed a Black pediatrician, Dr. Rodney Powell, to serve as the "face" of the clinic and stabilize its day-to-day operations. Powell's leadership helped USC's leaders engineer steps for another Black physician, Dr. Clifton Cole, to take the reins as the clinic was now to be funded independently without USC's oversight as a federally funded neighborhood health center.

As he relinquished his leadership to Black physicians, Tranquada indicated his strong belief that the use of medical services to conjure an independent self-sufficient citizen did not adequately anticipate the Black Power movement's ability to capture the imagination of Black residents. Tranquada, writing alongside the white sociologist Milton Davis, argued that "the Black people of Watts" were "not [the] apathetic, alienated hicks" most associated with the Southern civil rights movement but were engaged citizens who had a "growing sophistication in understanding the ways of the white power structure."[43] Although Tranquada and Davis saw some versions of Black Power as disruptive and menacing (such as those that promoted "violence" and generated "further racial hatred"), they saw Black people's "call for freedom from white colonial policies" as producing the desiring subject they had exactly hoped for from antipoverty programming. That is, narratives of Black Power appeared to be more successful in engaging citizens to participate in antipoverty programming than traditional civil rights narratives of integration.

In contrast, both Tranquada and Davis recognized that the perceived white orientation of the project only helped fuel what they referred to as a "self-fulfilling prophecy," where the community's "attitudes of futility about involving community, affect the actual outcome." They argued that "if it is believed that cooperation between OEO, CHC, and the university is impossible, people representing the organizations become progressively alienated, and eventually the anticipation of conflict helps create what they predicted was inevitable." Such conclusions posited that Tranquada and Davis did not believe that the community had a problem with the clinic's overall antipoverty *program* but had conflict with the program's white *authority*. In short, "because of the overriding problems of power," they believed, "any attempts to resolve the conflict through traditional problem-solving techniques were unsuccessful." Indeed, white oversight proved to be such a problem that both administrators argued that "rational problem solving was not always feasible in the Watts neighborhood health center."

THE BODY, THROUGH THE MIND

Tranquada and Davis's comments about the resurgence and popularity of Black nationalist discourses pointed to the success of Central City Community Mental Health Center, a Black-led clinic originally opened in 1961 by Dr. J. Alfred Cannon on the premises of the Church of Christian Fellowship, a three-hundred-member congregation in West Adams. In 1966, the National Institutes of Mental Health awarded Cannon a $900,000 grant to help the clinic move into an abandoned furniture store in the heart of Watts's Broadway district. By 1969, Central City's services had expanded to include a new service branch that later served as the basis for the nonprofit Kedren Community Mental Health Foundation.

In a similar manner to the history of neighborhood health centers, the community mental health movement sought to check physician authority by taking the brunt of care responsibility away from superintendents in state hospitals and giving it to psychiatrists, family members, and community caretakers situated in the "free market." In theory, the presence of mental health clinics aimed to prevent the onset of mental illness in poor patient populations by catching mild forms of mental distress before they developed into more serious conditions or to divert the diagnosed mentally ill from state hospitals by assigning them care options set within the community. For mental health leaders in Los Angeles, the problem of prevention and diversion appeared particularly troublesome in Black neighborhoods because the Short-Doyle Act (1957) had failed to incentivize enough providers to build services in those neighborhoods. As one 1967 study observed, Black men diagnosed with schizophrenia admitted to the county's psychiatric emergency wards were more likely to be sent directly to state hospital care, the most punitive and carceral of mental health services, partly because of the absence of community mental health services in their neighborhoods.[44]

As suggested by how USC's Watts Clinic leaders hid mental health services behind primary care services, most clinicians also understood that Black people feared directly utilizing mental health services because the stakes of being diagnosed as "crazy" were known to be high. As historians of psychiatry have observed, Black people's presence in asylums and state hospitals remained relatively scant until Emancipation.[45] After Reconstruction, Southern state officials deployed, alongside punitive penal work programs, the threat of committing to state hospital care any Black worker unable to labor or be cared for by a wage-laboring breadwinner.[46] Once incarcerated, Black "inmates" often found psychiatric commitment to be a lifelong sentence because most psychiatrists tended to regard mentally ill Black people as "incurable" and as having little to no psychiatric research value.[47]

Central City's reputation as a mental health service center thus represented the latest manifestation of a much longer and circuitous mental hygiene movement that sought to separate psychiatry's deep social associations with punitive disciplinary power by promoting its ability to draw citizens to normality and health through their own individual desire and free will. Whereas USC's leaders sought to coerce Black people into mental health services through the deployment of bodily health services, Cannon's approach at Central City sought to entice Black people to use mental health services by drawing on their well-established desire to stabilize their own lives through social services centered on housing, employment, and childcare.

According to Gerald Grob, the mental hygiene movement's roots can be traced to the late nineteenth century, when psychiatrists increasingly began to believe that "they possessed the requisite knowledge to prevent as well as to treat pathological behavior" and in the process forge a "new social order" by fusing emerging scientific and administrative knowledge to reshape policy in realms far beyond the state hospital.[48] Instead of relying on shackles, psychiatrists began to subject state hospital "inmates" to "moral therapy" training in vocations believed appropriate for their race and class under the belief that the repetition of perceived appropriate behavioral practices conditioned healthy minds from the "outside" in.[49] By the early twentieth century, faith in these practices made psychiatrists believe that their insights could "lead the way in research and policy formulation" for broad applications outside asylum and state hospital care "in such areas as mental hygiene, care of the feebleminded, eugenics, control of alcoholism, management of abnormal children, treatment of criminals, and to help in the prevention of crime, prostitution, and dependency."[50]

State reform schools in California and New York, for instance, were early sites for practitioners to experiment with mental hygiene approaches on poor youth of color incarcerated in juvenile justice programs. Juvenile justice reformers combined moral therapy's cognitive behavioral therapy approaches with mainstream discourses of gender, sexuality, and hygiene under the belief that both would reduce the burden of welfare, prisons, and state hospitals on society by creating citizens of color who could be trusted to live independently under white middle-class Victorian values, rules, and social order. California's Whittier State School for Boys, for instance, strove to create "manly, productive citizens" capable of being future male breadwinners; New York State's Reformatory for Women at Bedford sought to mold girls into proper housewives and mothers.[51] These reform programs, in turn, entwined discourses of race and sexuality to mark individuals within a continuum of "normal" and "degenerate" based on the polarities of heterosexual and homosexual.

Although reform schools demonstrate how adherents of the mental hygiene movement still held racist psychiatric notions that "disease was a product of environmental, hereditarian, and individual deficiencies," such approaches marked a significant break from older racial scientific theories that people of color were incapable of inhabiting the same intellectual complexity, psychic interiority, and gendered evolutionary distinctiveness as white heterosexuals.[52] As Siobhan Somerville argues, the psychiatric order of American slavery did more than just valorize white heterosexuality and the two-gender binary as evidence of white straight people's minds and bodies as supposedly more complex, sexually restrained, and "evolved" than the minds and bodies of people of color.[53] It also gave birth to an entire field of inquiry dedicated to investigating the intellectual difference between white subjects deemed "inverted," "homosexual," or "abnormal" and people of color also similarly believed to have supposedly un- and underdeveloped minds and bodies.

Somerville's investigation into modern sexology points to how by the early twentieth century the focus of mental health inquiries began to diverge, placing white sexual subjects on an axis between "heterosexual" and "homosexual" that was entirely separate from an axis that placed all people on a spectrum between "civilized" and "atavistic." Whereas, as Benjy Kahan argues, many sexologists at the beginning of the early twentieth century began their inquiries about sex by accepting homosexual behavior as one of several "minor perversions" unrelated to same-sex attraction or gender presentation, they settled by the 1930s on the idea of homosexuality as a natural mutation in human beings.[54] Increasingly, for those committed to racial scientific theories of difference, like Havelock Ellis, Edward Carpenter, and their followers, the task for sexologists was how to differentiate white homosexuality from the homosexuality of people of color without undermining racial science's investment in white people's evolutionary superiority.

As chapter 5 of this book shows, sexologists used psychiatry's power to differentiate race and intellect to argue that white people's homosexuality served as a different but equally evolved stage of human development as white heterosexuality. At the same time, they also argued that homosexuality in people of color still served as an indication of their race's gender and sexual atavism. That is, as Jules Gill-Peterson argues, whiteness helped account for white children's "plasticity," or susceptibility to evolutionary change, while Blackness helped account for Black people's inability to inhabit any gender and sexual distinctiveness.[55] Accounting for racial difference when it came to questions about sexuality thus pushed early twentieth-century white mental health researchers to try to maintain the racial boundaries of intellect and gender complexity through the use of psychoanalysis, a new method that departed from older biological theories and methods.

As scholars have shown repeatedly, many psychiatrists used the belief that people of color lacked the "psychic interiority" of white minds to exclude them from psychoanalytic research on homosexuality.[56] By midcentury, however, proponents of racial psychiatric sameness increasingly used psychoanalysis toward opposite ends by using it to prove that homosexuality, across racial groups, served as the human species' most exemplary form of scientific evolutionary atavism.[57] As Dennis Doyle argues, it was thus important, by the 1950s, for proponents of racial sameness to believe that "the psychological nature of African Americans could not truly be thought of as racially indistinct from that of whites until psychiatrists presented black men and women as fundamentally male and female in nature."[58]

Doyle's work on proponents of psychiatric universalism in Harlem shows that by the 1960s researchers mobilized discourses of gender distinctiveness to posit that the pathological figures they associated with dysfunctional Black families were not inherent to racial biology but were "suspended" or "deformed" psychic states brought on by a Black individual's exposure to racism, segregation, and discrimination. Some researchers, such as Judge Justine Polier and Dr. Viola Bernard, believed that Black children's lack of access to the same opportunities as white children accounted for high rates of sexual maladjustment in Black subjects as adults. Others, such as Drs.

Fredric Wertham and Hilda Mosse, argued that Black people's status as an oppressed class exacerbated what they referred to as a "catathymic crisis," a psychic crisis developed from a traumatic social basis experienced early in life.[59] Along with psychiatric intervention, both approaches assumed that Black subjects could be integrated into "mainstream" white society through capitalist assimilation or class revolution in ways that would reduce or eliminate the appearance of mental disorders in Black populations.

The belief that scientific racism's most devastating legacy was not simply that it ordered Black people as intellectually inferior to white people, but that it had rendered them without either a distinct gender or a stable sexuality, greatly influenced Cannon while attending Columbia University Medical School. As a psychiatrist, he dedicated his research to proving the gender distinctiveness and sexual stability of Black men and women.[60] By the mid-1960s, Cannon's research as an assistant professor of psychiatry at UCLA joined an emerging cohort of Black mental health researchers, such as Kenneth Clark and Mamie Clark, who tended to condemn homosexuality indirectly in Black communities by focusing on sexually maladjusted individuals—such as single mothers, pregnant teens, and absentee fathers—understood to be on the "margins of heterosexuality."[61] Although still queer in a broad sense, such a focus on marginalized heterosexuality drew the public's attention to Black people's supposed closer deviation from accepted social norms than that of homosexuals.

His 1964 article "The Psycho-Social Aspects of Segregation" shows Cannon believed that without the ability to properly challenge segregation and white supremacy, Black individuals projected the psychic tension engendered by discrimination and class-based oppression onto family members through "defenses such as denial, reaction formation, somatization, projection, and acting out."[62] Rather than help lubricate and strengthen the expected gender roles between breadwinning men and obedient wives and children, he described the "matriarchal anti-male atmosphere" induced by society's racist anti-Black male employment practices as robbing Black children of their proper identification with their expected gender roles as adults. Unable to occupy the role of breadwinning men and regarded as weak and irresponsible by Black women, he argued that Black men "displace [their] anger versus the dominant group on women," and Black women, in turn, visit "displacement of [their] anger upon [their] children, especially [their] sons."

Cannon's writings show, however, that he departed from Harlem's integration-based and class-based psychiatric approaches by building on the work of

Dr. Abram Kardiner and Dr. Lionel Ovesey. In *The Mark of Oppression* (1951), Kardiner and Ovesey argued that violent behavior in Black populations was the result of personality maladjustments developed by Black children forced to identify and strive toward white norms but denied the ability to achieve them because of racism and prejudice.[63] Rather than posit the existence of psychiatric universalism, Kardiner and Ovesey argued that American culture created two different "basic personalities" in Black people and white people. In their analysis, unhealthy amounts of anxiety, hostility, desire for status, and sexual maladjustment developed within Black individuals because they must "identify [themselves] with the Negro, but [also] initiate compensatory identification with the white, who is also hated."[64] Such an argument suggested that society neither needed to integrate (as Polier and Bernard believed) nor needed class revolution (as Wertham and Mosse did) but simply needed to develop a separate set of psychiatric approaches that recognized Black culture as distinct and different from that of white people.

Cannon found Kardiner and Ovesey's work more compelling than other approaches because he increasingly believed that economic advancement and assimilation into mainstream middle-class society did not release Black people from the psychic stress of white supremacy. Rather than make Black people feel more normal and accepted, Cannon argued that the tendency of Black elites to "ape white middle class standards" to "correct any doubt of the validity of the racial myths erected [against] them" demonstrated that doubt and worry continued to haunt the psychic space of Black elites despite their relative economic security and social status vis-à-vis the poor.[65] Such observations pointed to mental health problems that integration-based and class-based approaches to racial psychiatry assumed would cease once Black individuals successfully availed themselves of "opportunity" and class advancement. Indeed, by the 1970s Cannon believed that the imposter syndrome induced in Black psyches under white supremacy was leading to "problems of child delinquency, drug problems, high divorce rate and other evidence of stress and social fragmentation" in Black subjects who were "widely regarded as 'having made it.'"[66]

The sum total of Cannon's research thus posited that effective therapeutic interventions in Black people had to produce not only a proper sense of one's "relatedness" to other genders and sexualities but also an appropriate sense of "relatedness" to one's supposedly proper race and culture. By linking gender and sexuality with race and culture into one interlocking psychological matrix, he posited that forcing Black children to psychologically develop under so-called white cultural norms led to the sexual maladjustments believed by culture of poverty theory to prevent Black individuals from economically advancing. To unlock Black people's supposedly natural and healthy psychological development as African-descended people, he argued for the rebirth of African cultural practices that would help Black individuals "to understand, relate to and accept their ancestral 'core.'"[67]

As his activities at Central City show, however, reconnecting with one's African-ness did not mean refusing capitalism or heteropatriarchy. In fact, a 1968 newspaper article demonstrated that getting people to work and live self-sufficiently was a major objective of Central City. Reporters described it as a facility with two doors—one to "deal with the mental ills found in city slums," and another marked "Community Service Center."[68] Cannon and other administrators, however, admitted the latter door mattered more because most residents feared walking through a door potentially labeling them as "crazy." CMHCs were thus essentially small psychiatric clinics "disguised" as Community Service Centers—or, as they are commonly called today, Community Based Organizations (CBOs)—and were primarily understood by residents as places to receive assistance with employment, housing, childcare, and temporary welfare services to help people get back on their feet.

Similar to how USC's leaders disguised efforts to reform the psychology of patient participants through the deployment of bodily health services, Central City used its social welfare services as a ploy to get the poor into therapy. As Richard Sanville, a Central City administrator, explained: "Many times we find that people who need economic aid also need mental or emotional treatment and we walk them through corridors to our consultation rooms."[69] And just as USC's leaders argued that mental health services were necessary to reduce costs around illness in hospitals, Sanville argued that social services helped prevent costs related to severe mental illness by closely tying poverty to mental illness. "After all," he asked, "what is mental health? If you're so poor you can't feed your kids, you're under a stress that often leads to mental illness. If a child is so hungry he can't pay attention in school, he falls behind and can become either a delinquent or mental case."

Once referred, Cannon revealed that he used a form of psychoanalysis tailored to Black working-class individuals he referred to as "instant therapy," which suggested that he deployed the method as a way to signal to other psychiatrists that Black people were as psychologically modern and sexually complex as white middle-class patients. The therapy Cannon preferred and used more widely appeared to be a modernized form of cognitive behavioral therapy. Central City's hallmark programs, for example, were a "Teen-Queen" club for Black girls and a karate class for Black boys.

More behavioral therapy sessions than youth programs, the "Teen-Queen" club and karate class exposed Black children to positive adult role models early in life to prevent the development of sexually maladjusted personalities. Cannon remarked, for instance, that Central City's "Teen-Queen" girls' club was "based on the idea that black is beautiful," and that its "stress [on] Afro-American standards of beauty, grooming, and conduct . . . help[ed] the young Negro girl build an image of herself that relates to her environment."[70] Cannon also defended the instruction of boys in karate as a "virile sport" that conveyed ideas of "discipline and proper diet" to young Black men.

Central City's referral services, and especially its youth programs, illustrate what made Cannon's research interventions so dynamic in comparison with previous psychiatric studies on race anchored by criminal justice systems. By rooting his research in community settings, Cannon's work focused psychiatric studies on "normal" race populations not assumed to be either criminal or pathological. Thus, rather than place clients on a spectrum that pegged them to a position between "normal" and "degenerate," Central City placed patients on a continuum based on the polarities of being "mentally well" and "at-risk" (of developing a mental illness).

According to Dr. Harry Brickman, director of the Los Angeles Department of Mental Health Services, the architecture of Central City formed the overall programmatic agenda of the county's community mental health program in racialized neighborhoods across the city. Brickman explained that the county's vision was to create a network of CBOs "'riding on the shoulders' of established community caretakers," a term he used for mental health professionals of color (psychiatrists, psychologists, and social workers) working in their own communities.[71] By "enrich[ing] their capacity to deal with mental health programs of their essentially non-mental health caseloads," Brickman argued that county resources would help CBOs "deal directly and more effectively with the emotional problems of their welfare recipients, probationers, students, etc.," but empower them to refer a client to "definitive mental health professionals in the community" for treatment and research.

That Central City's activities might have appeared to be unremarkable, unscientific, and normal to the untrained eye is exactly what made Cannon's mental health clinic so successful. Cannon offered Black residents a vision of normality and health pinned to their normative participation in the economy as waged workers and properly gendered and sexual subjects that was already familiar and widely regarded in shared cultural discourse as "common sense." It was also a vision of health and normality not unlike the one offered by USC's Watts Clinic. What made their directives different, however, was the continuing and haunting suspicion that white-led antipoverty programs hid an ulterior motive of sustaining prevailing racial hierarchies in new guises and a growing new belief that Black-led antipoverty programs centered on narratives of Black nationalism and capitalism had the capacity to finally authenticate Black communities as modern and developed.

Whereas USC's clinic struggled at the end of 1968 to even advance its antipoverty programming, Central City boasted more than five thousand patients a year. So popular and widely successful were Central City's programs in carrying out antipoverty objectives that Cannon and other Black mental health professionals broke ground in late 1968 for a new $3.7 million seven-story mental health center with funding from the Department of Health, Education, and Welfare and private donations. The diminishing returns of integrationist-based approaches to antipoverty programming and the perceived success of Black-led antipoverty programming, however, hid how many Black community members interpreted Black Power differently than Cannon and his peers.

THE DIFFERENCE A MAN MAKES

The architecture of Black mental wellness Cannon built to reinforce his research shows that he managed to capture the hearts and minds of many Black community members, but not all. Like many Black mental health professionals at the time, Cannon did not limit his psychiatric interventions to clinical spaces. In fact, throughout the 1960s and early 1970s, he argued that connecting Black individuals to an "ancestral core" required mental health professionals to go "beyond the narrow confines of psychiatry and other health disciplines" to recruit others into the work of making spaces beyond clinics conducive for healthy Black psychological development.[72] As this section shows, Cannon directly helped shape the direction of the Black Power movement in Southern California by founding, leading, and operating a suite of Afrocentric community centers and programs not explicitly named as mental health institutions and services.

As Cannon's late-1970s writings reveal, his efforts around normalizing work and family life as "natural" aspects of Blackness were not just intended to unlock individual health but to help Black Americans cultivate a deep-enough shared "race-feeling" with other African and African diasporic peoples in a process he referred to as "re-Africanization."[73] To him, "re-Africanization" reignited Black people's cultural connection with Africa in order to create an "economics" based on a "supportive spiritual-cultural matrix" of Blackness, whereby Black Americans marshaled the fruits of their work and family life away from white society and toward Black America, Africa, and the African diaspora.[74] Cannon believed that the more deeply and widely Black Americans recognized "their shared 'ancestral' cores and the mutuality of destinies" with each other and with African and African diasporic peoples, the more effective the therapeutic effect of his approach would be

Such an approach effectively asked Black working-class people to overlook tensions within the Black community along the lines of class in a similar manner to how, as W. E. B. Du Bois put it, white elites encouraged white workers to overlook their "practically identical interests" with Black workers in the years after Reconstruction.[75] According to Du Bois, it was precisely the cultivation of a white "racial-feeling" among the "poor white and planter" that helped "the political success of the doctrine of racial separation" produce such "astonishing economic results" for white American society by the end of the nineteenth century. Whereas Du Bois lamented a missed opportunity for Black workers to unite with white workers to overthrow capitalist elites in the aftermath of Emancipation, Cannon saw the 1960s as an opportunity for the Black working and middle class to unite against white supremacy by marshaling their resources to build an economy that he believed could counterbalance the "economics" and "supportive spiritual-cultural matrix" built between white elites and white workers since the 1880s.

To prove that it was possible for non-Anglo-descended people to be successful as a racial "class" in "mainstream" America, Cannon pointed to Jewish and Japanese Americans, "two formerly 'abused' ethnic groups," who by the 1960s, he perceived, were "not only surviving, but [were] prospering, because of their comprehension and recognition of the essentiality of 'core identity' enhancement" programs."[76] Just like the cultural and economic connection of many white Americans to European nations, Cannon attributed Jewish and Japanese American success to their "constant contact, acceptance and involvement" with "ancestral lands," particularly after the establishment of the state of Israel in 1948 and the rebirth of Japan's economy after World War II. He argued that the psychic connection each group maintained to their "home of homes" through language courses, cultural schools, and community celebrations allowed each to safely navigate white spaces because it "nurtured and replenished" their sense of self no matter their class or social location in society. This connection helped American Jews, for instance, avoid the psychic tension of double consciousness by allowing them to "safely identify with *both* Israel and America" while recognizing the "dangers of 'over' assimilation and consequent 'loss' of identity in adopted homelands."

Rather than limit the work of "identity enhancement or African 'core' clarification and construction efforts" to mental health professionals, Cannon demanded that his re-Africanization efforts "be joined by historians, archeologists, economists, artists, architects, business experts, spiritualists, educators, behaviorists and health workers."[77] His work to manifest a psychologically therapeutic landscape for African Americans began in earnest in 1967 when he founded the Mafundi Arts Institute, a Black arts center in Watts, with fellow UCLA academic C. Bernard Jackson and Ron Karenga (leader of the Pan-Africanist *US* Organization and creator of Kwanzaa). The center forwarded the objectives of re-Africanization by presenting positive representations of Blackness and African heritage through a slew of "identity enhancement" and "ancestral 'core' clarification" programs centered on dance, art, film, photography, and acting classes for youth at the Mafundi. As James Taylor, a Mafundi staff member, explained, the center was intended to complement antipoverty objectives because "Dr. Cannon thought that social and economic reforms would not work unless people had self-worth [and he] thought that the way to do that was through the arts."[78]

Having begun an arts organization located near and connected to Hollywood, Cannon ventured to broadcast respectable and dignified representations of Black people at a scale large enough to reach every person of color who owned a television set. Mafundi served as a proving ground for talent—a conduit between producers and executives from Hollywood looking to fill casts with people of color and a job creation engine for citizens from different communities of color. The centers also became well known for showcasing theatrical works for, about, and by people of color, hoping they would be picked up in larger more established venues. Mafundi, in particular, housed youth art programs in "art, drama, music, dance, film making, fencing, and modeling," which all exposed Black children to African aesthetics and political art.[79]

Cannon's explicit recruitment of Black professionals and his skepticism about achieving "social and economic reforms" without a cultural dimension shows that he believed any attempt at re-Africanization would fail without the leadership of Black middle-class men. His fears were exacerbated by the writings of Black social scientists like E. Franklin Frazier and Nathan Hare, who by 1965 criticized Black middle-class professionals for their insufficient participation and growing disinterest in the Black freedom movement. In *The Black Bourgeoisie* and *The Black Anglo-Saxons*, Frazier and Hare, respectively, took issue with the propensity of many Black middle-class members to see their economic and social interests as more aligned with the white middle class than the Black working class.[80]

A closer look at Cannon's own thoughts on the imposter syndrome induced in Black professionals shows that he was concerned about the psychological impact integration had on Black middle-class people's fitness to lead the race. He intimated, for instance, that the appropriation of white cultural norms led Black men and women to overcompensate in ways that alienated them from the Black masses. He criticized, for instance, how Black professionals spent time and money on cosmetics, cars, and clothes to produce an "attractive appearance."[81] These projections not only created "an intensely paradoxical phenomenon" when it came to ideas of racial progress but also created "deep widespread resentments" within Black working-class people who considered Black middle-class people "uppity."[82]

Cannon's plan for the "re-Africanization" of the Black middle class did not necessarily mean wearing dashikis or an Afro haircut. Ironically, having mastery over one's cultural connection to Black people and to Africa by following the supposedly normal gendered and sexualized scripts of breadwinning manhood mattered more to his ideas than wearing African garb or styles. His championing of teaching karate to Black boys as a "virile" sport was thus less about imparting an authentic African art to children and more about preparing boys to think of themselves as the proper actors to defend and care for their families and communities.

His ideas of who fit the criteria of being a normal middle-class Black leader therefore tended to be reflections on whether or not individuals demonstrated enough self-mastery to exhibit sexual restraint and channel their psychic energy towards strengthening a shared racial feeling with other Black people. For instance, he championed civil rights ministers for marching with the Black masses in Selma, Alabama, but criticized the absence of most members of the Black middle class.[83] He also lauded personal actions to present Blackness as positive, dignified, and sexually respectable by railing against the rise of "so-called Blaxploitation films" which represented Afrocentric Black characters and subjects as "super sexed, super violent and super dumb."[84]

Cannon and Karenga, however, increasingly felt threatened by an alternative approach to Black freedom posited by the Black Panther Party, an antiracist, anticapitalist, and anti-imperialist organization founded in Oakland in 1966, with a Los Angeles branch established in 1968.[85] Unlike Black cultural nationalists, who focused on forging racial cohesiveness around heterosexuality and Black capitalism, the Panthers argued for a complete overthrow of capitalism by working with oppressed and working-class people regardless of their racial, gender, and sexual identities. For instance, the Panthers worked with single mothers of the National Welfare Rights Organization to develop free health clinics and community survival programs.[86] They also worked with gay liberation and disability rights organizations who shared the Panthers' critiques of the psychiatric community and the police as being the Black, gay, and disabled communities' "biggest oppressors."[87]

These alliances signified the organization's shift away from more militant and masculinist confrontation models of organizing toward what its leaders called its "survival pending revolution" programs focused on feeding, clothing, housing, and providing healthcare for all poor people. According to Ashley D. Farmer, this new organizing agenda led to a public endorsement of women's equality in 1970 and reflected the organization's deeper recruitment of women into its ranks and leadership.[88] These alliances and their association with Black Panther Party leader Huey Newton, however, marked how these new positions took place amid an internal split between Newton and Eldridge Cleaver that diluted his ability to enforce ideological discipline over the party's new positions. As Jared Leighton argues, many Panthers thus continued to make homophobic and sexist statements out of line with the Party's official doctrine.[89]

Scholarly focus on the Panther split has helped to obscure how Panther leaders essentially offered a different version of Black manhood that did not prioritize the need to rehabilitate Black men back into patriarchy through capitalism. Although imperfect in practice, the Panthers' evolving ideological line posited the importance of redefining a manhood that did not simply reproduce the attributes of manhood commonly associated with white patriarchy's ableist, sexist, homophobic, and transphobic characteristics. As Audre Lorde later phrased it, such an approach recognized that "our sons must become men" but "such men as we hope our daughters, born and unborn, will be pleased to live among."[90]

The Panthers were also influenced more directly by the writings of Frantz Fanon, a Black psychiatrist from Martinique who argued in *Black Skin,*

White Masks (1952) and *The Wretched of the Earth* (1961) that the psychic tension induced by colonialism could be resolved only through violence against one's oppressor.[91] The Panthers interpreted colonialism as the entanglement of the historical processes of racism and capitalism and saw Fanon's identity as a Black Caribbean clinician working toward revolution as an armed member of the Algerian independence movement as a more apt therapeutic model than the one offered by Cannon. As Newton phrased it, "As far as returning per se to the ancient African Customs, we don't see any necessity in this. We say the only culture worthwhile holding on to is a revolutionary culture. The only way we're going to be free is by seizing political power which comes through the barrel of a gun."[92]

Cannon regarded the Black Panthers' growing influence in Los Angeles as alarming because it threatened the imagined "cohesiveness" of his therapeutic model by mobilizing the Black working class toward futures that eroded the "relatedness" of normative ascriptions of gender and race underpinning his re-Africanization theory. By 1969, Cannon felt increasingly alarmed after his attempts to seat Charles Thomas as director of UCLA's Afro-American Studies Center appeared to be undone by the influence of two student leaders, John Huggins and Alprentice "Bunchy" Carter, on the university's Black Student Union (BSU). As students, Huggins and Carter helped popularize approaches to Black nationalism rooted in anticapitalism at the same time that Cannon and Karenga had hoped to direct the BSU's and Afro-American Studies Center's ideological direction as advisory board members. The ideological battle was so heated that two members of Karenga's armed "Simba" patrol carried out the assassination of Huggins and Carter after it appeared they stood poised to ascend as the Black Student Union's newest elected leaders.[93]

The activities of Black politicians near and around their murders, however, shows that Cannon was not the only community leader worried about the Black community's seeming lack of cohesion. Just as concerned with the Black Panther Party as he was with the interracial tension of USC's Watts Clinic, Black congressman Augustus Hawkins admitted that he felt "it necessary to organize a special impact group" after witnessing the interracial turmoil of USC's Watts clinic.[94] Although he admitted that the clinic proved to be "a difficult project to straighten out," he believed that the energy of the Black Power movement could be better marshaled away from a critique of capitalism and colonialism toward community projects focused on Black consumerism and Black capitalism.[95]

In 1967, Hawkins empowered his deputy Charles Knox to establish and lead the South Central Improvement Action Committee (IMPAC), a business-oriented umbrella organization for Black political, business, and activist leaders and organizations interested in marshaling antipoverty programming money to make Black neighborhoods more conducive to Black entrepreneurialism. Although IMPAC mostly showcased President Richard Nixon's small business loan programs, its most well-known and successful project was the construction of Ujima Village, a low- to moderate-income housing development of three hundred townhomes and apartments on 121 acres with a planned onsite mall of seventeen shops. By the time the first residents moved into their homes in 1972, the project involved over fifty named Black organizations and individuals and boasted the financial support of several banks and insurance companies, including Prudential, Bank of America, and Broadway Federal Savings and Loan.

Built a mile from the construction site of King-Drew and on land formerly occupied by a petroleum "tank farm," Ujima Village was originally designed as a place that community leaders hoped future workforces could live in. It was sited near the soon-to-be opened King-Drew Medical Center, a new highly anticipated postal service distribution center, and a new industrial park also slated nearby. According to Florence Vaughn, Ujima's lawyer, the development was imagined as a "city within a city" by situating a community center on a ten-acre plot near the shopping mall. This would house a "24-hour child care center, a center for handicapped children, library facilities, gymnasium, mental health referral service, movie theater, hobby center, community meeting rooms, outdoor recreation, and swimming pool."[96] Vaughn, however, argued that the real significance of the development was its ability to translate the individual psychological significance of "Black is beautiful" in making "positive everything that has been negative about black ghettos" by providing Black residents "a real sense of community [and] racial pride" through individual and collective ownership of Black property.

As the inclusion of mental health services indicates, the project notably served as the most exemplary demonstration for Cannon's "re-Africanization" theory. Cannon initially served as the chairman of IMPAC's housing committee and later as director of the Ujima Village Community Development Corporation before becoming chairman of IMPAC's board. After winning an appointment as King-Drew's chair of psychiatry, Cannon sought to demonstrate the benefits of his Black nationalist approach to mental health services. He launched a "large scale, 3-year program focused on preventative mental health services" at Ujima to "identify, develop and mobilize the Human Resources of Ujima Village residents [by] training them as Mshauri ("counselor" in Swahili) or community linkers between Ujima and the resources of the larger Los Angeles region."[97] Describing the Mshauri as "family health facilitators or family extenders," the program was to ready residents for work either in King-Drew's newly planned "Community Mental Health and Mental Retardation Center" or in community mental health–inspired CBOs elsewhere in the city. As research assistants, Mshauri were also expected to help Cannon and Dr. Rose Jenkins compare the mental health of Ujima residents with another master-planned community for Black residents called Alondra-Wilmington Plaza. According to Jenkins, such a study would document "the effect that residence in each location has on developing social responsibility, awareness, and leadership behavior in young Black children."[98]

Alongside increased police violence and state-sanctioned counterintelligence operations against the Black Panthers, the Ujima Village project helped isolate and ostracize the Panthers by serving as a vehicle to bring together elected Black civil rights political leaders with Black cultural nationalists to outcompete the Party for the hearts and minds of the Black masses. In fact, police intervention helped draw the contrast between the Panthers' own version of community health services—the Alprentice "Bunchy" Carter Free Clinic (one of a rare set of Panther clinics to include mental health services)—and the mental health services associated with the Black cultural nationalism of Cannon, Karenga, and Thomas.[99] After a police raid on the Bunchy Carter Free Clinic in 1970, Panther medical volunteers felt compelled to operate out of two mobile vans parked outside the tear-gassed building. Such a scene made Cannon's approach to "revolution" appear safer and more palatable than the growing association of the Panthers with violence and radicalism.[100]

IN BED WITH THE STATE

From the perspective of federal antipoverty researchers, the discourses of a culture-based approach to Black nationalism in Cannon's community mental health clinics appeared to succeed in unlocking the shared objective of producing desiring self-governing individuals that had eluded Giorgi and Tranquada in their similar deployment of health services. Whereas Giorgi and Tranquada's appeals to coax Black individuals into normality and health through work and respectable family life were interpreted as "once again" an instance of the white community "imposing its own solutions on the Negro area," the same exact appeal coming from the voice of a respected Black clinician could make work and respectable family life seem not only desirable and alluring but also made these practices somehow more naturally "Black" or "African." As evident in the number of projects carried out and people who participated in institutions led by Cannon shows, the call to define health and normality through universal work, respectable family life, *and* Black nationalism helped keep the viability of antipoverty projects alive when many federal and local authorities considered them ineffective and redundant.

Such an observation demonstrates that the spirit of antipoverty programming did not die with the end of Johnson's administration but was reborn under Nixon as initiatives of "Black capitalism."[101] Indeed, replacing USC's white clinicians with Black physicians allowed federal authorities such as John Veneman, Nixon's undersecretary of health, education, and welfare, to once again uphold the Watts Clinic as a shining example of how to control hospital costs.[102] Such a focus on the skin color of program leadership shows how antipoverty program policies moved away from citizen participation mandates and toward identifying Black America's future business leaders. As Cannon's programs show, the presence of a Black boss or a Black elected official helped obfuscate the relations of racial capitalism that permitted inequality to persist.

To claim that race alone was the central factor in determining the different levels of success between Giorgi and Tranquada's and Cannon's antipoverty approaches, however, elides the multitude of competing visions of Black freedom that emerged in the late 1960s and early 1970s that did not prioritize change on capitalism and heteropatriarchy. Thus while Cannon, Karenga, and Hawkins appeared successful in containing the threat that the Black Panther Party posed to their vision of community "cohesion," they appeared unable by the opening of King-Drew Medical Center in 1972 to thwart the voices of Black women leaders who increasingly drew the connection between the discourses of breadwinning manhood underlying antipoverty programming and their marginalization and oppression as Black women in this regime.

Initially drawn into efforts to "take back" control of USC's Watts Clinic, a group of Black woman leaders associated with antipoverty and welfare rights organizing, including Johnnie Tillmon, Caffie Greene, Lilian Mobley, Mary Henry, and Nona Carter (informally named the "mothers of Watts" by Kofi-Charu Nat Turner), increasingly turned their attention to the rest of King-Drew's health system by the hospital's opening in 1972.[103] Many of the women, including Greene, had not only previously led their own popular and successful youth programs in the neighborhood but had also fostered the future leaders of the Black Panther Party under it. Greene was also responsible for introducing her sister Johnnie Tillmon, future national leader of the welfare rights movement, to the landscape of political organizing in Los Angeles when Tillmon first arrived in the city from Arkansas in the 1950s.

The irony that antipoverty clinic leaders aimed to produce independent and sexually responsible economic actors by creating practices that extended the surveillance and maintenance mechanisms of the state was not lost on poor women of color. The intense scrutiny of the private and sexual lives of poor people of color drew a deep contrast with the practices that white middle-class people had developed by the 1960s to evade detection for sexual practices the state deemed troublesome.[104] By the 1960s, strategies of racial and gender conformity helped a class of "straight-passing" and "straight-looking" white middle-class men and women avoid the most punitive aspects of the White Straight State.[105]

As scholars of the history of sexuality observe, white middle-class men and women could generally hide instances of same-sex intimacy and non-normative sexual practices by conforming their comportment and behavior in public to match mainstream racial and gender norms. Their ability to obtain jobs and own homes, in turn, provided them an ability to pass as "normal" by the simple fact that owning property provided them privacy rights that poor people were generally unable to enjoy. As this chapter shows, owning property and health insurance also gave them the ability to consume healthcare on demand, in any manner, and no matter the cost burden they and other consumers faced.

The idea that poor people deserved the same privacy and consumer rights as white middle-class people motivated poor women activists in Watts to win the same rights for themselves. As early as 1969, Black women antipoverty advocates like Greene and Lilian Mobley had begun to counter-organize against Cannon over his direction of the community's mental health programs. By 1971, Mobley and Greene had self-organized the "King-Drew Mental Retardation Committee" as a community group, which sought to influence the plans for King-Drew's yet-to-be-built acute psychiatric unit.

Whereas both women leaders were willing and ready to contribute to planning mental health services, Cannon was unwilling to yield his authority to them.

Cannon refused to recognize Mobley's and Greene's self-organized committee. He accused both women of being "aggressive and hostile" and argued in a letter to Mobley that their "small gang" had "abused about every courtesy and privilege" afforded them within community organizing spaces.[106] Attempting to speak on behalf of others, Cannon went as far as to state that "our community, and certainly me, is fed up with your community disruption and divisiveness." More than just demonstrating the animus that Cannon held for women leaders, his correspondence with these Black women antipoverty advocates reveals just how formidable many Black women leaders had become by the early 1970s.

As the next chapter demonstrates, the intervention of Black women, especially welfare rights activists, on King-Drew's master plan played a definitive role in reshaping the mission of the health system. However, as opposed to meeting every demand of Black women activists, the conflict they engendered with the Black physician leaders of King-Drew helped Black political leaders surreptitiously and quietly assert a new direction for the health system. Like Cannon, Black political leaders like councilman-turned-mayor Tom Bradley recruited the discourses of racial normality and health to advance new ideas of economic development in urban policies to create ideas of community "cohesion" contingent on emerging ideas of multiculturalism.

FOUR

Profiting from Working Poverty

BY LATE 1971, local activist Johnnie Tillmon was ready to change the direction of the welfare rights movement. Shortly after founding one of the nation's first local welfare rights organizations—Aid to Needy Children (ANC) Mothers Anonymous in Watts—Tillmon had joined forces with civil rights activist George Wiley to form the National Welfare Rights Organization (NWRO), a national confederation of local welfare and antipoverty advocacy organizations. Since its founding in 1966, the NWRO had successfully leveraged the federal government's prevailing labor policies of supporting women's roles as homemakers to improve benefits for women on welfare. Frustrated, however, with legislative progress in the quest to help poor women and mothers on welfare win true autonomy for themselves and their families, Tillmon saw new opportunities to change the direction of gendered federal antipoverty policies by tackling their problematic manifestations in King-Drew Medical Center's master plan.

Tillmon was not the only Black community leader in Los Angeles seeking to change the medical center's purpose and mission. Councilman Tom Bradley, a migrant from Texas who had arrived in LA as a young boy in 1924, had witnessed how poverty deepened as jobs and capital moved away from the inner city toward racially exclusive suburban developments. Since his election to the city council in 1961, all efforts enticing large-scale employers to return and hire workers of color had largely failed except for an urban revitalization program moving the old Spring Street financial district to a downtown neighborhood known as Bunker Hill. The willingness of employers to move just a short distance from the city's overcrowded neighborhoods of color inspired Bradley to think differently about King-Drew's ultimate purpose in poor Black communities.

Both Tillmon's and Bradley's visions for social progress brought them into conflict with a slightly older vision for change embodied in King-Drew's master plan. Since the Watts Uprisings, politicians, health policy leaders, and residents had designed King-Drew as an antipoverty program that sought to match the health and income levels of white neighborhoods by first prioritizing the education and employment needs of Black male heads of households. However, by 1971, Drew Medical School's leaders Dr. Mitchell Spellman and Dr. M. Alfred Haynes had only enough money on hand to finish the proposed health system's hospital. Cost overruns, inflation, and construction delays plagued their ability to build a series of Black-led neighborhood health clinics integral to the system's design as a "community action program."

Hoping to win the support of the nation's two largest health policy funders, Spellman and Haynes opened up the master plan to scrutiny by the Department of Health, Education, and Welfare (DHEW) and the Commonwealth Foundation. From mid-1971 until six months after King-Drew's official opening in February 1972, both agencies jointly funded three research consulting firms—Lester Gorsline Associates, Arthur D. Little Inc., and the Urban Workshop (hereafter collectively referred to as the "study team" or "consultants")—to assess how effective the master plan had been in engaging local residents to use the medical center as an antipoverty program. The Master Plan Study brought King-Drew's original vision into open conflict with welfare rights activists and local politicians.

As this chapter shows, Tillmon and other welfare rights activists sought to manifest a vision for social change that did more than just address the various forms of unfreedom facing poor Black women. Unlike other antipoverty approaches centered on male breadwinning manhood, by the early 1970s many Black welfare rights activists stood at the forefront of an ongoing poor people's campaign seeking to maximize autonomy for women of color by normalizing housing, healthcare, childcare, food security, and guaranteed basic incomes as human rights for all citizens. Although they presented their policy position as an alternative to breadwinning manhood, they sought to free men of color as well as variously gendered people of all racial backgrounds from gendered patriarchal kinship patterns to choose lives and care arrangements that fit their individual needs rather than the state's predetermined outcomes.

This dream clashed with a different vision for racial inclusion offered by a growing coalition of racially liberal progressive politicians like Bradley. Instead of supporting measures giving poor women of color more individual autonomy, Bradley's multicultural coalition of Black, Asian, Spanish-speaking, gay, and liberal white politicians saw poor women of color's labor and proximity to Bunker Hill and downtown districts as pivotal to securing LA's new position in the US economy as a "global city" for financial trade. To entice global financial firms that elites thought were needed for Southern California to survive in a new emerging "global" economy, Bradley sought to guarantee new profit margins for employers willing to "risk" relocating to downtown Los Angeles by subsidizing working poverty through robust public health, housing, and transportation programs in the center city's surrounding neighborhoods of color.

For downtown employers, this approach created a "business-friendly" landscape and an immense cheap workforce whose healthcare and housing needs were addressed by municipal programs funded by the city and county. For Bradley, providing his constituents with accessible modern healthcare, plentiful low-rent apartments and public housing, and an abundance of low-wage jobs easily accessible by public buses offered better alternatives than facing an economic future where poor people of color voted with their feet. By the late 1960s, politicians representing Black, Asian, Spanish-speaking, and gay neighborhoods feared that overzealous "slum clearance" programs and the absence of jobs were causing their constituents to seek jobs and homes elsewhere.

To prevent a complete loss of LA's identity as a multiracial, multiethnic haven, Bradley allied himself by the late 1960s with downtown elites organized through the Community Redevelopment Agency of Los Angeles (CRA-LA), a city agency imbued with extraordinary powers to raise public capital for private development. The combination of these relationships would help Bradley become mayor of Los Angeles in 1973. With CRA-LA, Bradley before and after his election led the urban revitalization of Bunker Hill and nearby neighborhoods by supporting measures to "conserve" and "enhance" the identity of certain neighborhoods just outside Center City to "preserve" their character as low-income neighborhoods of color. As the next chapter shows, preserving some neighborhoods as "family friendly" working-class and low-income communities required deliberately earmarking other neighborhoods for further deterioration in order to make neighborhoods like Bunker Hill exciting places for mostly elite white financial workers to "live, work, and play."

The DHEW's and Commonwealth Foundation's recommendations facilitated these new spatial relationships by encouraging county officials to build comprehensive care clinics and childcare centers in the same low-income neighborhoods earmarked by city officials for "preservation" as neighborhoods of color. Despite being built in response to welfare activists' demands, county planners saw these institutions as vital for economic programs that turned welfare policies away from longer-term support for women on welfare and their children toward practices that coerced women back into working motherhood. Such policies reflected society's growing dependency on women workers given the economy's shift to a "service" economy based on labor often associated with "women's work." At the same time, a trend emerged among employers to seek and valorize women workers for the profit margins "women's wages" produced for bosses in a turbulent economy that Diana Pearce has termed the "feminization of poverty."[1]

These policy objectives were not intended to gentrify neighborhoods of color by replacing poor Black residents with higher-income white residents or to achieve antipoverty objectives of raising the poor into the middle class but were designed to harness and manage poverty's productive capacity to drive economic change elsewhere. These measures demonstrate what Clyde Adrian Woods calls the "resilience of plantation relations" through capitalism's capacity to renew itself with regional alliances that emerge in response to capitalist crisis.[2] In Los Angeles, a new crop of inner-city political leaders allied themselves with downtown's financial elite to "restore and reproduce their profitability and power" by arresting the economic development of neighborhoods of color. Together, their tactics managed poverty's capacity to make other neighborhoods and regions productive.

As scholars of the feminization of poverty and working poverty phenomena argue, this shift from one stage of racial and sexual capitalism to another illuminates how politicians and employers all looked to successfully restructure the economy by exploiting the power and labor of poor women of color. Scholars examining this period argue that these processes inaugurated a "race to the bottom" that is better known in social science circles as "globalization." By the 1990s, the labor arrangements led by Bradley's multiracial and multicultural coalition inspired unscrupulous employers to hire workers more vulnerable than citizens of color to exploit, like undocumented workers, or relocate to where labor and environmental regulations were more lax, like the US-Mexico border, to undercut the standards common in Los Angeles.

The clash between welfare activists, Drew Medical School leaders, and politicians in the midst of global economic restructuring thus illuminates how leaders in Los Angeles rejected two differently gendered sets of economic proposals for Black freedom—one pinned to Black breadwinning manhood and another centered on the autonomy of poor women of color—to support policies renewing old patterns of racial segregation under new racially liberal discourses associated with a global economy. After witnessing decades of capital flight from inner-city neighborhoods, politicians like Bradley welcomed the return of investment in the form of a new financial district downtown because it offered constituents a job and income, however temporary and low paying these might be. This approach, however, not only made the health and economic power of communities of color more dependent on the vitality of a racially exclusive financial district downtown but also reinforced older spatial relationships of power under a benevolent belief that such arrangements were crucial for respecting the racial and class character of neighborhoods of color.

Bradley believed that these relationships gave Black and Spanish-speaking residents an opportunity to challenge widespread beliefs that people of color were lazy and unproductive by helping to highlight their contributions to LA's reinvention as a global city. Similar to Booker T. Washington, Bradley sought to engineer an "opportunity economy" that called upon Black citizens to temper their dreams for a speedy and comprehensive process for social and economic inclusion by demanding they "cast down their buckets where they are" in order for the race to "prosper in proportion."[3] Following the principle that waged labor—no matter how low-paid or strenuous—dignified people's attempts to feed, clothe, and shelter their families, Bradley hoped that citizens would see LA's working-class neighborhoods of color as hardworking, family-oriented, and sexually respectable, just like the city's white suburbs.

The irony of this vision, however, is that most observers witnessing LA's rise as a "global city" failed to see how important workers of color were to LA's new political economy. The city's policies neither challenged racial segregation nor altered society's widespread acceptance of labor practices that paid workers of color less than white workers and women less than men. The combination of these relationships kept the contributions that communities of color made to LA's survival hidden in plain sight because most citizens continued to associate race with poor health, deteriorating infrastructure, and lower real estate values. In short, rather than consider LA's working poor as "assets" to capitalism's revival, most citizens continued to regard poor people of color as liabilities requiring more police and more prisons to contain them.

GLOBALIZATION

King-Drew's Master Plan Study provided welfare rights activists, health policy experts, and politicians with early evidence of how social science experts were beginning to interpret trends in the flow of capital. Social scientists began describing these shifts as "globalization," a phenomenon naming the increased interrelatedness of regional economies across the globe. In the United States, scholars have variously described the relocation of manufacturing firms in the late 1960s that once served as the nation's economic base to new markets abroad as "deindustrialization" and the emergence of a labor market characterized by the selling of one's skills as the growth of a new "service" economy.

The term *service economy* is often used by scholars to highlight the importance of highly paid, highly educated workers in an economy based on the transaction of capital between regions in the United States and markets abroad. A "financial class" of insurance, real estate, and financial workers, a "creative class" of artists, entrepreneurs, architects, and designers, and an "intellectual class" of academics, doctors, nurses, and engineers all point to highly desirable service-sector jobs that rose in importance as the number of middle-class jobs for autoworkers, machinists, and construction workers dwindled. Unlike most postwar manufacturing jobs, which did not require a college degree, the high threshold related to high-end service-sector jobs made it hard for manufacturing workers to easily retool and retrain themselves so their incomes could keep pace with a shifting labor market.

The term *service economy*, however, also describes the numerical growth of low-wage, "unskilled," seasonal, or temporary service-sector jobs that historically were associated with immigrants, women, and poor people of color. Employment opportunities in home and personal services (housekeeping, laundering, and landscaping), food services (farming, cooking, serving, and event planning), retail (selling food, clothes, and goods), and entertaining (hoteling, performing, and making art) all grew in number and density after the 1960s. In response to deindustrialization, many municipal leaders turned to the presence of large retail conglomerates to generate tax revenue and counteract the loss of property taxes associated with manufacturing.

Like the Great Depression, the crisis provoked by global economic restructuring created precarity in all sectors of the US economy, including in white neighborhoods. According to Jefferson Cowie, "the mid-1970s marked the end of the postwar boom," with 1972 marking "the apex of earnings for male workers" and the years 1973 and 1974 signaling when "real earnings began to stagnate and then slide."[4] By the end of the decade, white residents began to see signs of social disorder in their communities that they had only previously associated with neighborhoods of color and the inner city. For many poor people of color living in the inner city, the same events produced the frequency of "working poverty," a phenomenon where wages routinely fail to cover the costs of living.

Social science scholars tracing these shifts in capital, however, tended to frame the global economic restructuring unfolding across the nation as a benevolent and inevitable force, largely because it was seen as a natural next step in the United States' development as an international economic superpower. It made logical sense to many leading economists that American firms and diplomats would seek new ways to generate profits after aiding Japanese, British, French, and German leaders and business owners to rebuild their economies after World War II using US goods, talent, and capital. By the 1960s, regionally dynamic cities like New York, Los Angeles, Chicago, and Houston became important nodes for operatives in Tokyo, London, Paris, and Berlin to facilitate the flow of goods, talent, and capital between their "markets" and the United States.

Securing the distinction of being a global city was increasingly understood by many municipal leaders as a strategy for survival. Living in a global city ensured that the capital from other global cities flowed to its residents first before anywhere else in a particular region. The terms *global* and *service economy* thus do not signify the birth of radically new economic relations but describe the socio-spatial concentration of global-facing finance, real estate, and insurance workers whose services facilitate the flow of capital, talent, and goods within one large multinational "free trade" zone. In spatial terms, the economic hierarchy subordinated certain regional cities, like San Diego and Santa Barbara, to internationally significant cities like Los Angeles. Likewise, neighborhoods once considered self-sufficient and independent during the 1940s and 1950s increasingly found themselves, by the late 1960s and 1970s, dependent on economic activity made possible by international financial districts, like Bunker Hill, under a waning manufacturing economy.

The problem facing LA's city leaders by the late 1960s was that they had encouraged every community to center urban development around employment schemes that would make every neighborhood independent and self-sustaining.[5] In fact, King-Drew was envisioned as an alternative to the energy, aerospace, defense, and entertainment industries that had anchored employment in the "liberal" westside districts of Beverly Hills, Century City, Hollywood, Westwood, and Mid-Wilshire. It was also built as an answer to the "conservative" power brokers of Pasadena and downtown who razed Bunker Hill to rebuild the city's old financial district because they "viewed property values in the old Broadway core as irreversibly eroded by the area's very centrality to public transport, and especially by its heavy use by Black and Mexican poor."[6]

As the next few sections show, the need to subordinate all neighborhoods in Los Angeles to a new financial district in Bunker Hill was a problem for welfare rights activists as much as the city's elite downtown boosters. Since the Watts Uprisings of 1965, politicians, health policy leaders, and activists, including Bradley, believed that the problem of Black poverty demonstrated that poor Black neighborhoods like Watts were too dependent on other neighborhoods for work and employment. They had devised King-Drew as a vehicle to organize employment and labor in the Black community along mainstream ideas of gender and sexuality. The underlying hope of this plan sought to demonstrate the close cultural association with the economic development of independent and self-sustaining neighborhoods by producing a community of individuals as supposedly distinctly gendered and sexually complex as those living in white neighborhoods.

The problem with this approach is that it prioritized the employment and education of Black male heads of households and healthcare workers over the immediate health service needs of poor Black women and children. By upholding the belief that Black women's and children's needs were best met through the care and consumer power of Black male breadwinners, King-Drew's master plan demanded that married women and their children wait for the economy to improve in order to get better health services and income security. It also implicitly asked women on welfare to get married in order to access health services and income security not available through welfare.

For elite downtown boosters, however, the problem by the late 1960s was that there were *too many* independent self-sustaining neighborhoods. This idea manifested in the fact that several neighborhoods had downtown office and shopping districts competing with the city's historic downtown financial district. In fact, by 1969, a study commissioned by the CRA-LA revealed that Bunker Hill's financial district not only competed with other cities, such as New York, Chicago, Atlanta, and San Francisco, for the business of multinational firms but also competed with other "prestige" office districts in LA.[7] Examinations of tenants in the luxury office districts outside Bunker Hill,

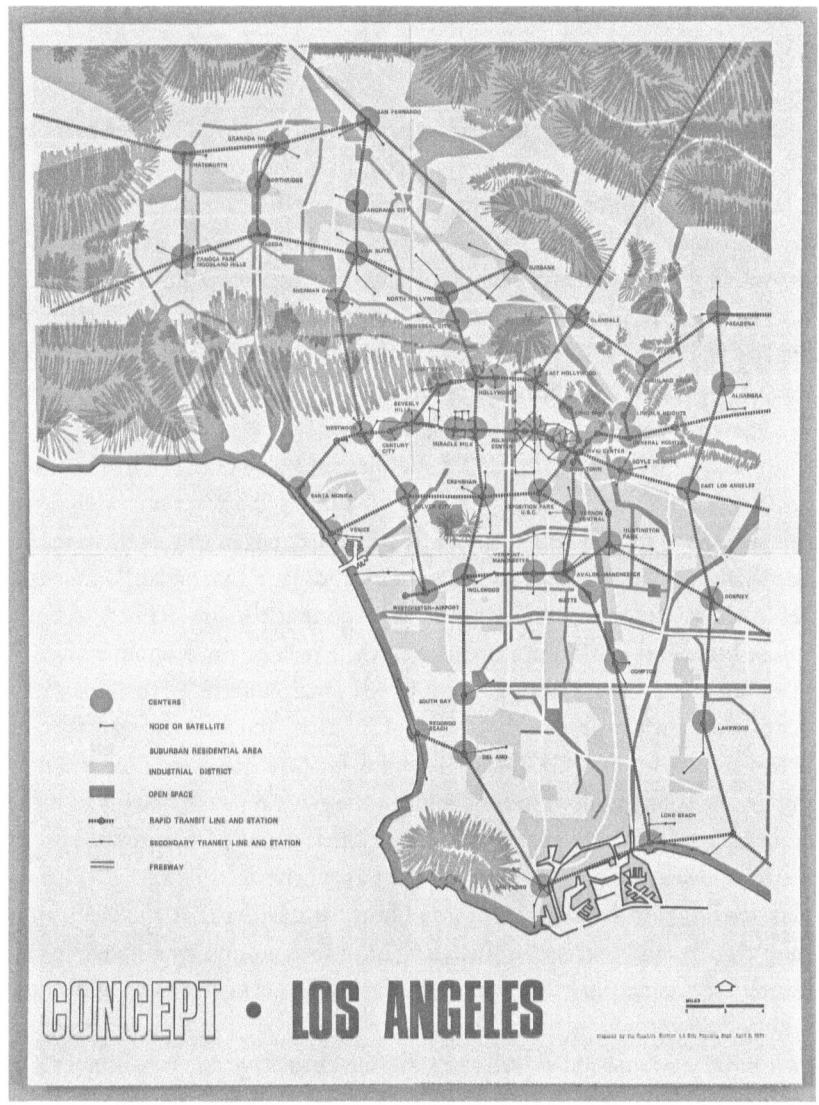

FIGURE 3. A megalopolis broken into "bite-size pieces," with downtown being "the biggest bite of them all"

The city of Los Angeles's regional approach to urban planning took shape in its general plan, briefly known as "Concept Los Angeles." This pinned all regional economic growth to a dense cluster of economic functions in center city. Newly minted in city documents as the "Central Business District," the center city region consisted of a new multinational finance district (Bunker Hill), a revitalized Eastside industrial district full of warehouses, factories, and distribution centers, and several tourist and entertainment destination sites, such as Little Tokyo, Chinatown, and Olvera Street. Source: "Concept Los Angeles" (1974) Bunker Hill Development Records, Box 13, Folder 4, Special Collections Library, University of Southern California.

like Century City, had shown that they had been able to attract only firms of "regional," "secondary," and "local" relevance to Los Angeles but very few with international significance.

The prospect of losing international business to other cities pushed LA's elites by the late 1960s to target Bunker Hill as the region's premier luxury office space for multinational finance firms. As one *Business Week* article in 1970 reported, studies like the 1969 survey of competing office districts were part of a five-year process to develop a city-wide master plan.[8] According to LA's chief urban planner, Calvin S. Hamilton, the "general plan" called for the city to invest in the growth of the region's existing "high-activity urban centers" by "breaking [the megalopolis of Los Angeles] into bite-size pieces," with downtown being "the biggest bite of them all."

In the twenty years since CRA-LA's founding in 1948 that it had taken to raze and develop Bunker Hill, city elites managed to attract several international firms to its new financial district. But they began to worry that planners had been too zealous in building a landscape that Mike Davis later described as "fortress L.A."[9] Critics observed that the city's efforts to build "office buildings and shopping centers, while needed for economic vitality, [did] not add up to a bustling, night-time downtown life."[10] To attract residents who "are just tired of the lax life of suburbs" and are looking for "some urban hyperactivity," CRA-LA's Richard G. Mitchell hinted at the new importance of neighborhoods of color in the general plan by saying that the city was now moving toward revitalizing Little Tokyo, Chinatown, and its historical Mexican plaza of Olvera Street as tourist destinations. The urban planner Edgardo Contini was more blunt, suggesting that the city's aims should go beyond tourism by including initiatives around jobs, housing, and healthcare. As he put it, the problems facing Los Angeles as a region now required downtown's elites to become "involved in the *problems* and *needs* of its minority population as well as its middle-class, day-time inhabitants."

A CONTENDING VISION OF BLACK FREEDOM

Mitchell's and Contini's comments underline how urban planners understood that developing Los Angeles into a "global city" required reexamining past practices of racial exclusion. Their comments about making LA a major tourist destination and dealing with the problems and needs of "minority populations" posited the need to not only celebrate racial and ethnic diversity

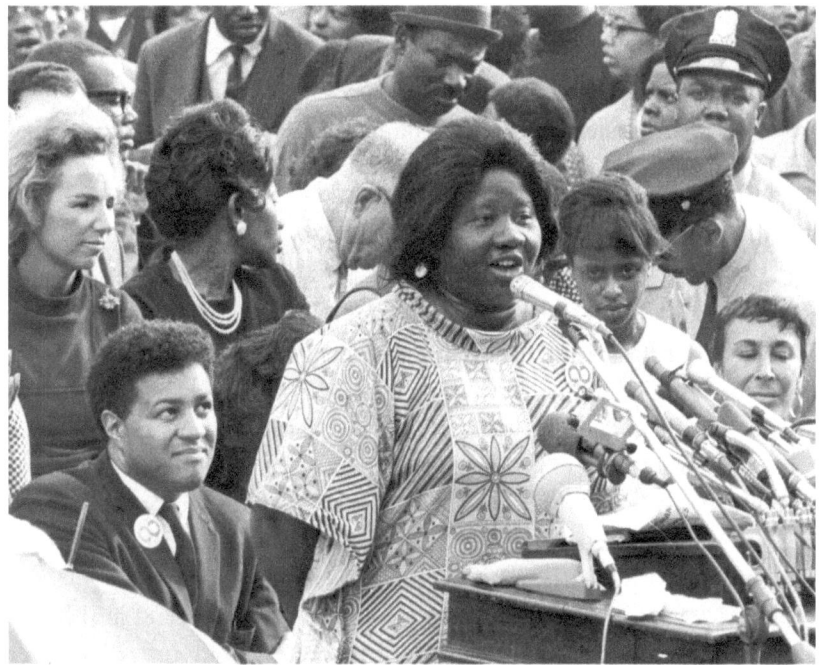

FIGURE 4. Johnnie Tillmon
Johnnie Tillmon speaks at the Mother's Day March in Washington, DC, in 1968. Sitting behind her and looking on are George Wiley and Ethel Kennedy. Source: George Wiley Papers, Wisconsin Historical Society (WHI-8771).

but also include those populations in the region's newly restructured economy. At the same time that city elites looked for leaders of color to assist them with making LA's emerging political economy a reality, poor residents looked to leaders of color to help them challenge the terms of inclusion manifesting in the city's antipoverty projects.

By 1969, Johnnie Tillmon had been engaged in a successful battle over community control of USC's Multipurpose Health Clinic, an antipoverty clinic built ahead of King-Drew's opening with the idea that it would serve as the health system's first exemplary clinic. As the former chair of ANC Mothers Anonymous and NWRO president, Tillmon had been appointed to the clinic's advisory board. Since its opening in 1967, she and a group of Black women antipoverty advocates had helped rally local residents to demand better community accountability from the clinic's leadership by replacing its white leadership with an all-Black medical staff.

As the last chapter shows, King-Drew's leaders initially interpreted the conflict at USC's clinic as a problem of race and not as a problem with the clinic's antipoverty programming agenda. By 1969, relations were so poor between USC's leadership and the community that Spellman and Haynes severed the planned relationship between the medical center and the clinic. The effort to win funding from the DHEW and Commonwealth Foundation in 1970 thus came out of Drew Medical School leadership's belief that its mission would still be a success so long as the clinics they built for Black residents were led by Black physicians.

By the time the master plan study team assembled to assess what local residents thought about King-Drew's overall plan in mid-1971, it was already too late for Spellman and Haynes to realize that most residents did not agree with the health system's theory of change. Welfare rights activists, for instance, used the first listening session held at Jordan Downs, a public housing project, to contest the master plan. As one consultant observed, those who attended believed the medical center was designed to provide "jobs and other economic services rather than primarily educational and health care services."[11] As the consultant explained, this was a "substantive issue" for poor women because it implied that King-Drew's leaders were hesitant to develop and distribute high-quality medical services to women in the community unless they themselves, or the men they were married to or had children with, earned better incomes to pay for it.

The challenge issued by welfare rights activists pushed at the boundaries of the NWRO's official approach to welfare policy since its founding in 1966. Under Wiley's executive directorship, the NWRO successfully leveraged the federal government's prevailing discourses of gendered divisions of labor to win better benefits and services for women on welfare. According to Premilla Nadasen, the NWRO argued that welfare benefits were necessary to assist mothers with raising future citizens and helped expand the franchise of stay-at-home motherhood to working-class women and women of color who—unlike most white middle-class women—worked and mothered at the same time.[12] Although effective in contesting mainstream depictions of poor and working-class women as immoral, sexually promiscuous, and unruly, the NWRO's early rhetorical strategies were largely successful because they conformed to the state's promotion of women's roles in properly gendered and propertied male-headed nuclear households.

As Margot Canaday argues, federal provisions since the New Deal were "less about meeting absolute need than about securing the gendered underpinnings of certain familial arrangements."[13] Federal programs thus sought to reserve jobs for white married men in order to "put a 'brake on [white] women's eagerness to be the family breadwinner.'" Welfare benefits, in turn, sought to preserve a woman's capacity to re-enter society as a (re)married woman under the belief that her needs were best met by marriage to a man, regardless of his earning power. Welfare administrators thus designed benefits, such as food stamps and household furnishing grants, around traditional gender roles for white women like childrearing and tending to the home. They ensured, however, that welfare rates paid below prevailing rates of poverty in order to encourage women to remarry.

The problem facing poor women of color by the 1960s was that welfare administrators regularly denied extending eligibility to them, although not to most poor white women, due to pressure by local employers. According to Annelise Orelick, politicians and welfare administrators often worked hand-in-hand with Southern employers to make it difficult for Black women to avoid working in agriculture and domestic services.[14] As Sarah Haley argues, the idea that a Black woman's gender or her motherhood did not exempt her from working was reinforced by common practices of policing and incarceration that used Black women's unemployment as a context for revitalizing forced labor through penal imprisonment.[15] The NWRO's assertion that poor Black women were eligible and deserving of benefits was thus a radical political move to assert Black women's status as equal to white women.

Wiley also cultivated the NWRO to serve as a vanguard unit for a larger Poor People's Movement, which included liberal progressives, academics, trade unionists, and leaders in the Democratic Party. Wiley's commitments to this broader movement sometimes subordinated the desires of poor women of color by prioritizing actions that advanced poor women's interests only when they overlapped with the interests of a larger ungendered conception of the "working class." Wiley's vision often placed the needs of poor women second to more abstract ideas about social justice in ways that differed from Tillmon's approach to prioritizing the immediate day-to-day needs of women on welfare.

Wiley, for example, worked closely with Richard Cloward and Frances Fox Piven, two white urban sociologists, to promote a theory of change centered on welfare that they presented in their 1966 article, "The Weight of the Poor: A Strategy to End Poverty."[16] Cloward and Piven argued that the welfare rights movement's ultimate aim was not to improve welfare benefits per se but to manufacture a "profound financial and political crisis" that would transform society completely. By instituting a "massive drive to recruit the poor *onto* the welfare rolls" to implode it, not improve it, they believed that the resulting "internal disruption," "furor," and "collapse" of an overburdened welfare system would eventually generate "major economic reforms at the national level" that would result in a more equitable system for the poor.

Like many burgeoning social advocacy organizations in the 1960s, the NWRO represented the professionalization of community and political organizing made possible by the infusion of philanthropic funding into member-driven dues-paying community organizations made popular by Ella Baker and Saul Alinsky.[17] While having paid organizers enabled the NWRO to extend the scope of its advocacy and reach, it also made its organizational goals susceptible to co-optation and influence by funders. The NWRO's mission thus tended to reflect goals that brought together the interests of members, funders, and paid organizers.

The most radical and socially transformative demand out of the convergence of NWRO's political coalition was its fight for a universal basic income. By 1972, the NWRO's campaign around an "adequate income" manifested in a congressional proposal known as the Family Assistance Plan (FAP). Tillmon believed that the implementation of a universal basic income without regard to gender and race would free all poor people, not just poor women, from "the threat of starvation and other economic threats."[18] Yet, despite their central role in getting the concept considered in Congress, Nadasen argues that women on welfare continued to be "an exception to the consensus around the guaranteed income."[19] Leading politicians and supporters of passing FAP consistently set income rates well below the NWRO's recommended level of $5,500 and suggested stipulations requiring recipients to enroll in work programs to receive benefits. These proposals put welfare rights leaders at odds with other antipoverty advocates.

These structural constraints tested both Tillmon's resolve and her leadership style. Tillmon later admitted that she had always resented Cloward and Piven's thesis because—just like King-Drew's master plan—their theory of change subjugated the immediate needs and desires of poor women of color to an abstract idea of a "common good." She also explained that the battles between ANC Mothers Anonymous and USC's clinic leadership in 1969 and King-Drew's leadership in 1971 exemplified what Wiley famously referred to as the "Johnnie Tillmon model," a model that prioritized collective decision-making based on an open and involved democratic process where concerned parties "[do] things on a day to day basis."[20]

In contrast to Wiley's strategy of achieving a preconceived notion of broader economic change by leading poor women of color to it, Tillmon believed that poor women of color needed to be engaged in an open and transparent process of defining what meaningful and lasting economic change looked like and who needed to be empowered to lead society to that change. Although she did not disavow strategies requiring paid staff to organize large demonstrations and protests, the power she preferred to develop was having a social organization so strong and highly respected that it dealt "directly with the Administration and our welfare department" without having to "do a lot of demonstrations and hollering in the streets."[21] In short, her leadership approach believed that the "people 'who are hurting' do it themselves" and "don't depend on organizers to come and do things for them."

For Tillmon, the battle over health services tested welfare administrators' commitments to reform the sexual behavior of poor women by withholding or denying health services to women on the belief that such services more properly belonged to those who had access to them through marriage or work. More important, it also tested the NWRO's own resolve to fight for feminist objectives that did not conform to the state's preexisting policy objectives or curry immediate favor among the NWRO's funders. By the late 1960s, Tillmon increasingly found herself leading efforts within the NWRO to push for policies supporting poor women's rights to use healthcare as a human right and use public assistance programs to free them from the interlocking forces of racism, sexism, and poverty.

Especially after the legislative failure of FAP in 1972, Nadasen argues that this conflict led to an organizational split in 1973 and the dissolution of the NWRO's national office in 1975.[22] Other scholars, however, such as Annelise Orelick, Rosie Bermudez, and Alejandra Marchevsky, have shown that many local chapters—such as those in Las Vegas, Watts, and East Los Angeles—continued to organize late into the 1970s and beyond.[23] Some leaders close to Tillmon, such as Catherine Jermany, argue that the organization's internal division always reflected the fact that some chapters, like Tillmon's ANC Mothers Anonymous, had been built by poor women who self-organized themselves using their own resources, while others, like Dorothy Moore's Welfare Recipients' Union, had been formed with the assistance of paid NWRO organizers.[24] Tillmon thus tended to narrate the closing of the NWRO's national office as the rebirth of a diffuse heterogeneous movement of autonomous local chapters.[25] Tillmon took it as a point of pride that she had a personal hand in developing the leaders of many of the chapters who continued to work with each other after 1973.

Her strategy to decentralize decision-making freed chapter leaders to mount campaigns, craft rhetoric, and form political alliances based on the organizing conditions facing women on welfare in their local contexts. For Tillmon, the NWRO's reprioritization of organizing methods permitted her to work on issues that motivated her and other Black women to create ANC Mothers Anonymous in the first place. She argues that ANC Mothers Anonymous was first formed as a way for Black women to enter the workforce to earn wages that matched the earning power of men. In fact, the organization's first action included setting up resources to help members make their answer to the question "What would you do if you had an opportunity to go back to school and be retrained for a job?" a reality.[26] Tillmon recounted that the entire chapter's first success was securing an apprenticeship for a mother with six children facing denial of welfare benefits, whose dream was to become a mortician.

That women lost benefits when their children turned of age and that welfare benefits were regularly denied or suspended pointed to the myriad of dangers facing poor Black women when they were set adrift in an employment landscape animated by racial and sexual coercion. As scholars of working-class Black womanhood have argued, seeking public assistance was one of several survival strategies for poor Black women that included working as a maid, laundress, or cook in the formal economy or working as a sex worker, "number runner," or psychic in the informal economy.[27] Although going on welfare did not make Black women rich, independent, or release them from stigma, it did permit many to avoid the sexual predation that frequently accompanied work in the formal and informal economy and mitigated the threat of policing and imprisonment associated with being out in public as a Black woman.

The belief that welfare was an imperfect solution to the dangers facing poor Black women helps account for why welfare rights activists fought so hard to craft benefits to help poor women of color accomplish things that were considered impossible or just out of reach. In addition to giving poor mothers of color the right to raise their children with the same attention and care as middle-class white mothers, Tillmon saw welfare as a potentially empowering tool for women of color to use to improve themselves so long as a woman's choice to mother was not contingent upon returning her to work as quickly as possible.

The local skirmish between welfare rights activists and USC in 1969 and King-Drew in 1971 illustrated how welfare agencies began to conflate the two by requiring women to exchange their participation in reform programs for benefits, like health services, needed for survival. Tillmon was clear that any woman who met local eligibility criteria for enrollment on welfare should be given "categorical" benefits outright and that women who desired a chance to work, get training, or get an education should be allowed to voluntarily enroll in what she called "self-help" programs.

These distinctions between categorical aid and self-help programs were important to welfare rights activists because King-Drew's vision of withholding health services to reform Black women reproduced the logic behind California Governor Ronald Reagan's proposal to enroll all "able-bodied" welfare recipients in work programs to get welfare. More popularly known as the Work Incentive Program (WIN or WIP), WIP initially enrolled women into work training and employment programs on a voluntary basis when it began in 1967. Tillmon and others initially celebrated WIP because it promised education, job training, and employment programs that made it possible for women to better themselves and their lives without jeopardizing their ability to eat, feed, and house themselves and their families.

Reagan's 1971 proposal, however, undercut the program's most empowering aspects by making enrollment in WIP mandatory for most women on welfare. Although the program initially included enrollment in university courses or into high-paying jobs, many activists grew frustrated by the fact that the only employers willing to participate were not interested in educating women or in paying them wages above the poverty line (or even above welfare rates). By the early 1970s, Tillmon and others came to regard it as a "slave labor" program in disguise because it undermined poor women's ability to make choices about their labor (both reproductive and otherwise) and coerced them into labor that did not better their lives or their children's.[28]

By 1971, rumors that King-Drew's services might require a "nominal fee" and a physician referral to get public hospital care exacerbated fears that the hospital was designed to criminalize and reform poor people rather than address their immediate health needs.[29] However, as opposed to emerging out of the imagination of white conservatives, the fact that King-Drew's plan was a product of biracial support from medical leaders and urban policy experts associated with the Democratic establishment only helped motivate Tillmon to break from the strategies, tactics, and rhetoric of respectable stay-at-home motherhood that had defined the NWRO's early period of organizing. Her move thus joined a long history of Black activists who not only rejected white supremacy's new manifestations in conservative politics but also refused to consent to their reproduction, as Daniel HoSang argues, in the emerging terms of 1960s and 1970s racial liberalism.[30]

Tillmon's opposition to King-Drew's master plan thus served as a vehicle to clarify the political vision of the Black women who had formed the first welfare rights organization in the nation. It allowed Tillmon to defend access to public health services as a human right and to win rights that advanced the interests of poor working women like childcare. According to her, "Child care was an issue [for all the women who founded ANC Mothers Anonymous in 1963] because we didn't advocate staying on welfare."[31]

Although it was "one of our first priorities," she admitted that the issue was subordinated until 1971 because most of the NWRO's organizers were "male" and "ninety-nine percent white," and because its day-to-day operations were overseen by Wiley, the NWRO's executive director. Above all, NWRO staff appeared reluctant to take on the issue because sending children to be looked after by other women appeared to undermine the NWRO's prevailing narrative about the central importance of supporting women's roles in the home. Speaking to the activist scholar Guida West in 1974, Tillmon explained that the campaign for childcare "took seven years to get somebody to hear me" and "took four years after, to get the thing off the ground" because Wiley and NWRO's mostly white staff "were not mothers" and "couldn't understand my situation [as one]."

For Tillmon and many Black women on welfare, childcare was a tool "to move ourselves off welfare" because it freed them to determine a future without the coercive forces of racism, capitalism, and patriarchy. In her experience, "unless you got a relative or something, [childcare] was too expensive." She also, however, implied that poor women should not have to trust their children to just any provider. In addition to the fact that women on welfare needed childcare to make it to medical appointments for themselves and their children, Tillmon demanded that the care children received be molded by science. As she recalled, "We wanted to go beyond [just advocating for basic childcare]—we wanted the young children to have more than custodial care so that is why we wanted a childcare center [attached to the medical center.]"

Tillmon's campaign around King-Drew permitted the NWRO to create political networks driven by local needs rather than those determined to be important by power brokers in Washington, DC. The work around King-Drew's master plan brought ANC Mothers Anonymous into a political orbit larger than that formed by the Democratic Party. Black welfare rights activists worked with other Black women activists in Watts, Chicana welfare rights activists in Spanish-speaking neighborhoods, and political leaders often depicted as the Democratic Party's opponents and adversaries.

Among those working with Tillmon on transforming King-Drew's mission was Caffie Greene, Tillmon's sister. Before focusing on King-Drew, Greene operated a youth center known as Teen Post, a community organization eventually funded by the Economic and Youth Opportunities Agency of Greater Los Angeles, the city's official antipoverty funding board. As director, Greene mentored several prominent Black Panther Party members, such as Bunchy Carter, Ray "Masai" Hewitt, Gael Davis, Tommy Lewis, and Wayne Pharr.

Tillmon also worked with Alicia Escalante of the East Los Angeles Chicana Welfare Rights Organization. Tillmon mentored Escalante and in 1966 encouraged her to form a chapter to represent the interests of Chicana women living in East Los Angeles. By 1971, Tillmon engaged Escalante in hopes of helping the Master Plan Study's consultants better understand the plight of recently arrived immigrants from Mexico and Central America to a neighborhood in King-Drew's health service district known as Florence-Firestone.

By the 1970s, the activities of welfare rights activists in Los Angeles show that they were unafraid of talking with Republicans and making deals with those that both political parties were prone to label as "radicals."[32] Activists successfully navigated the growing violence between Black cultural nationalists such as Karenga's US and anticapitalist Black organizations such as the Black Panthers, and continued to work within Black coalitional spaces such as the Black Congress, which brought together organizations that had survived the violence of that ordeal.[33] As Jermany argued, the organization's nonideological position reflected a belief that "there was no such thing as an enemy... only people to play games with to juggle to get your space on the green."[34]

Tillmon clearly used the lessons learned in Los Angeles to reshape the NWRO's national agenda. By 1972, the NWRO's annual meeting prioritized educational discussions around healthcare policy and mounted workshops around organizing daycare centers and neighborhood health centers and gaining "community control of hospitals."[35] All these subjects also formed the backbone of the NWRO's contribution to the Children's March on Washington in 1972, which served as a renewal of the NWRO's leadership in the Poor People's Campaign of 1969.

The successful demonstration of the "Tillmon Model" helps explain Wiley's departure and Tillmon's ascendancy as executive director of the NWRO in 1973. Wiley's resignation roughly coincided with the exit of several chapters and key leaders, resulting in the formation of a competing national welfare rights organization aligned with trade unions and progressive academics. By the 1980s, Tillmon noted that "most of the groups I organized [were] still doing something," while "most of the groups [that Wiley and NWRO staff had] organized collapsed."[36]

RENEWING JIM CROW

For Tillmon, the Master Plan Study presented an opportunity for activists to renew the welfare rights movement by prioritizing a vision for Black Freedom that did not hinge on breadwinning manhood. In their opinion, winning direct access to health services and childcare services was a better alternative to making all communities independent and self-sustaining by empowering poor women of color to make decisions about the future without coercion or force. Tillmon and others knew, however, that the public's willingness to meet their demands stemmed from the recognition that a crisis of jobs continued to plague Black neighborhoods. Speaking in late 1971, Tillmon argued that "if [municipal leaders and private employers] couldn't come up with jobs, then they should leave us [welfare recipients] alone, and put some more money in the [income assistance] checks. It's just as simple as that."[37]

The actions of Bradley, however, show that most Black politicians did not interpret such criticism of the economy as a reason to support welfare. They tended to interpret such demands as a call for local politicians to solve the crisis of jobs in Black neighborhoods by any means necessary. For Bradley, the pathway to supplying poor people of color with job opportunities rested with Bunker Hill. Instead of focusing on welfare rights activist campaigns around USC's clinic and King-Drew's master plan in 1969 and 1971, Bradley focused on partnering with downtown elites to engineer the spatial relationships needed to revitalize downtown Los Angeles as a "global city" using the labor of poor people of color. As Mike Davis argues, Bradley's move unified the "multicultural" elites of the city's racial, ethnic, and gay neighborhoods with white conservative business interests by making downtown redevelopment the "showpiece program" of his leadership agenda.[38] That agenda began in earnest right around his first run for mayor in 1969.

Although unsuccessful, that mayoral campaign allowed Bradley to better represent himself as a broker between the city's leaders of color and downtown elites. His leadership was crucial in helping CRA-LA leaders address the perceived corporate sterility and unattractiveness of Bunker Hill by working with community leaders in Little Tokyo, Chinatown, and Olvera Street to extend community redevelopment programs to include their neighborhoods. Given that many downtown firms had financial interests in Asia and Latin America and that many Asian and Latin American corporations were beginning to have financial interests in Los Angeles, CRA-LA planners hoped that "the charm of ethnic diversity" found in these neighborhoods would foster the city as a "tourist" destination and a location amenable to global financial trade.[39]

CRA-LA's investments in these neighborhoods differed from its past "slum clearance" approach in Bunker Hill. Rather than raze and displace residents in Little Tokyo, Chinatown, and Olvera Street, Bradley pushed CRA-LA's leaders to support what city planners later referred to as "incremental development."[40] These policies regarded the spatial concentrations of poverty and old infrastructure created by racism and segregation as temporary assets that could be exploited to lubricate the emergence of a regional economy pinned to the new financial district.

By 1971, Bradley helped CRA-LA leaders see the importance of preserving and investing in the real estate represented by the deteriorating Eastside's downtown warehouse districts. Whereas Little Tokyo, Chinatown, and Olvera Street supplied the "ethnic charm" to make Bunker Hill more attractive and friendly for multinational firms and their workers to relocate to, the warehouse districts would serve as a central supplier of restaurant, entertainment, and special event goods to make Bunker Hill a playground for the rich. For generations, the warehouse districts housed several key industries related to wholesale produce and flower distribution and were home to the city's fashion and apparel firms.

Bradley's advocacy for the nondescript and easily overlooked warehouse districts showcased what leaders of color could finally do with access to capital and control of major employment centers like Bunker Hill. For politicians from the Black and Brown neighborhoods, investment in the wholesale food, flower, and apparel companies helped them reverse the flow of businesses and people to other competing cities and locations. By the late 1970s, the CRA-LA's efforts to consolidate and update the city's wholesale food distribution center helped secure downtown as a destination site for the entire region's restaurant, catering, and event firms. Its efforts to do the same for apparel manufacturers by subsidizing their ability to update their factories helped make Los Angeles a larger producer of clothes than traditional locations like New York.

As scholars of labor have shown, closer relationships to downtown elites made many politicians of color, like Bradley, were more willing to overlook business practices that were detrimental to workers of color. According to Ruth Milkman, part of the success in efforts to shift the financial district from its old location along Spring Street to Bunker Hill hinged on new labor arrangements centered on subcontracting building services, such as housekeeping, landscaping, and security services, that were once paid in-house by building owners.[41] This shift occurred right as the ending of price supports, land consolidation, and the devaluation of the peso in Mexico fueled migration to the United States.

The combination of these factors transformed not only the nature of work but also who did the work itself. Unlike the union-protected jobs that characterized building service work in the Spring Street corridor, new janitorial subcontracting firms operating in Bunker Hill, such as Aramark, ABM, and ISS, were nonunion, offered no healthcare, and paid wages under the region's prevailing labor standards. More important, employers used the shift to Bunker Hill to hire immigrant workers and women of color to fill low-wage jobs once held by unionized Black men. Rather than focus on these shifts, Bradley and other city officials used the profit margins associated with lower overhead building costs to encourage corporations to relocate to Los Angeles rather than other cities.

In the Eastside industrial districts, the CRA-LA's investments helped apparel manufacturers compete with lower-cost manufacturing firms in Asia and Latin America by reproducing "third world" labor conditions on domestic soil.[42] As Edna Bonacich, Lucie Cheng, and Paul Ong argue, the city's investments in supporting the needs of light-manufacturing firms helped the region buck national trends by growing the number of manufacturing jobs during a period when most regions of the United States were losing them.[43] As they argue, the ability of these manufacturing firms to maintain profits and stay in the United States rested on their ability to find people willing to work for lower wages.

Similar to shifts in the building service industry, apparel manufacturers looked to undercut fashion importers by turning to immigrant women of color to fill jobs once occupied by unionized white women. By exploiting the fact that women's wages were generally less than men's and that white workers' wages were generally more than what most Black workers earned, employers in downtown Los Angeles were able to produce profit from garments made in the United States that were otherwise profitable only if made by workers in Asia and Latin America. Such investments and support were particularly critical to apparel manufacturers who took advantage of the district's proximity to the Port of Los Angeles and the national railway system to produce textiles that were as affordable as foreign-made textiles because they were made closer to American consumers than those abroad.

FEW SOLUTIONS FOR GLOBAL PROBLEMS

The multiple discourses around labor arising out of the welfare rights movement and Bradley's partnership with downtown elites showcased how most politicians and health policy experts who had supported King-Drew's original master plan had moved on by 1971 to other priorities. Rather than support the medical center's original mission, the Master Plan Study was an opportunity for the region's politicians to repurpose the medical center's mission towards responding to welfare rights activists' demands and advancing the interests of downtown's new multicultural alliance. The effect transformed an antipoverty project centered on rehabilitating men of color into a vehicle that helped reinforce new racist cultural representations of men of color as "absent fathers," regardless of their employment status or presence in the home.

This conclusion manifested in the findings of the Master Plan Study.[44] Conducted in two phases, the study issued an initial report in late 1971. That report, known as Phase I, surveyed all the medical center's partners and stakeholders on the viability of King-Drew's "community medicine" plan. The consultants issued a report disagreeing with King-Drew leadership's assumption that most poor Black people needed the guidance of Black male physicians to know how to navigate healthcare's bureaucracy. As the study team's interactions with welfare rights activists demonstrated, most residents demonstrated "a considerable level of sophistication in coping with the representatives of public agencies and private institutions" because of a long "history of involvement in community action organizations including neighborhood councils, welfare rights organizations, civic clubs, churches, and fraternal and labor organizations."[45]

The study team also agreed with welfare rights activists that the medical center's public hospital and health services could not be used as a way to reform patients' sexual behavior. By extension, such a recommendation also ruled that its health services could not be used as a way to address the neighborhood's poverty. While "high rates of unemployment, low income, poor transportation, and depressing physical decay" might represent the basic problems facing patients in King-Drew's health service area, the study team argued that Drew's "principal focus" ought to be "on health" rather than being "principally a community action or economic development agency."[46] There were "few solutions" that Drew could provide for "these global problems."

To defend this position, the study team cited research refuting the belief that public investment in the education and employability of men of color would result in higher incomes and greater health coverage for families of color. In fact, using research generated by King-Drew's own Department of Community Medicine and by labor experts at UCLA, the study team concluded that most male laborers of color in Los Angeles were ineligible for the medical center's employment opportunities and ineligible for admission to its medical school and allied health training center because of their perceived extremely low educational levels and labor skills.[47] Citing the dropout rate for local high schools, which averaged 39 to 43 percent, new economic studies also found that Southern California's Black and Brown men took longer than normal to find work, and when they did find job opportunities, these were often underpaid and temporary.[48]

The problem with such studies is that they elided how the structural dimensions not only made work so hard to find but also made paid work unable to cover higher costs of living. The study team's conclusions let racism and capitalism off the hook by hiding the persistent refusal of most employers and unions to hire men of color. It also obscured new employment trends encouraged by the city's own leaders of color, who sought to help employers hire more immigrants and poor women of color to produce higher profit margins.

The effect thus framed unemployment in communities of color as a failure of poor men of color to exercise the necessary amount of individual responsibility and vigilance to secure employment. The irony of such conclusions is that many members of poor households, including men, did work but still found it hard to cover basic living costs. As ideas about men of color being "absent fathers" took deeper root, Black and Chicana feminists felt compelled to refute ideas about racial manhood based on white supremacist ideas of breadwinning manhood as it became increasingly common for leaders of color to blame both men and women of color for what employers and politicians ultimately had the power to fix.

Chicana feminist Adeljiza Sosa Riddell, for instance, argued that the application of breadwinner discourse in Chicano communities through the concept of machismo was just "a myth propagated by subjugators and colonizers who take pleasure in watching their subjects strike out vainly against them in order to prove themselves still capable of action."[49] Her influential 1974 essay eloquently argued for the recognition of working poor men of color who "had little time for concern over masculinity" because of the care work they shared alongside women in working long hours and keeping their families alive, united, and dignified.

Black feminist bell hooks also signaled the growing fact that many men of color were deliberately kept from fathering because of growing rates of incarceration. She wrote, "Fathers who are not present all the time can still be a loving presence," and "the presence of biological fathers matters less than the presence of loving black male parental caregivers."[50] All these statements pointed to a belief that men of color were never redundant or expendable in communities of color because they continued to contribute to the reproduction of life in ways that did not require them to always contribute earnings or leadership.

By measuring men of color against mainstream ideas of breadwinning manhood, however, the study team encouraged readers of the report to accept poverty and working poverty as facts. As the study team phrased it, the medical center "has relatively few jobs to give out" and consequently "can only have a marginal impact on the economy of the service area."[51] While they acknowledged that supporters of the original master plan have "remarked, not entirely facetiously, that the greatest health need in the service area is jobs," the study team argued that "providing jobs and opportunities for training... cannot be the central reason for [King-Drew's] existence."[52]

Black and Chicana feminists also understood that racist perceptions about women of color were tied to racist perceptions about men of color. They felt the urgency of critiquing mainstream notions of breadwinning manhood because growing social acceptance of "absentee fatherhood" as a structural feature of racialized manhood accompanied a growing conservative belief that women of color were less interested in being good mothers than in living extravagantly and fraudulently off welfare. As scholars of welfare policy have shown, the growing disillusionment with male-centered antipoverty programs directly contributed to new policy positions centered on forcing more women off welfare.[53]

Growing acceptance of absentee fatherhood as a feature of racialized poverty and the need to police the number of women of color on welfare manifested in the second phase of King-Drew's Master Plan Study. The study team referred to this phase informally as the hospital's "shakedown period" because it reformulated the medical center's mission to managing rather than alleviating poverty.[54] Using the data and statistics gathered by Haynes, the second phase gathered medical center staff and community activists from March 1972 to March 1973 to streamline services to address the most frequently observed biomedical health concerns of poor people in the community: maternal and infant mortality, hypertension, alcohol and drug abuse, "accidents," and "homicides."[55] The study team convened task force groups dedicated to each ailment. Each task force was charged with incorporating the input of welfare rights activists and community leaders into action plans balancing the needs of poor consumers against the cost concerns of taxpayers.

In contrast to King-Drew's leaders who argued health could not be detached from "isolation, poor housing, and economic deprivation" or, as physicians today refer to it, the social determinants of health, the study team ruled that bodily health and its epidemiological influences could be discretely separated.[56] Essentially, their recommendations expected physicians to limit their interventions to the biomedical realm and refrain from intervening in poverty itself. This limit, however, did not divorce the relationship between biomedicine and poverty but instead racialized certain biomedical services under the sign of poverty. That is, it made maternal and infant mortality, hypertension, alcohol and drug abuse, accidents, and homicides *normal* and *expected* features of doctoring for physicians working in poor urban neighborhoods.

The programmatic result of these discussions empowered the County of Los Angeles to appropriate the Drew School's original vision of focusing "consumer friendly" health services on mother and infant care, hypertension, and drug and alcohol abuse in large-scale ambulatory care clinics they referred to in planning documents as "comprehensive health clinics." Instead of building these new clinics under the Drew Medical School's leadership, in 1972 the county applied to the Department of Health, Education, and Welfare for construction grant funding to build and pilot a demonstration clinic capable of carrying out the wishes of welfare rights activists and meeting the needs of newly arrived Spanish-speaking residents.

Originally dubbed the Southeast Multipurpose Comprehensive Health Clinic until it was renamed the Hubert Humphrey Comprehensive Health Clinic when it opened in 1976, King-Drew's first demonstration mega-clinic sat at the corner of Slauson and Main, an intersection close to four of the county's largest public housing units. Like previous antipoverty clinic designs, the Humphrey clinic provided preventative and low-cost health services in one location away from the more expensive acute-care services found in the hospital. Unlike the original plan, the clinic tailored its architecture and services to the demands of poor women on welfare by functioning as the main point of service for mother and baby care. It not only housed social services programs such as food stamps on the same premises as exam rooms, an X-ray machine, a blood laboratory, and a pharmacy but also featured an auditorium for health education classes and a childcare center to help mothers attend health education courses and social service appointments.

County officials also used the time before the Humphrey clinic's opening to retrofit older facilities into smaller "neighborhood healthcare clinics" and built a childcare center named after Johnnie Tillmon on the premises of King-Drew Medical Center. Both projects were designed to test out and eventually implement best practices in the rest of the county health system's institutions. In 1974, the county repurposed a building into a health clinic catering to the "Spanish-speaking" Florence-Firestone neighborhood within King-Drew's health district. By the end of the decade, lessons from the Humphrey clinic had not only helped reorient the purpose and function of the rest of the county's extended public health systems but—as the nation's first-ever federally funded "comprehensive health" clinic—became the template for building similar clinics elsewhere in the nation.

All these actions signaled the county's eventual adoption of what it referred to in 1971 as its "regionalization" plan.[57] The plan marked the county's pivot away from using its county hospitals as antipoverty machines towards their use in a larger system of managing poverty. The policy also reflected the county's response to private healthcare providers' lackluster reaction to federal incentives to enter poor and working-class medical markets since the implementation of Medicare and Medicaid in 1965. The refusal of private health providers to help shoulder the burden of caring for the poor had devastating consequences for poor people living throughout Los Angeles County.

A general belief that Medicaid reimbursement rates were too low to sustain a successful practice coupled with fears that treating poor patients would drive away paying patients and ruin provider reputations produced a deeper crisis of providers in low-income neighborhoods before 1965.[58] For poor people living in middle-class neighborhoods, the refusal by private hospitals to accept Medicaid-eligible patients required them to seek care in facilities further away from their home communities. For poor people living in poor neighborhoods, Medicaid's failure to properly incentivize providers to serve low-income communities exacerbated the fact that its success at punishing providers who failed to meet new federal standards worked to eliminate many who had served low-income patients for generations. The combined effect severely limited access to healthcare for all poor people regardless of where they lived in the county.

"Regionalization" sought to fix the growing need to identify an access point for every poor and medically indigent citizen in the county by assigning every resident to a geographically determined set of public health and hospital institutions. Whereas the county's hospitals before 1971 were generally understood to serve the poor neighborhoods immediately around them, the "regionalization" plan enlarged the service boundaries to account for poor residents living in neighborhoods where private hospitals refused to admit patients enrolled in Medicaid. Such practices gave birth to the term *safety net hospitals*, signaling which hospitals within a particular regional market regularly accepted the least profitable patients.

BETWEEN A ROCK AND A HARD PLACE

The county's regionalization plan signaled much more than a rejection of King-Drew's original master plan. It represented the willingness of county officials to align the mission of all its existing public hospital and health infrastructure with the City of Los Angeles's goal to anchor all regional economic activity to Bunker Hill's development as a global center for finance capital. In this respect, the master plan study served as a device that bolstered support for Bradley's mayoral election campaign in 1973. Whereas Bradley's vision for racial inclusion had garnered a handful of powerful downtown leaders to support his campaign in 1969, Bradley's mayoral campaign featured the near unanimous support of a group of downtown elites known as the "Committee of 25."

Bradley's election as mayor allowed him to expand the spatial relationships he helped engineer in the city center area to neighborhoods outside it.

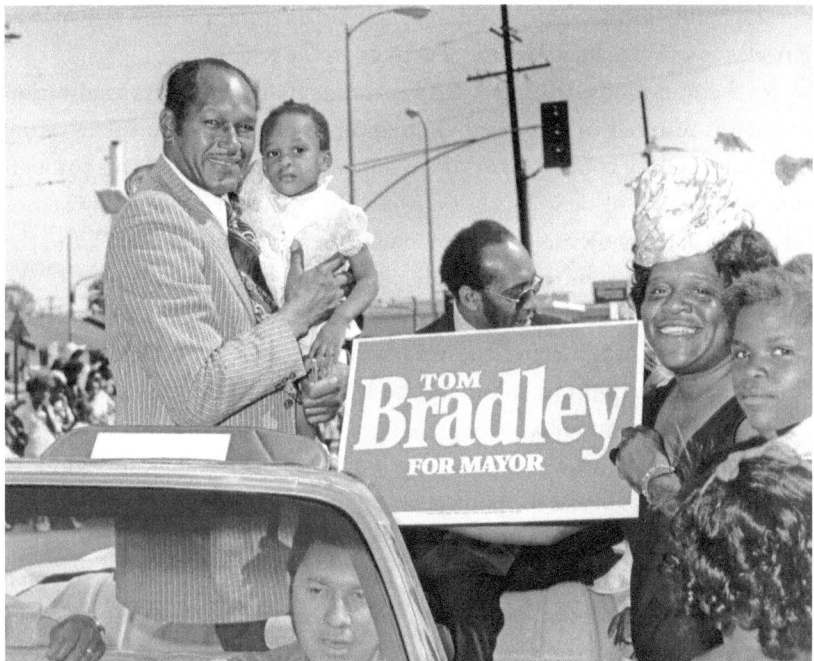

FIGURE 5. Tom Bradley

Tom Bradley campaigning for mayor of Los Angeles in 1973. Source: Guy Crowder Collection, Courtesy of the Tom and Ethel Bradley Center at California State University at Northridge.

His actions to develop public housing and improve public transportation routes to and from the city's neighborhoods of color gave more meaning to the Master Plan Study's explicit recommendation that King-Drew's leaders accept poverty as a fact of providing health services in Watts. The city's redevelopment plans show that accepting poverty in the neighborhoods of color around city center was necessary to contain poverty in order to supply downtown's employers with cheap labor.

Plans to lubricate downtown's special relationship with neighborhoods of color began in earnest by easing the movement of workers of color to and from Bunker Hill and between Bunker Hill and other neighborhoods within the Central Business District. City planners understood that improving public transit would not "by itself solve all of the economic and social problems downtown," but they realized that "transportation access (*particularly access to the substantial labor pool located in close proximity to the Central Business District*)" (emphasis mine) was necessary to "reinforce existing development, attract new development, and maintain a downtown Los Angeles as a viable, major center of activity in the region."[59]

By the mid-1980s, the CRA-LA's investments in public transportation initiatives resulted in improved circulation to and from the surrounding neighborhoods of color to downtown. Regional elites achieved this through the introduction of rapid bus lines (Metro Bus), the revival of a downtown bus service later known as the Downtown Area Short Hop (DASH), and the construction of a subway that Bradley referred to as a "people mover." To connect these public transit systems with the suburbs, County Supervisor Kenneth Hahn engineered the return of the regional streetcar system through a new rapid rail commuter network (Metrolink) via a successful ballot proposition in 1980.

To solidify downtown as a place to work and downtown's surrounding neighborhoods as places for poor people of color to live, Bradley worked in tandem with the CRA-LA to rechannel revenue from Bunker Hill's corporate tax base toward constructing and rehabilitating low- to moderate-income housing in neighborhoods of color. In addition to adding over 3,900 residential units from 1976 to 1980 in Watts, Pico Union, and Little Tokyo, Bradley's administration launched a five-year plan in 1980 to build 6,900 more low- to moderate-income housing units in Normandy, Chinatown, Watts, Monterey Hills, Adams, Boyle Heights, and Lincoln Heights.[60]

Where new housing construction projects appeared unfeasible, the CRA-LA funded redevelopment through individual home ownership programs. It used new federal Community Development Block Grants centered on low-interest loans and services, such as financial counseling and assistance with property and termite inspections, to encourage homeowners and landowners to improve existing properties. It also encouraged individuals to do so by investing funds to improve streets, sidewalks, and landscaping.

The county's health services served as the keystone to these efforts because it gave working-class workers an incentive to live in neighborhoods with public hospitals and clinics. Although county-run, the county's health services bore Bradley's mark based on his influence in pushing city and county services to share locations and better coordinate services with each other. His ideas were informed by his experience working closely with the leaders of the nonprofit Avalon Carver Community Service Center. Testifying to the McCone Commission in 1965, he observed that it was "our experience that people ... would go for an appointment to see their social worker in connection with relief from the county, and at the same time, would find they had to go some-

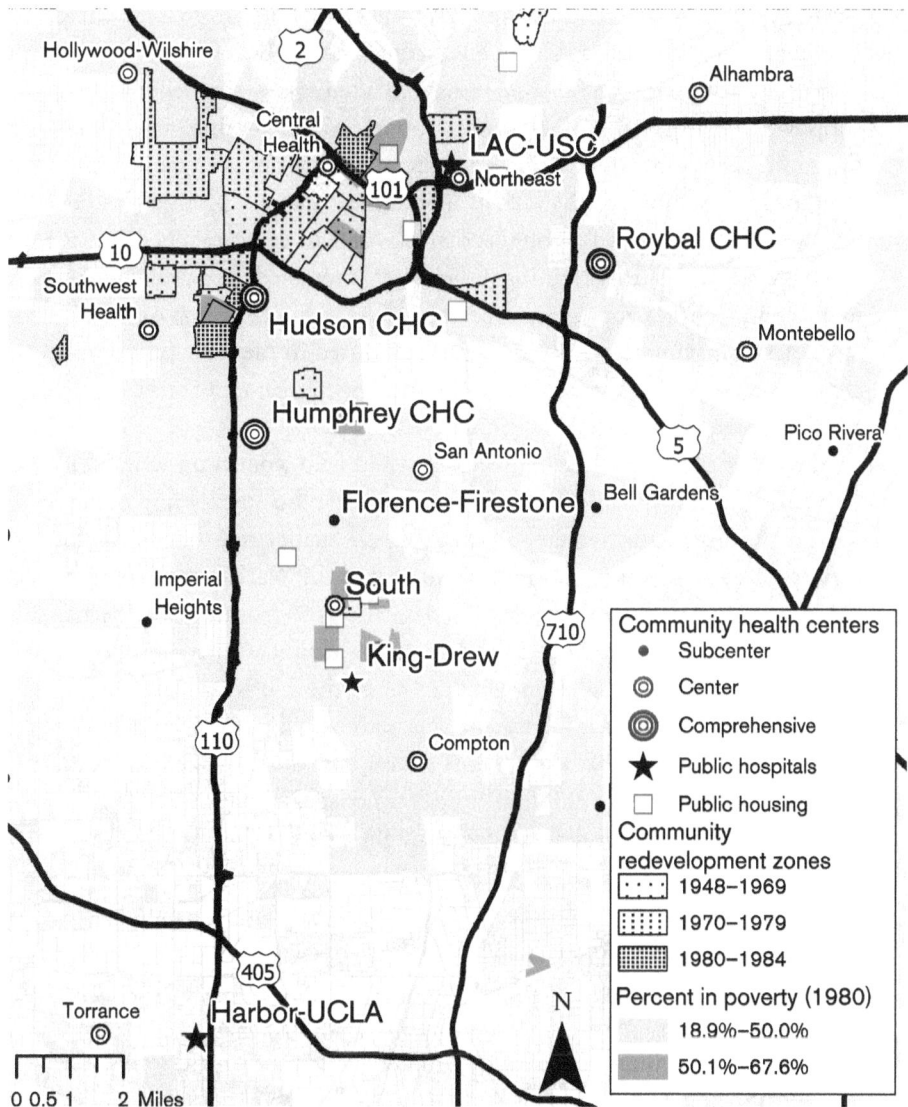

MAP 9. Anchoring working poverty

From the late 1960s onwards, the city and county of Los Angeles worked in tandem to shift the region's labor-capital relationships towards new global financial relationships by anchoring working poverty in poor neighborhoods of color through housing, health, and transportation services. Regional leaders avoided the population and economic decline associated with overzealous slum clearance programs by instituting what they called "incremental development." Map: Tyler Munn.

where else to make an application for a job [and] would have to go somewhere else for information dealing with a number of other problems."[61]

By the early 1970s, these observations marked a growing belief among antipoverty advocates that the greatest obstacle to overcoming poverty was the government's inability to make welfare an efficient bureaucracy. Rather than spend time coordinating various appointments at multiple sites, Bradley suggested that poor people would actually be able to dedicate more time to finding work and getting training if they were "provide[d] a central location for all these facilities, for all of these services." As he put it, "What we have in mind here is having some of these agencies housed in the same building—county, state—employment, social welfare, the whole gamut of services that are usually required in such a community."

The belief that consolidating services would help women on welfare, in particular, find work and acculturate themselves more quickly into society was put into action in January 1975 in a small facility refurbished by the county that sat two miles away from the center of Watts—the Florence-Firestone Multipurpose Neighborhood Center.[62] According to internal memos from Dan Grindell, deputy director, to County Supervisor Hahn, Florence-Firestone's racial demographics since the Uprisings had shifted away from being a majority–African American neighborhood to the point where a "vast majority of [its] patients [were] now Spanish-speaking" and were "mainly women and children" who "cannot speak English."[63]

Observing that many new residents sought care for their recorded biomedical afflictions of "rabies, lice, TB, ear-nose-throat infections, worms and parasites, and obesity" but were fearful of being "deceived, cheated, and taken advantage of by landlords, merchants, etc. because they are unaware of legal rights [and are] not taking advantage of public education for their children and themselves," Grindell relayed how the county used its clinics to do more than just administer healthcare. In addition to twice and sometimes thrice daily offerings of forty-five-minute in-lobby public health education sessions on "family care," "family planning," "women's care," and "pediatric care," Florence-Firestone staff also prioritized programs designed to "teach usable English phrases using a Berlitz method," "inform residents about available resources in the community," and "provide information regarding legal rights and responsibilities" related to renter and consumer rights.

The point of expanding services in health facilities to include educational courses on law, language, and family planning was not to encourage greater dependency on government services but to promote greater economic independence and self-responsibility among Florence-Firestone's residents. Instead of residents becoming more dependent on government health services, Grindell argued that the clinic's educational approach kept citizens from becoming a "burden on society and to the school system" by helping them to "seek further education, to help their children function in the schools, and to be responsible residents in their community."

As classes on better motherhood and family planning also indicate, the educational approach sought to reduce welfare rates in ways that avoided the controversy of *Madrigal v. Quilligan*, a case that shed light on a forced sterilization program at Los Angeles County General Hospital.[64] Although the filing of the lawsuit in 1975 brought an end to the county's attempt to reduce welfare rates through forced sterilization, Florence-Firestone demonstrates how the county sought to achieve the same ends through more liberal approaches centered on ideas of patient choice and education.

The apparent success of Florence-Firestone's clinic as a demonstration of the county's regionalization program led to scaling up operations to fit the needs of larger poor neighborhoods closer to downtown Los Angeles through the Hubert Humphrey Comprehensive Health Clinic. The clinic's two-story building featured 125,000 square feet of space and was designed to serve the nearly forty thousand people living within four miles. In keeping with Florence-Firestone's focus on population control, the Humphrey clinic's health education programs called on welfare rights activists to craft an array of public health education courses promoting family planning, especially for Black teenage youth.[65] Unlike Florence-Firestone, the center featured an in-clinic childcare center, open to children of all patients with an appointment. It also housed a staff of "Nutrition and Home Economists" responsible for overseeing the community's Women, Infant, Children (WIC) food stamp program.

Touted by Secretary of Health, Education, and Welfare Caspar Weinberger as "the first comprehensive health care center to be constructed in the nation," the Humphrey clinic was designed to be the "first county project of its kind where multiple health services [are] provided in one facility."[66] It was much larger and more costly than a small neighborhood clinic, and federal and municipal officials were careful to let taxpayers know that the entire purpose of the facilities was not to encourage welfare dependency but to consolidate in one place health and welfare services to free up women's time to find work. According to Liston Witherill, a county health official, the whole point of the county's "unification program" was to enable government to "use our tax dollars more effectively by ending duplicated and fragmented services and decreasing costly hospitalizations."[67]

The close monitoring of the Humphrey clinic's services by federal and local officials fed into new policy formulations at both the national and local levels by not only guiding national policy decisions about federally funded comprehensive healthcare clinic programs in the nation but also serving as the model to reorganize the county's entire healthcare system. The apparent success of the Humphrey clinic and its smaller neighborhood health clinics led the county to reproduce it in all of the largest neighborhoods of color nearest to downtown. Three years after the Humphrey clinic's opening, the county opened two large comprehensive healthcare centers in South Central and Boyle Heights, two densely populated neighborhoods of color on the edge of downtown.

Records from welfare rights activists and local community members show that they initially regarded these developments by city and county leaders as positive responses to their longtime demands for better municipal services and infrastructure. Since intervening in King-Drew's Master Plan Study, welfare rights activists had successfully participated in the construction and operation of the Johnnie Tillmon Child Care Development Center, a childcare center on the premises of King-Drew Medical Center and had instituted a five-year program named "Early Teenage Pregnancy" that paired young mothers with older mothers who also had children at a young age. According to Tillmon, both victories assisted Black mothers with navigating modern motherhood and making care for their children more scientific and less "custodial" by having medical professionals help mothers "in the areas of social emotional growth, independent living skills, sensory-motor development and intellectual development" while also furnishing children with "lessons designed to help them develop a positive ethnic identification and a potential to succeed at their own pace."[68]

As a 1980 "Progress Report" recorded, residents called upon to participate in the community boards also celebrated the city's initiatives as evidence of a collective commitment to producing sexually respectable neighborhoods regardless of class and color. Spared the bulldozer and practices of displacement that characterized development in Bunker Hill and South Park in the 1950s and 1960s, the city's decision to "preserve[e] neighborhoods with minimal disruption to residents" in the communities around downtown was seen by residents of color as an investment in rebranding neighborhoods of color as hardworking, sexually respectable, and family-oriented places.[69] In particular, city planners strategically used citizen board meetings to rally low-income residents around the idea of preserving single-family homes as a way to achieve the "preservation of the City's traditional single-family life style" and to support the construction of housing designed for various rehabilitation initiatives, such as "in-fill housing" and "move on" housing, as commitments to helping residents achieve their moral strivings.

As the next chapter shows in greater detail, Bradley defended the city's investments to literally and figuratively anchor working poverty in neighborhoods just outside the Central Business District as neighborhood "preservation" campaigns that "maintained and reinforced" the "ethnic flavor" of districts like Little Tokyo.[70] The effect of these positive discourses allowed Bradley and the leaders of the CRA-LA to claim that the city's emerging global economy worked for everyone because it managed to draw participation in work of every neighborhood in the region, including those long neglected. Board members appointed by Bradley, such as CRA-LA's Chairman James Wood, were quick to argue that the city's new "impressive" and "positive" look had much to do with "the signs of vitality" in "Chinatown, many parts of East Los Angeles, and the inner city" brought about by the "housing rehabilitation programs and the development of many needed facilities."

Claiming that his quest to "save Los Angeles" as mayor began "with the revitalization of our neighborhoods and increasing housing opportunities for all our citizens," Bradley declared that the CRA-LA's investments in neighborhoods of color proved the "commitment to serving all of the city [by] fulfilling the unique needs of each community in which it works." Such statements sought to erase the once antagonistic association of Bunker Hill with white elitism and replace it with the image of a multiracial downtown that equally served the interests of white citizens and citizens of color.

Reports by the CRA-LA often backed up assertions about the city's new multicultural identity by noting the number of jobs saved or grown by the city's and county's unique engineering of spatial relationships between downtown, its neighborhoods of color, and its mostly white suburbs. Indicative of early anxieties about securing a finite number of workers in the industries of international real estate, finance, and insurance, reports focused on the development of Bunker Hill could not help but boast how "a high proportion" of jobs downtown brought "well trained, professional or executive type workers" who were "well educated, middle and upper middle income workers."[71]

The same reports, however, also pointed out that "for each new professional job that comes downtown, any number of lower level non-professional jobs may be created." In this regard, efforts to help "downtown flower and produce markets fix up their decaying facilities, instead of leaving the city," reportedly led to saving an "estimated 7,000 jobs"—"a high percentage of [which were] held by skilled or semi-skilled minorities."[72] Other observations reported similar efforts in the city's apparel district, where an astonishingly "dynamic and diverse composition" of twenty thousand workers were employed, of which "72% are women."[73]

Narratives of job creation, however, belied how downtown employers were motivated to situate their businesses in and near downtown because they knew that the city's and county's investments in healthcare, welfare, and housing relieved them of their responsibility to pay wages high enough for workers to cover housing and healthcare costs. In fact, the reliance of employers on publicly funded services to house and care for workers often manifested in glowing reports of how relatively "cheap" land and labor was in Los Angeles compared with other competing regional markets. Indeed, according to Gaylord Milbrandt, an executive vice president of a firm providing cost-of-living information to corporations looking to relocate, "San Francisco finishes almost at the top of the ladder at every economic level," but "Los Angeles finishes several thousand dollars cheaper—8% to 10% lower, even in the most expensive areas."[74] Although three hundred dollars per square foot of luxury office space in Los Angeles may have sounded "breathtaking," real estate experts described it as "pocket change" compared with the one-thousand-dollar average in San Francisco and as still cheaper than Chicago, New York, and Denver, whose real estate costs started at and averaged above three hundred dollars. By the 1980s, the use of public funds to drive down wages for workers not only helped "stabilize" the number of manufacturing firms in downtown's Eastside industrial districts that required access to low-cost space and low-cost labor but also helped attract foreign companies, especially those from around the Pacific Rim drawn to do business in Los Angeles based on its growing reputation for "predictable returns" and "relative cheapness of land."

Whereas city leaders were once worried about Bunker Hill's prospects as the city's new financial district, city planning documents heralded it by the late 1970s as not only being "the heart of the region" but also being "physically and commercially the center of the Western United States."[75] Such phrasing demonstrated how municipal leaders and city planners began to argue that Bunker Hill's health reflected the "region's health" and that "the two are tied irrefutably, one to the other."[76] In this way, city documents revealed how city leaders and planners imagined every neighborhood, both Black and white, as having a "special responsibility" to downtown and, downtown, in turn, as having a special responsibility to every neighborhood.[77] By the late 1970s, city planners began to imagine that center city's "special responsibility" not only extended to other luxury office districts but also stretched far beyond county boundaries to encompass the entire "megalopolis" of Southern California, including "Santa Barbara on the north, to San Diego to the south."[78] By the mid-1980s, city officials went even further, celebrating the city as a global financial center for the Pacific Rim.

WORKING MOTHERHOOD AS FALSE CHOICE

For welfare rights activists, the city's rebirth by the early 1980s as a global city turned out to be neither a triumph over racism nor a triumph over patriarchy. Their activism to change the direction of King-Drew's master plan did win them access to healthcare benefits and services they would have had to wait for or never receive under the original plan, but it did not gain them the autonomy of choice they had so diligently sought to achieve. Instead of having healthcare and income security organized around breadwinning manhood as King-Drew's leaders originally envisioned, Tillmon and other welfare rights activists in Los Angeles wanted to distribute health and welfare benefits through King-Drew's health system as one campaign within a larger strategy to organize access to life's most basic necessities in order to empower women to live a life of their choosing. A surface reading of all the policy initiatives by the City and County of Los Angeles during the 1970s suggests that municipal leaders responded to the demands and criticisms of welfare rights activists in ways that appeared to carry out their vision to win poor women of color more freedom.

By the 1980s, however, the waged labor of poor women of color represented an even more crucial role in the region's political economy, as city and county officials increasingly organized the entire region's employment and economic productivity around spatial relationships that encouraged the suppression of wages and benefits in the city's neighborhoods of color. In a context in which antipoverty advocates increasingly demanded better wages and benefits for men of color, the actions of the City and County of Los Angeles show that municipal leaders helped private employers find new ways to make profits by completely bypassing the employment of men of color and relying on society's widespread willingness to pay women "pin money" instead of living wages.

Against the rising tide of activism by women on welfare, the effect of these structural phenomena made the demand by welfare rights activists to live beyond the reach of waged labor, patriarchy, and racism through the achievement of universal basic income and universal healthcare a threat to the region's new political economy. As the orientation toward freeing up women's time for employment and work training by the county's comprehensive healthcare and neighborhood health care centers demonstrates, the ultimate goal of consolidating health and welfare services in public clinics was not to have these services work *for* women but to work alongside expanded workfare programs to coerce mothers back into waged work.

As Chicana welfare rights activist Alicia Escalante observed in 1973, "forced work" for women on welfare did not just affect families on welfare but the lives of all working people. She argued that "forced work" was a "real threat to all working people" because it served as a way "to manipulate the labor market to the advantage of only the employers, the owners of industry, business and finance."[79] By creating a class of workers forced to accept wages lower than prevailing labor standards, Escalante argued that "forced work" disadvantaged "not only those out of work, on relief, and unprotected by unions, but also those employed and organized. [It] does not create jobs nor enable people to become self-supporting. On the contrary, forced work has the effect, the intentional effect, of driving wages down, of increasing the competition for already scarce jobs."

Escalante's observations about the true impact of the county's health and welfare policies and the city's redevelopment plans reveal that efforts to transition women off of welfare did not lift them out of poverty as intended. Instead, policies purporting to prevent poverty and dependency actually ended up doing the opposite. By the 1980s and 1990s, the privatization of social services and the increasing amount of public subsidies provided to private corporations made more and more working people in the United States dependent on public services. Some corporations, like Walmart, even began demanding employees enroll in food stamp programs.[80]

Rather than combat employment and occupational discrimination, then, the effect of Bradley's supposedly more inclusive economic policies intensified the processes of racism and patriarchy around poor women of color's labor by expanding the available number of low-paying "unskilled" jobs. Ultimately, for poor women of color this expansion rendered the significance of being on or not being on welfare meaningless, as the jobs offered via work incentive programs were increasingly practically the same jobs available to women of color before becoming mothers. Indeed, a large reason why NWRO activists opposed the renewal of WIP programs in 1972 had to do with the fact that women enrolled in workfare programs earned less money in the same low-paying jobs they would have worked if not on welfare. Work incentive program jobs neither provided wages above regular welfare checks nor offered any career advancement. Moece Palladino, for instance, complained in 1977 that she was offered a job "crushing bottles in a glass recycling center."[81] When she inquired about what job training might arise from such an opportunity, she was told "there would be some persons put in training to crush bottles."

Despite winning many of the services activists fought to include in King-Drew's health system, Tillmon continued to reiterate the true objective of their vision around health and welfare programs. She bemoaned that the jobs offered to people of color continued to be jobs that did not provide "adequate wages, cost of living increases, decent child care and supportive services" and that "for too long women have been limited to dead-end low-paying jobs."[82] In her opinion, the only way to improve poor people's lives was to expand the number of "non-sex-stereotyped jobs which have permanency and the opportunity for advancement." By the 1990s, Tillmon lamented that the revitalization of employment and occupational discrimination around women of color only led to a larger and "younger generation of welfare recipients" who face "far more obstacles than she faced."[83]

FIVE

An Asylum Without Walls

NEARLY A DECADE AFTER TAKING office as mayor of Los Angeles, Tom Bradley used the 1984 Olympics to showcase how LA's unique embrace of multiracial and sexual tolerance had made it a "global city." By coupling the city's existing sports infrastructure, such as the publicly funded Los Angeles Coliseum, with the private corporate sponsorship of the United States' largest and most profitable multinational corporations, LA's hosting of 140 nations was the first-ever modern Olympic Games to be financially successful. By staging the games in historic neighborhoods of color and visibly themed neighborhoods, Bradley and his unique governing coalition of white business elites and Black, Brown, Asian, and gay community leaders sought to show the world how capitalism centered on racial and sexual "pride" made cities both healthy and productive. Compared with LA's previous turn hosting the Olympics in 1932, the 1984 games helped rebrand the city's reputation as the nation's "white spot" toward a "global city" of multicultural neighborhoods for multiracial and gay people.[1]

There was, however, one neighborhood that municipal leaders strove to keep hidden. In the shadow of the new financial district, shrouded by large warehouse districts and hemmed in by freeways and the Los Angeles River, stood a neighborhood that city and county leaders colloquially knew as "Skid Row" and had renamed in official documents as "City Center East." Since the 1880s, and especially after sprawl dispersed populations farther from downtown after World War II, Skid Row's density of single residency occupancy hotels (SROs), taxi dance halls, and nearby rail yards made it a secluded haven for so-called vagrants, ex-offenders, addicts, prostitutes, and the mentally disabled. Unlike other areas, city officials erased Skid Row on city maps while redirecting tourists to iconic beaches, Disneyland, and the Watts

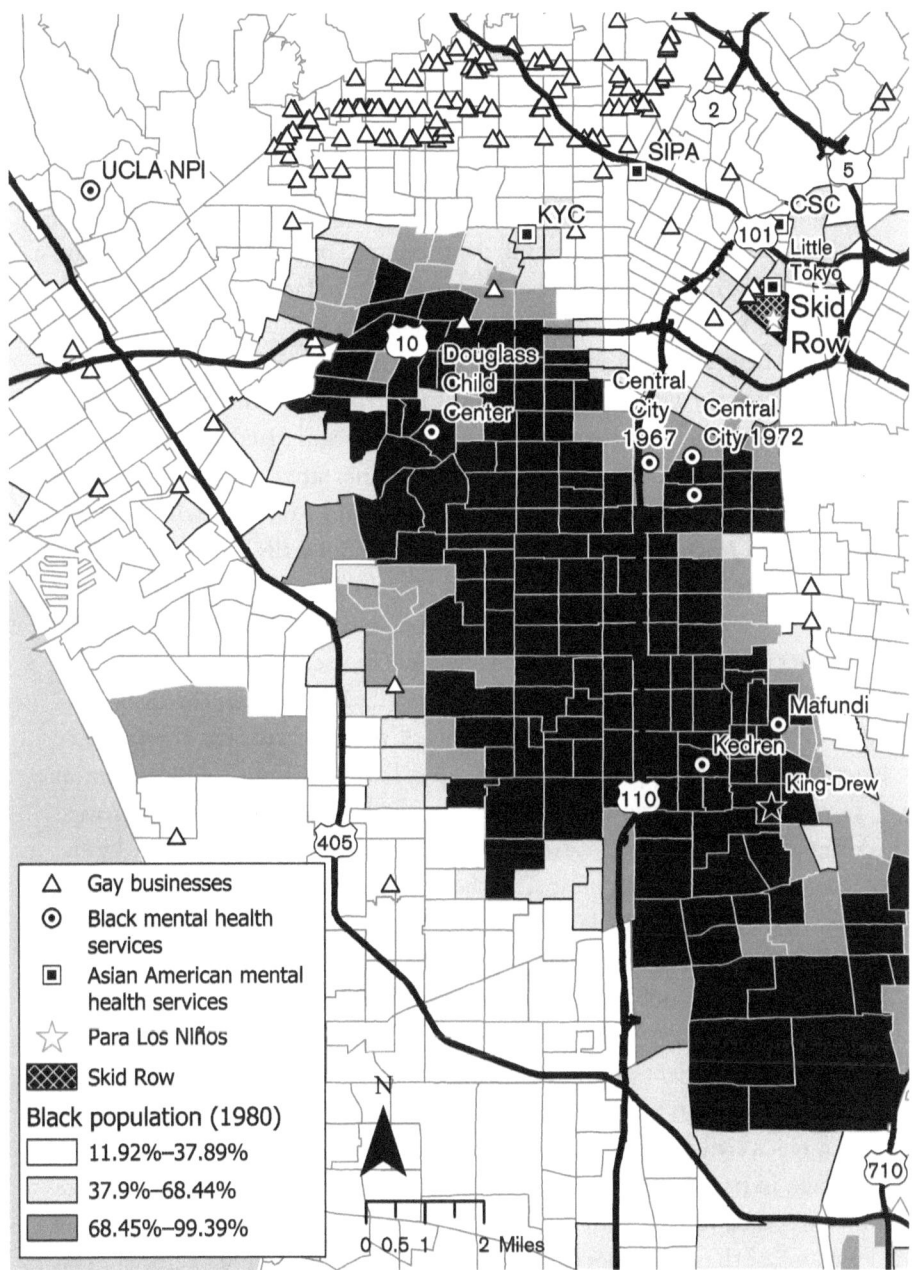

MAP 10. Skid Row's relationship to Black, Asian, and gay neighborhoods

The gay business points mapped are 1984 listings of bars, restaurants, bathhouses, bookstores, and sex shops from a popular guidebook series called Damron's Address Book. Map: Tyler Munn. Source: Damron's Address Book, 1984, One Archive, University of Southern California.

Towers on event maps. They even went as far as publishing the Olympic Organizing Committee's main hotline in popular gay guidebooks and highlight gay establishments in West Los Angeles to discourage Skid Row's discovery during and after the Olympics.[2]

As opposed to the carefully curated images advertising LA's diverse neighborhoods, depictions of Skid Row could not hide the growing importance of prisons and policing in managing the thousands of people unable to secure employment in the city's new political economy. In fact, standardized police sweeps surveilled Black and Brown neighborhoods to "clean up" inner-city districts before, during, and after the games. It used the Olympics to solidify a new city ordinance to police Skid Row differently from the rest of the inner city.[3] Whereas policing *outside* Skid Row led to regularized arrest protocols, tactics *within* Skid Row targeted homeless and other suspect citizens for open-air capture rather than arrest, turning Skid Row into what Jennifer Wolch and Michael Dear term an "asylum without walls."[4]

These strategies resulted in the *Los Angeles Herald Examiner* reporter Tony Castro observing that pre-Olympic sweeps seemed to increase the number of Black and Brown trans women and sex workers in Skid Row, people the Los Angeles Police Department (LAPD) named "the Dragons."[5] Strangely, however, "the Dragons" tended to evade arrest, although they reportedly solicited patrons "virtually just feet away from LAPD's Central Division Station" and were suspected to be behind Skid Row's increased drug-related homicides. Patrolmen argued they were "handcuffed" by the Dragons' ability "to disappear . . . at the sight of a 'suspicious' car" and because they could not "get a male police officer to dress up in women's clothes." In reality, the LAPD's ineffectiveness had nothing to do with slippery suspects or cross-dressing policemen but had everything to do with a new city ordinance called the *containment and mitigation policy*.

The containment and mitigation policy formed the nucleus of a larger strategy to detain a range of queer subjects like "the Dragons" who, under post-1960s civil rights and mental health law, could not be immediately incarcerated in prisons or involuntarily committed into state hospitals but were not welcome to return to their "home" districts in Black, Brown, and gay sections of the city. More than an account of population management systems outside prisons and state hospitals, this chapter approaches the enforced segregation of queer, homeless, trans, and mentally disabled people of color in Skid Row as part of a broader inquiry about the shared relationships between multiculturalism and policing after 1965. Multiculturalism and policing grew to be significant to the city's governance, especially after the election of Bradley in 1973, an event that brought racial and gay elites formerly excluded from city governance into positions of power.

As the last few chapters show, Bradley's election occurred during an intense period of global capital restructuring that replaced California's manufacturing landscape with a larger service-sector economy. Although Bradley attempted to broker deals to secure employment for as many workers of color as possible within a restructuring job market, the number of available workers always far outpaced the number of available jobs. As Ruth Wilson Gilmore argues, rather than invest in full employment, housing, and universal healthcare, voters by the 1970s interpreted the crisis's local dimensions—crime, homelessness, drug trafficking, and mentally disturbed "street people"—as reasons to increase prisons and police outfits targeting urban neighborhoods.[6] Gilmore, however, cautions against accounting for the carceral phenomenon solely through the race and sexuality of those incarcerated, even though this helps explain the persistence of racism, homophobia, and classism in *one segment* of a fearful electorate (the white middle class). Such narratives obfuscate racial capitalism's inner workings and, more important, fail to account for how and why Black and gay voters also consistently voted for increased policing measures.

Gilmore's work is a part of a larger body of scholarship interested in the contradictions of racial and sexual liberalism that Cathy Cohen terms crosscutting issues, processes that fold some members of minority communities into the promise of modernity and state protection by renewing violence and exclusion on others of the same social category.[7] Examples of cross-cutting deepen distinctions within and between historically marginalized groups. Christina Hanhardt and Mike Davis, for example, have detailed in their respective studies of community change in 1980s San Francisco, New York, and Los Angeles that gay and Black elites mobilized discourses of law and respectability against trans, queer, and gang youth of color perceived to be outside the bounds of supposed gay and Black "community norms."[8] As Robert McRuer and Jasbir Puar argue, even after psychiatry's removal of homosexuality as a mental illness (1973) and the passage of the Americans with Disabilities Act (1990), law and medicine still reified the exclusion of trans, queer, disabled, and debilitated people through the entwined discourses of compulsory "heterosexuality" and "able-bodiedness."[9] These crosscutting logics sustain exclusions based on the intersections of race, sexuality, and disability by obscuring how racial capitalism and economic dispossession underwrite the enlargement of carceral spaces and normalize surveillance and policing as a common good.

This chapter offers another account of cross-cutting by highlighting the influence of the community mental health movement on LA's urban politics after deinstitutionalization, especially the legal and psychiatric movement to abolish involuntary commitment in state hospitals. Although a broad goal of the community mental health movement from its inception, deinstitutionalization renewed urgency among community mental health leaders in gay and racialized neighborhoods to end police brutality and normalize race and homosexuality through a new set of identity-based community institutions and actors who brokered city issues related to crime, homelessness, and economic development under the representative signs of race and homosexuality. To salvage this vision, municipal officials designed and implemented Skid Row's containment and mitigation policy as a way to transform the neighborhood into an "asylum without walls" that served as a necessary but unacknowledged mental health institution within King-Drew's health system.

This chapter begins by deconstructing the containment and mitigation policy as the product of the sometimes contradictory, sometimes conjoined, trajectories of community mental health, deinstitutionalization, deindustrialization, and urban redevelopment phenomena facing Bradley after he assumed office. These convening factors explain the policy's reinvention of spatial dynamics *between* inner-city districts that privileged Black and gay neighborhood development over Skid Row by dividing the inner city into a large ring of multicultural neighborhoods earmarked for economic revitalization and aggressive policing and a "homeless district" to concentrate and detain "undesirables." In theory, if the city pushed all "undesirables" within Black and gay neighborhoods into Skid Row or prisons, the normality of remaining Black and gay residents would delink associations of race and homosexuality with criminality, pathology, and poverty. Although the policy produced new spatial differences by making a "homeless" district distinct from Black and Gay districts, this division subjected Skid Row residents to the logic of racial and sexual liberalism governing the rest of the city because the policy intended to incubate self-identified "homeless" activists and advocates who could broker issues pertaining to homeless "issues" in the same way that Black and gay leaders were expected to in their districts.

The policy reveals the kinds of neighborhood architecture believed necessary to forge community change based on ideas of personhood and identity. This chapter thus revisits the Community Redevelopment Agency of Los

Angeles's "incremental development" policies to show the city's 1970s efforts to incorporate subjects formerly excluded and stigmatized into the new emerging political economy that expanded ideas, approaches, and practices first propagated by a community mental health movement led by Black elites in the 1960s. By the 1970s, community mental health activists in other neighborhoods also came to similarly invest in community mental health clinics as part of a much broader group of institutions designed to produce "normality" and mental wellness in racialized and sexualized people and places that included, but were not limited to, youth programs, community-based organizations, and even gay bars. Although the normalizations produced within each community promised inclusion for all individuals under the banner of race or homosexuality, the re-invention of Skid Row as a city ordinance-enforced "homeless district" shows that Black, Asian American, and gay activist commitments to respectability politics necessitated the re-use of its historical association with homelessness to spatially contain its excess.

THE CONTAINMENT AND MITIGATION POLICY AS IDENTITY POLITICS

As the history of the Black-led community mental health movement of the 1960s reveals, deinstitutionalization was not exclusively about mental disability. Community mental health professionals like King-Drew's Black psychiatrist Dr. J. Alfred Cannon supported deinstitutionalization because its vision to release the mentally ill from treatment in state hospitals to community settings also furnished funds hoping to end the belief that people of color were inherently pathological. As chapter 3 demonstrates, however, this did not mean acting as if mental illness did not exist at all. Cannon and others in the community mental health movement believed mental health funds dedicated to showing that most people of color were "normal" and that most mental illnesses were preventable would eventually help to direct funds towards people of all racial and class backgrounds who were, in his opinion, severely mentally ill.

As this chapter shows, by the 1970s, assertions of psychiatric normality and community pride throughout LA's Black, Brown, Asian, and gay neighborhoods challenged mainstream society's deep association of postwar "vice districts" as hotbeds of mental illness. Assertions by community mental health professionals that most people of color and gay people were normal and not mentally ill at all supported a growing concern among California's politicians and bureaucrats that state hospitals were improperly detaining citizens, such as the elderly and the poor, who were neither mentally ill nor dangerous to society at all. According to Gerald Grob, this belief fueled what he calls an "unholy alliance" between liberals and conservatives, who supported deinstitutionalization because they were eager to relieve taxpayers of the burden of caring for the mentally ill.[10]

This perception underlies California's signature deinstitutionalization law, the Lanterman-Petris-Short Act (LPS) (1967), which empowered patients deemed not dangerous to themselves or to others to seek treatment in a less- or nonrestrictive setting of their choosing. LPS thus allowed citizens unfairly detained because of their race or sexuality to avoid psychiatric commitment. However, since the law permits any patient to refuse care and ask for unsupervised release without legal recourse, deinstitutionalization is mostly remembered as a failed movement that resulted in severely mentally ill "street people."[11]

Grob argues that most of psychiatry, including community mental health providers, participated in the "wholesale neglect" of the severely mentally ill, "especially the chronic patient and the de-institutionalized," because most providers saw deinstitutionalization as an opportunity to treat the most profitable or least difficult diagnostic cases.[12] Indeed, providers who rushed to treat poor populations—such as Cannon in South Los Angeles, Royal Morales in Filipino Town, and Evelyn Hooker in West Los Angeles—contributed to this phenomenon. While they did not contest the existence of severely mentally ill patients in their communities, their research and therapeutic agendas aimed to treat those who had never been institutionalized or diagnosed with a mental illness. Their interest in diverting individuals deemed "at-risk" for severe mental illness from institutionalization stemmed from a belief that the stress and anxiety of racism and homophobia could be successfully managed to prevent incarceration. Up until this point, a majority of research on race had been relegated to controlled populations in juvenile detention centers and prisons.[13]

From the perspective of community mental health professionals, Bradley's election as the first Black mayor of a majority-white city was thus seen as a major victory because it demonstrated that people of color could be seen as leaders by society and because his strong relationships with community mental health proponents ensured citywide support for their programs. His election, however, forced community mental health activists to confront the "street people" problem with greater urgency. The crisis of homelessness also presented a major obstacle to an emerging economic consensus among regional politicians that metropolitan growth needed to restructure the economy away from manufacturing toward facilitating new flows of capital between global marketplaces abroad by anchoring financial conglomerates in a revitalized downtown.[14]

Bradley hoped that downtown's rebirth would economically raise, rather than physically displace, poor people of color in downtown and near downtown neighborhoods. He believed that any attempt to improve the economic status of the inner city, however, would not have any appreciable effect without a homeless policy that successfully advanced community mental health objectives in a manner that mitigated deinstitutionalization's negative effects without reversing or invalidating LPS law. In 1976, he formalized a policy to redesign Skid Row as a neighborhood for the mentally ill to live freely and away from society *by their own choosing*.[15] The policy accepted and enhanced Skid Row's character as a proper place for the homeless and severely mentally ill so that areas outside it could economically develop unobstructed. City officials hid its enforced segregation policy in plain sight by trusting that citizens would not worry about Skid Row because they remembered it as a place for the homeless and because they had generally avoided downtown since the 1950s.

The city also expected Skid Row eventually to contain more than the mentally ill and homeless. Since 1967, city-funded social science investigations helped planners understand that deinstitutionalization was not the only phenomenon creating homelessness.[16] Observations of presumed substance abusers, ex-felons, and women living alone confirmed suspicions that Skid Row was being used as a "half-way" home for those unwanted in formal custodial institutions (state hospitals, jails, and other detention centers) and in their own "home" communities.[17] Urban analysts interpreted the increased number of the chronically mentally ill, workers unable to find stable work, and the working poor as proof that the neighborhood was growing because of deinstitutionalization's entanglements with deindustrialization.

These reports provided a glimpse into the root causes of homelessness that urban planners were less willing to acknowledge. Whether intentional or not, urban policy reports on homelessness downplayed the region's growing crisis of affordable housing and working poverty. The combination of gentrification, a lack of public and low rent housing, and jobs paying under the poverty line drove displaced citizens into Skid Row. As homeless advocates at Los Angeles Community Action Network (LA CAN) recently pointed out, the higher frequency of displacement and evictions increased the number of people living in Skid Row who were gainfully employed as dishwashers, street vendors, restaurant workers, janitors, and even healthcare workers.[18] The loss of housing, food, and income security associated with life in Skid Row, in turn, exposed a growing number of its residents to greater policing and health risks (both physical and mental in nature).[19]

Instead of addressing these root causes, Bradley used these reports to focus on the idea of homelessness as a "personal choice" by crafting what planners initially referred to as Skid Row's *rehabilitation and mitigation policy*, which enriched funding to SROs and shelters and encouraged the development and concentration of indigent services. City technocrats characterized their position as an enlightened alternative to past policies. "Slums were things to be 'cleared' . . . [but] today, this approach is generally considered short-sighted, and inhumane," since it would leave no viable housing option for the "adult Los Angeles resident who will either be forced to or prefer to live in what most of the citizenry would regard as unacceptable conditions."[20]

"Prefer to live as" and "forced to" live as homeless signaled how Bradley's administration defended the concentration of homeless in Skid Row as a method to enhance their rights as a newly protected citizen class. In fact, city officials argued, "a policy focused solely on making a geographic area like Skid Row the site of more prosperous and economically productive activity *undervalues the social productivity involved in preserving and improving the living places* of very poor people, many of whom are also afflicted by a host of other debilitating problems" (emphasis mine). Here, the city encouraged Skid Row residents to identify, desire, and self-fashion an identity as "homeless" so that the city might produce advocacy mechanisms and services to recognize their needs as such.

These statements reveal that urban planners saw the policy as an incubator of "identity" that matched individuals to space through programs oriented toward target populations. In Skid Row, SROs, shelters, and soup kitchens were prioritized for funding and preservation over businesses not catering to the homeless. Additionally, special subsidies and grant assistance programs were devised to entice social service providers working in the fields of mental health, social work, and law to relocate and ring the perimeter of Skid Row, with the intention that these actors would empower the homeless to advocate for themselves and the neighborhood.

The city knew that this strategy would increase crowding and the rate of violence in the neighborhood. From 1970 to 1986 Skid Row's nighttime population doubled from about six thousand to more than eleven thousand residents. In 1975, a new police substation built on Skid Row's southwestern

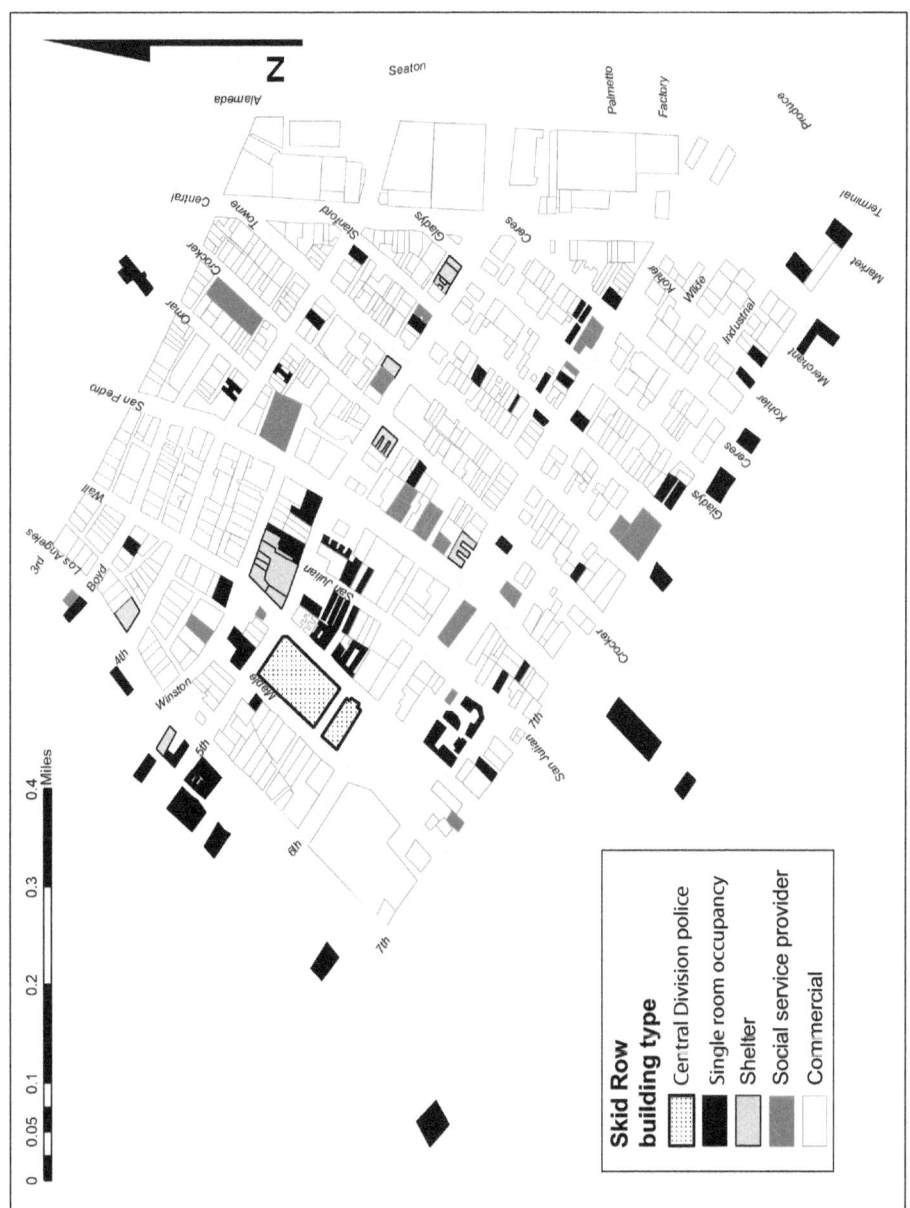

MAP 11. The containment and mitigation policy

By 1991 Skid Row contained twenty-four social service institutions, seventy-three Single Room Occupancy Hotels containing 5,830 units, transitional living programs with 593 beds, and seven shelters with 1,754 beds. Map: Nic John Ramos. Source: Housing Map and Land Use Map 1991 Briefing Report, Bunker Hill Redevelopment Project Records, Collection no. 0226, box 5, folder 14, Regional History Collections (Special Collections, University of Southern California).

corner was supposedly intended to protect residents from each other, but as the policing of "the Dragons" demonstrates, the LAPD appeared more successful in containing residents to the fifty-block area between the substation and the Los Angeles River.[21] In this sense, the city's leaders used racially and sexually liberal discourses found in politics and medicine to deliberately craft what others have termed a "hyperghetto," a new type of "ghetto" that Eric Tang defines as a "site of punishment and confinement for the poorest, most underemployed (and often unemployable) residents."[22]

Those who did not qualify as a part of Skid Row's new homelessness policy found themselves unprotected and, in some cases, the target of relocation programs. Paul Huh of the Pacific American Fish Company, for instance, complained that the "Mayor and the City have tried cleaning up the city and cracking down on prostitution but I think all they may have succeeded in doing is driving it down here."[23] His business sat a block from Para Los Niños, "a day-care center for neglected and abused children and youths," which catered to a rising number of Central American families now living in SROs. Pressured to clarify that "Skid Row is no place for children," the city renamed its policy the *containment and mitigation policy* to highlight the intended character of the neighborhood as a place for single unattached adults.[24] In an unprecedented move to service a population that city officials suspected or knew was largely undocumented, the city authorized funding initiatives to relocate immigrant families outside the district into areas deemed more suitable for children.[25]

RACE AND COMPULSORY HETEROSEXUALITY

The policy to remove and relocate Mexican and Central American families from Skid Row underlined the importance of new urban zoning practices that sought to transform the city's "ghettos," "barrios," and "slums" into respectable "family-friendly" neighborhoods of color. Alongside the unfurling of the containment and mitigation policy, Bradley engineered a parallel scheme to revitalize downtown by using private and public funds raised through the Community Redevelopment Agency of Los Angeles (CRA-LA). These funds indirectly subsidized downtown employers by offloading their need to pay workers wages high enough to cover housing and healthcare by expanding publicly funded housing, hospital, and clinic services in neighborhoods of color close to downtown. Although the city's scheme deliberately manufactured working poverty in certain neighborhoods in exchange for the assurance of global commerce in downtown, Bradley believed that his policies offered workers of color jobs far closer than those available in other comparable cities and offered workers livelihoods in neighborhoods with modern "amenities" not likely to occur elsewhere. To counterbalance the effects of working poverty, Bradley marshaled the excitement of 1960s community mental health–inspired Black pride campaigns to drive economic development in other neighborhoods around downtown.

By his election, Bradley inherited a political infrastructure made up of mental health practitioners and community activists who all followed the pathway paved by Black Power and civil rights activists by fomenting their own versions of racial and ethnic pride campaigns in their own neighborhoods. The rise of Chicano Power, Asian Pride, and Gay Pride movements in the city's Spanish-speaking, Asian American, and white gay and lesbian neighborhoods all reflected the spatial patterns unearthed by the movement of white residents and capital out of inner-city neighborhoods after the New Deal and GI Bill. Community pride campaigns also reflected how inner-city activists—regardless of their racial, ethnic, and sexual makeup—all sought to contest the stigma of living in so-called "vice districts" full of crime, sexual promiscuity, and poverty.

According to Emily Hobson, racial redlining practices favoring racially homogeneous neighborhoods after 1955, combined with a policing culture enforcing a "thin blue line" between racial groups, encouraged the cultivation of mono-racial neighborhoods. As a consequence, by the 1960s, "Black and Latino people were increasingly isolated both from white Angelenos and from each other."[26] These patterns resulted in Chicano and Asian neighborhoods stretching north and east of downtown and a Black region of neighborhoods running south from downtown through Watts and Compton and west toward Baldwin Hills.[27] Practices of police entrapment, street harassment, and surveillance also drove a once extremely multiracial and visible homosexual landscape underground in new Black, Asian, and Brown neighborhoods and encouraged the movement of white gay bars, organizations, and gathering places "above ground" to areas west of downtown now policed as "white ghettoes."[28] These patterns of displacement solidified a visible mostly white and gay community that extended west from downtown along Sunset, Melrose, Hollywood, and Santa Monica Boulevards. This landscape made it possible to think of different city zones as having particular interests tied to identity by the time that Bradley ascended to office.

More than just the epicenter for new political thought centered on "Black pride," Cannon's work in South Los Angeles made the city a fertile ground for community mental health professionals in other minoritized communities to mount their own campaigns around the normality of race or homosexuality in their own communities. As I show in this section and the next, community mental health professionals were pivotal in building new community institutions centered on developing healthy identifications with race and homosexuality. These institutions oriented people of color and white gay citizens toward greater participation and ownership of their own identity-based neighborhoods that also prepared them for success in arenas outside their communities. Although community mental health professionals implemented their theories in community mental health clinics, they also invested equally in institutions outside community mental health clinics (CMHCs) to amplify their effect.

King-Drew's Cannon had played an integral role in shaping the local political machine that helped catapult Bradley to citywide office by constructing a network of community mental health professionals and infrastructure throughout the city. Unlike the anticapitalist Black Power politics of the Black Panther Party, Cannon's form of Black nationalism was premised on the same urban and mental health policy approaches underwriting Daniel Patrick Moynihan's culture of poverty theory. Like Moynihan's emphasis on the perceived dysfunction of Black family structures, Cannon's approach to Black mental wellness drew upon a shared prevailing belief within the burgeoning fields of ethno-psychiatry and social and community psychiatry: that racial and ethnic differences held little to no meaning so long as every race and ethnic group was shown to demonstrate the same gender distinctiveness as white men and women and the sexual complexity of white heterosexual couples.

Cannon's emphasis on gender distinctiveness mobilized well-worn racial scientific ideas of the ordering of human intellect that ranked people on the basis of observed racial, gender, or sexual appearances and practices against the presumed evolutionary complexity of white straight men and women. Instead of arguing that Black people were incapable of inhabiting the complexity attributed to the gender and sexual stability of heterosexuality, Cannon posited that Black people's lack of exposure to positive representations of Blackness and corollary overexposure to negative and abject representations of Blackness accounted for the manifestation of so-called arrested or maladjusted psyches exhibited in Black adults. Rather than reify mainstream psychiatry's view that the Black community's perceived high rates of welfare dependency, family desertion, homosexuality, and sexual promiscuity were signs of Black people's inherently inferior intellect, Cannon argued that consistent positive exposure to proud, heterosexual, and economically productive Black adults, especially before the onset of puberty, was necessary to turn Black children into healthy Black adults.

Cannon was clear that creating a world conducive to Black mental wellness required new kinds of mental institutions, as well as recruiting people beyond the formal scope of psychiatry, psychology, and social work to make it a reality. By the late 1960s, with the funding support of Bradley and others, Cannon managed to build an impressive array of institutions and workers dedicated to Black mental wellness. By the mid-1970s, he was responsible for the construction and leadership of several mental health institutions, including Drew Postgraduate Medical School's Department of Psychiatry, Kedren Community Mental Health, the Frantz Fanon Research and Development Center, the Frederick Douglass Child Development Center, and Central City Community Mental Health, as well as several para-mental health institutions and organizations such as the Inner City Cultural Center, the Mafundi Arts Institute, Ron Karenga's US organization, and the South Central Improvement Action Committee's Ujima Village housing project.

Mental health leaders in both academic and clinical settings took advantage of the Black Power movement's popularity and the optimism it brought to the community mental health movement by adapting and reproducing Cannon's practices and theories. Dr. Harry Brickman, director of the County Department of Mental Health, for instance, stated that Cannon's practice of combining mental health services with programming centered on welfare, probation, elderly, and youth services at Central City was the bedrock strategy to prevent improper psychiatric commitment of people of color throughout the county. By creating a network of community-based organizations (CBOs) "'riding on the shoulders' of established community caretakers,"[29] Brickman argued that department resources would not only help community mental health activists "deal directly and more effectively with the emotional problems of their welfare recipients, probationers, students, etc." but also empower them to refer a client to psychiatrists for treatment and research.

Under this plan, any CBO in the city's racial and ethnic neighborhoods could be transformed into a portal for the county's mental health system by placing a race-based community mental health worker in it. By 1971, the National Institutes of Mental Health (NIMH) decided to replicate the county's strategy by creating two separate task forces for Spanish-speaking and Asian American populations in order to transform Latinx and Asian

American CBOs into de facto CMHCs across the nation.[30] As Cannon explained, CMHC and CBO staff provided a way for providers to "reach the young and the old who need help but just won't come to a mental health center" because of the stigma associated with race and mental illness.[31] More important, such services infused the racial and ethnic pride movements in other neighborhoods of color with the same community norms of middle-class respectable marriage and family advocated by federal urban policy.

Cannon played a key role in helping to staff these new mental health–oriented CBOs by serving as a key leader in developing UCLA's Program in Social and Community Psychiatry.[32] The program allowed him to hone race-based psychiatric arguments by exploring different types of prejudice facing other racial, ethnic, and "outsider" groups.[33] In turn, Cannon's work to model his approach to Black mental wellness and help develop programs appropriate for other racial, ethnic, and outsider groups helps account for the rapid proliferation of community mental health infrastructure in the 1970s.

In 1972, the NIMH seeded the infrastructure to reproduce Central City's "community service center" model under the auspices of the Mental Health Task Force on Asian Americans and Pacific Islanders and the Mental Health Task Force on Spanish-Speaking Americans.[34] As Cannon did, these task forces affirmed certain racial identities centered on respectable marriage and family and productive participation in the economy as true expressions of race while regarding sexual promiscuity, homosexuality, homelessness, criminal behavior, drug abuse, and violence as evidence of pathology. They did not regard this pathology as biologically determined but instead referred to its manifestation as evidence of the role that white supremacy played in producing a "ghetto/colonial/barrio" mentality or as "internal colonialism."[35]

The Asian American and Pacific Islander Task Force, for example, implemented the Asian American Mental Health Training Center (AAMHTC) in Los Angeles under the direction of Filipino American Licensed Clinical Social Worker Royal "Uncle Roy" Morales, which ran from July 1972 to June 1982.[36] Unlike Central City, AAMHTC's goal was to act as a resource for Asian American and Pacific Islander mental health professionals to develop new talent and to place them in existing CBOs. The placement of trained mental health professionals in existing CBOs such as Search to Involve Pilipino Americans (SIPA), the Chinatown Service Center, United Cambodian Community, Korean Youth Center, and the Japanese Pioneer Center essentially remade each community organization into a CMHC. In so doing, the AAMHTC fulfilled Brickman's vision to "enrich" the Asian

American community's "capacity to deal with mental health programs of their essentially non-mental health caseloads" while identifying and referring new mental health cases to the appropriate service. It also allowed different ethnic groups to develop their own distinct ethnic identities while constructing a "pan-ethnic" Asian identity that mirrored broader multicultural paradigms.

Many CBOs directly borrowed from Central City's programming. Morales, for instance, described SIPA as a "Youth Diversion Model" that utilized a mix of "counseling services, job development projects, recreational activities, a summer employment program and a summer recreation program" to steer Filipino American youth away from gang-related activity.[37] The CBO achieved youth participation by developing a repertoire that upheld knowing one's ancestral past and good citizenship as desirable modes of mental wellness by combining workshops on cultural dance, music, theater, language, craft-making, and history with activities centered on do-gooding such as neighborhood clean-up days, graffiti removal sweeps, and soup kitchen service.

By 1973, Cannon's efforts built an entire infrastructure of mental health programs with NIMH funding that doubled as a political machine dedicated to elevating elected officials of color, like Bradley, into higher office. These relationships explain why Bradley continued to fund community mental health through city grants when NIMH gradually defunded CMHCs in the late 1970s. Bradley reconsolidated the power of CMHCs in new CBO funding streams through Model Cities Funding and city community development and community service grants.[38] Eventually, he engineered new public-private partnerships to fund CMHCs through the United Way.[39]

Ultimately, Bradley supported community mental health's racial and ethnic "pride" objectives because they shared in urban policy's ultimate goal of achieving full community participation in democratic and capitalist institutions. As Daniel Widener argues, "African American culture became one site where elected officials could demonstrate affinity with and support for black residents of South Los Angeles" because it celebrated Black culture without necessarily supporting "an insurgent form of urban politics."[40] Instead of criticizing the city's ongoing commitments to racial capitalism and policing as problems in the Black community as the Black Panthers did, Cannon's narrative pointed to the personal and cultural shortcomings of Black individuals to adjust to new ideas of Blackness to account for the continued presence of worklessness and working poverty in Black communities.

Bradley did more than support community mental health theory; he played an active role in shaping new urban policy based on it. In 1974, he adopted the

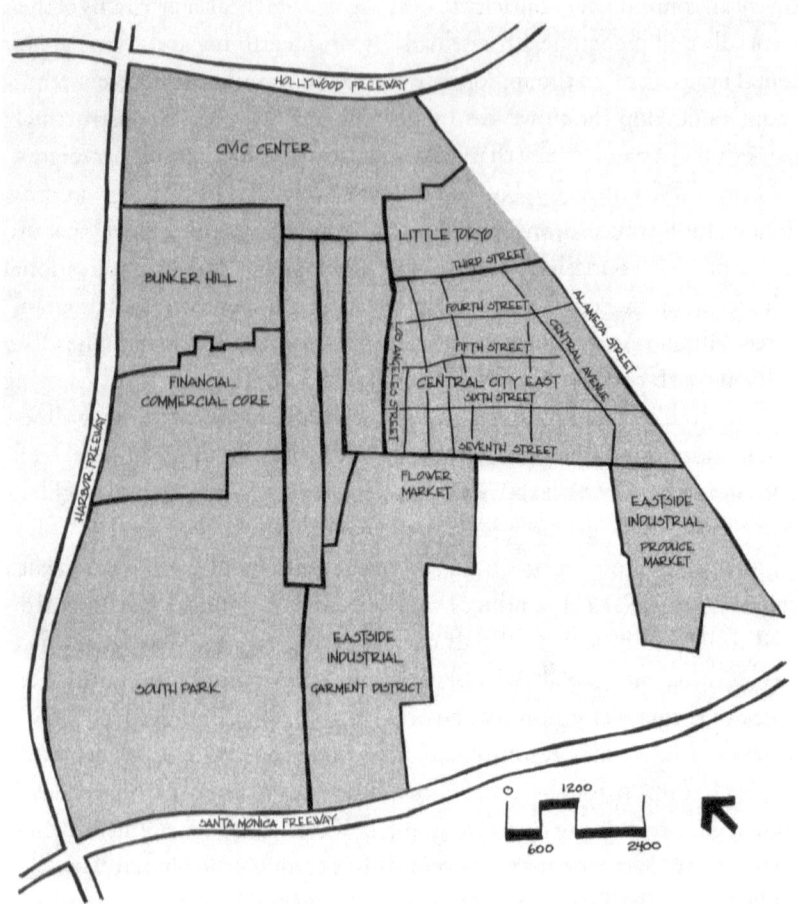

FIGURE 6. City center, Los Angeles

By 1974 the city renamed Skid Row "City Center East" in official city documents and maps. Here, Skid Row (depicted with greater street detail) is marked in relation to seven different "redevelopment zones." In turn, these zones cultivate a distinct neighborhood character oriented either to a sense of identity or industry. Source: "Central City East," Los Angeles Bunker Redevelopment Project Records, Box 5, Folder, 10, 7 (Special Collections, University of Southern California).

Skid Row rehabilitation plan and followed it with the Central Business District Redevelopment project in 1975 through CRA-LA, the city's public-private redevelopment agency. According to CRA-LA statements, these legislative ordinances achieved gentrification in downtown first by resolving the "human problems" associated with Skid Row's residents.[41] Rather than rely completely on policing, Bradley crafted a "humane" multicultural redevelopment scheme from lessons learned from psychiatry's productive power, particularly in affirming "identity" to stabilize "community" found in Cannon's work.

These policies reveal that Bradley's efforts to enhance and preserve the racial and ethnic character of neighborhoods of color outside Skid Row through "incremental development" were not just designed to integrate neighborhoods of color into the city's new political economy in ways that benefited business elites. They were also designed to enhance the social environment of districts toward healthy affirmed identity formations under the broader banner of economic development. Rather than erase the historical heritage of these neighborhoods, the CRA-LA's guiding policy preserved distinctive characteristics and a sense of neighborhood "identity" to drive new economic development. The promotion of the immigrant character of Little Tokyo and the loft space in the Arts District, for instance, sought to not only draw tourists and buyers of art to elements already present in these communities but also attract new capital from individuals seeking the global or artistic lifestyles assumed to come with life in these neighborhoods.

GAYNESS AND HOMO-RESPECTABILITY

By the early 1970s, the community mental health movement also shaped a burgeoning gay pride movement in Los Angeles. As with Cannon's race-based research, UCLA also supported positive research on homosexuality through Dr. Evelyn Hooker's work on the existence of nonpathological homosexuals. Although she did not directly organize people to action or form institutions like Cannon, Hooker provided gay activists with a framework to strengthen claims made in her research. As I show, Hooker laid a foundation from which gay activists built and defended an entire range of community institutions oriented toward normal homosexuality, consisting of gay bars, the Gay and Lesbian Community Services Center (originally the Gay Community Services Center), the Municipal Elections Committee of Los Angeles, and the Gay and Lesbian Police Task Force. Essentially, these institutions normalized homosexuality as white and middle class just as South Los Angeles institutions normalized Blackness as straight and middle class in ways that account for the policing of "the Dragons" into Skid Row.

Scholars generally cite Hooker's 1957 article "The Adjustment of the Male Overt Homosexual" as foundational to depathologizing homosexuality in the Diagnostic and Statistical Manual of Mental Disorders (DSM) in 1973.[42] Many of her friends were white gay men involved in the Mattachine Society, a homophile organization founded in 1950, who argued to Hooker that it was her "scientific duty" to research normal homosexuality, since they allowed her to "see [them] as we are," that is, "people who function in society and don't go to see psychiatrists because they don't need to."[43] The Mattachine Society was highly influenced by the civil rights movement, which inspired members to achieve a shared "dignified standard" with "the emerging cultures of . . . fellow-minorities" who forged a "disciplined, moral, and socially responsible" "homosexual culture."[44]

Hooker's research was groundbreaking because it accepted the existence of gay lifestyles in everyday settings as a fact, a point that departed from a predominant focus on situational homosexuality, a phenomenon drawn from studying homosexuality in asylums, the military, and prisons.[45] As she recounts, the NIMH funded her programs precisely because she studied homosexuals "in their social setting," that is, in what she called "homosexual community life."[46] In this way, Hooker did not depart greatly from Cannon and other community mental health professionals who made similar claims about the normality of people of color and who focused research and resources on subjects who were not mentally ill at all.

Similar to Central City's claim that its programs developed healthy Black minds, Hooker argued that certain gay institutions developed healthy gay minds. Based on her research from 1957 to 1961 in an area her friends referred to as the "swish Alps,"[47] Hooker argued that gay establishments, particularly the gay bar, functioned essentially as CMHCs—as community centers that helped gay men know "how to act, think and feel" as healthy homosexuals. Although she acknowledged baths, "gay" streets, parks, public restrooms, beaches, gyms, coffeehouses, and restaurants as part of the gay "scene," she singled out the bar as "the most important of these community gathering places" for its value as a "communication center" for exchanging leads on finding jobs, lawyers, and other everyday needs; as a place for "induction and training [for neophytes and those not-yet-'out']"; and as "integration centers for ['out' homosexuals transplanted from elsewhere]." In other words, gay bars functionally performed similarly to the poverty alleviation and mental health prevention programs being developed in CMHCs/CBOs.

However, Hooker did not argue that all spaces in the "scene" were equally productive for developing healthy gay psyches. She particularly feared that individuals risked developing maladjusted sexualities outside positive communal places such as gay bars. She favored bars because they promoted public and affirmative declarations of a stable sexual core of being either strictly homosexual or heterosexual. She was, in turn, antagonistic to sexual activity and gender expressions attached to street life that indicated sexual ambivalence or confusion (such as cruising, prostitution, hustling, and living in secret) that refused identification along this binary.

Like Cannon and other adherents of ethno-psychiatry, Hooker and those on the National Task Force on Homosexuality drew on racial scientific theories of psycho-development to argue that trans people, bisexuals, sex workers, and people living "in secret" were not normal and natural manifestations of human sexuality but signs of psycho-social maldevelopment and arrest. Hooker admitted, for instance, that she felt that people who refused to accept their assigned gender at birth and/or a stable sexual identity as gay or lesbian practiced a kind of "masochism"—"a self-inflicted pain"—that was "learned primarily through parental and other familial upbringing." Thus, while she defended homosexuality as a normal manifestation in human beings, she argued that childhood exposure to trauma could result in preventable adult sexual maladjustments.

Hooker embedded strict sexual binaries in her influential NIMH National Task Force on Homosexuality Report (completed 1968, published 1971),[48] which affirmed some forms of homosexuality as normal based on community productivity and safety while advocating for the prevention of some forms of homosexuality she considered "destructive."[49] As such, the successful homosexual depathologization campaigns supported by activists within and outside psychiatry purposely did not declassify "gender dysphoria" or distress with one's gender identity in order to discourage criminal behaviors associated with homosexual crime and street life.[50]

Hooker's work reinforced this division by arguing for the defense of one scene and not the other. She argued against harassment and raids of gay bars and patrons by arguing that they were a reputable part of the "market economy" and activities within them constituted a lawful form of "leisure" because the "negotiation of an exchange of sexual services" between two gay men in gay establishments was protectable under law since "the right to enter is determined by whether the buyer has the wherewithal."[51] Essentially, Hooker normalized participation in capitalist and public forms of homosexuality as prerequisite for healthy gay psyches and authorized renewed discourses of pathology and stigma related to trans people, bisexuals, gay sex workers, and people living in secret.

Hooker offered her diagnosis as a rejoinder to urban policy analysts and Black elites who saw sexual promiscuity and undifferentiated homosexuality as the root of all crime and poverty in inner-city neighborhoods. In offering evidence that some homosexuals—legally employed, involved in the community, and proud of their sexuality—were helping combat urban deterioration, Hooker sought to align gay activists' aims with urban policy agendas. As such, her Task Force Report called for community mental health funding to fold in homosexuality as a category eligible for public funding in order "to render service to a greater number of persons with homosexual problems and their families."[52]

Government funding for gay CBOs shifted the momentum of gay community politics away from liberationists and toward more measured forms of integrationism. For instance, although the Gay and Lesbian Community Services Center (GLCSC) was originally founded by militant Gay Liberation Front activists in 1971 to service gay neighborhoods from West Hollywood to Silver Lake, the largesse of funding changed the nature of its programming. A 1973 *Los Angeles Times* article detailed that the GLCSC ran a "Gay is beautiful" campaign in keeping with community mental health objectives that argued that homosexuality was "not a sin or sickness syndrome" and was geared toward politics "much like the black pride push of a few years ago."[53] As Ian Baldwin argues, however, although the center began by pushing large structural change related to gender and sexual norms, affordable housing, and street activism, the stipulations undergirding new funding streams emphasized working within prevailing mechanisms of social work, juvenile justice, and prison probationary programs.[54]

Thus, although GLCSC's executive director Don Kilfener explained that the center was interested in promoting gayness expressed as a "wide range of emotions, life-style and human possibilities," GLCSC staff did not agree.[55] Staff privately argued that the center was moving away from its militant origins and sacrificing the "identity of [the] agency and its own goals" by accepting "government money," and by leadership's purported focus on "placing straight-appearing gay people" in job programs.[56] The ensuing exodus of lesbian and militant-leaning staff members suggests that the center was changing because its remaining leadership not only was willing to narrow the definitions of which community members were serviced and for what reasons but preferred to reproduce the institution by mobilizing the new status that homosexuality enjoyed as an eligible public fund grantee equal to other race-based CMHCs and CBOs.

The status of the GLCSC as a major community mental health institution was bolstered by the rise of the Municipal Elections Committee of Los Angeles (MECLA), an organization originally founded as a consciousness-raising group of "A-Gays" named Orion.[57] MECLA's strategy was to "raise money and contribute that money to candidates who are favorable to gay people and their concerns, to defeat candidates who are not, and to educate all politicians and elected officials about the large number of successful and 'closeted' gay men and women who are not represented by the traditional gay leadership."[58] By "traditional," MECLA meant gay liberationists, and MECLA strove to represent those "who do not fit the stereotypes of 'gays' or 'homosexuals' and who have not been represented politically prior to this time." The irony of these statements is how quickly their organization came to replace liberationists as the mainstream voice for homosexuals in Los Angeles.

By 1978, MECLA's elegant black-tie dinners and "high priced pool parties" raised enough campaign money to gain the attention and protection of the city's biggest political players, including Mayor Bradley and his allies.[59] An LA-wide nondiscrimination ordinance, civic appointments of open and out leaders, and a successful 1984 West Hollywood cityhood campaign complete with an election of an all-gay city council soon followed. In 1982, *L.A. Weekly* described the "business persons, realtors, lawyers and therapists" of MECLA as having "helped steer LA gays on a course different from that taken by gays in other cities."[60] Unlike New York's "images of yet another sit-down protest in support of a doomed gay rights ordinance" or San Francisco's "massive street demonstrations," *L.A. Weekly* argued, due to MECLA's influence, the term *gay activist* in Los Angeles instead "mean[t] a black tie dinner at $100 a head."

Although GLCSC began receiving city grants as early as 1973, the amount of fiscal support it received grew exponentially after MECLA solidified relationships with Bradley's administration after forming in 1977 and after MECLA's emissaries made a habit of naming the GLCSC as the proper community partner to receive funds that they lobbied legislators to pass.[61] As the programs and accomplishments of MECLA and GLCSC demonstrate, Bradley supported their expressions of gay pride because they did not, as Abram J. Lewis argues, have the "revolutionary posturing, counter culturalism, and allegiances to anti-racist, anti-colonial, and radical feminist struggles" that characterized competing gay liberationist organizations.[62] Whereas the Gay Liberation Front, for example, contested the ongoing pathologization and policing of homeless, disabled, trans, and queer people of color,

MECLA and GLCSC had no qualms about assisting the city with policing them out of their neighborhoods.[63]

The significance of these divisions—between "normal" and "street" forms of homosexuality and integrationist and Gay liberationist perspectives—deepened in urgency with the AIDS crisis in the early 1980s.[64] In particular, the epidemic began to erode the civic image of gay sexual restraint and successful productivity that MECLA and the GLCSC had built and normalized over the 1970s. AIDS reintroduced underlying doubt about the pathology of gay men by conjuring a predatory and lustful sex-seeker, willing to put his own life and the lives of others in danger for the thrill of anonymous sex in risky settings. As Bruce Decker, Governor George Deukmejian's AIDS Task Force director, told reporter Linda Breakstone, "AIDS has resurfaced many of the natural doubts people had about homosexuals. What we're seeing in (polling) data is a shift that can be best epitomized in the phrase, 'Maybe I was right about those people in the first place.'"[65]

The effect made the county's 1985 Department of Health proposal to shut down bathhouses a political test for MECLA. According to Breakstone, "The bath house issue" gave "homosexual leaders . . . a chance to demonstrate their political maturity."[66] Fearing a loss of political clout and public influence, MECLA advocated for the voluntary closure of bathhouses, a measure that its co-chair Carol Childs defended as an "imperative symbolic gesture to demonstrate what we know—that the majority of the gay community is responsible." In doing so, MECLA tacitly framed bathhouse goers as irresponsible, like the forms of street homosexuality Hooker called "destructive" in 1971. Although gay militant groups, including the Lesbian and Gay Network and Lavender Left, protested MECLA and accused it of being "sell outs" and "self-appointed power brokers,"[67] GLCSC director Duke Comegys signaled to others in a community forum that his center "supports MECLA no matter what."[68]

Comegys's defense of MECLA revealed a deeper paranoia around the center's own survival. Movement toward conservatism in the general population and in the gay and lesbian community made GLCSC leadership and MECLA anxious about the future status of gay community issues in mainstream public policy. Pressured to act after Ronald Reagan's presidential election and Deukmejian's gubernatorial election, MECLA created a Republican outreach committee in 1982 to court conservative candidates and voters. In the same year, the GLCSC created the Gay and Lesbian Police Task Force (GLPTF), a committee of representatives from smaller constituent organizations.

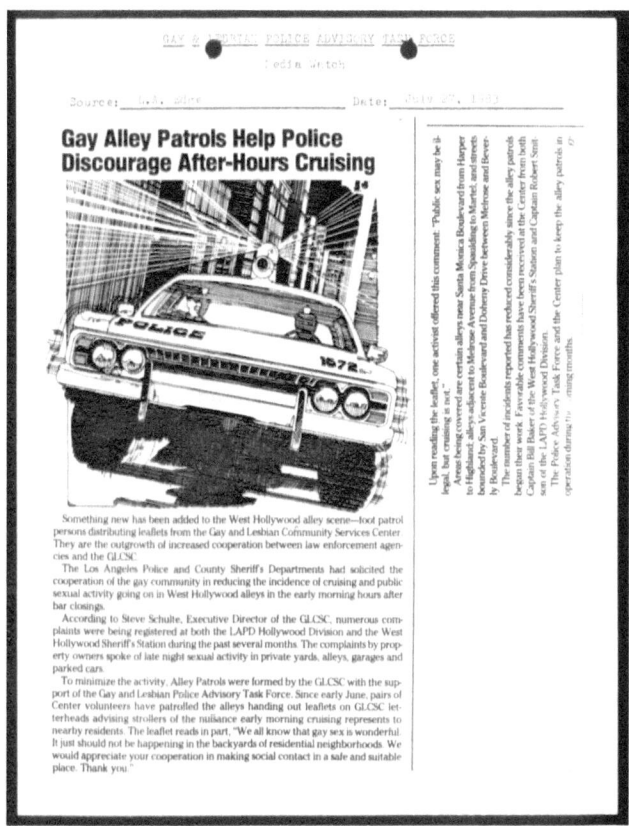

FIGURE 7. Policing through new community norms

In 1983, the *LA Edge* reported on the activities of the GLCSC and the Gay and Lesbian Police Advisory Task Force, whose volunteers had taken to patrol alleys with leaflets that read, in part, "We all know that gay sex is wonderful. It just should not be happening in the backyards of residential neighborhoods. We would appreciate your cooperation in making social contact in a safe and suitable place. Thank you." Source: "Gay Alley Patrols Help Police Discourage After-Hours Cruising," August 1983, Folder 5, Box 1, Gay and Lesbian Police Task Force Collection (ONE Archives, University of Southern California).

The GLPTF saw its interaction with city officials and the LAPD as an opportunity to reassert the normality of homosexuality in a new era of AIDS. Rather than be confrontational with the LAPD, the GLPTF prioritized changing the LAPD from the "inside" by making the hiring of gay and lesbian officers its main objective. This tactic was strategic because it enforced the idea that gays and lesbians were ready to, literally and figuratively, police their own streets. To cultivate an image of respectability, the GLPTF and the GLCSC advertised their ride-alongs in police cars and their formation of "gay alley patrols" to "discourage after-hours cruising" and "to minimize [street] activity" by imploring street passersby to note that while "gay sex is wonderful. It should not be happening the backyards of residential neighborhoods."[69]

Both MECLA's and GLCSC's actions were significant because former LAPD chief Ed Davis had reached out to MECLA for an endorsement for his upcoming election for US senator. Davis had once referred to homosexuals as "fruits" and "fairies" and oversaw LAPD policies that refused recognizing homosexuals as an "official minority" for fear of giving "recognition to the homosexual activists' perverted causes and provid[ing] them with a degree of credibility."[70] However, seeing his own successful bid for higher office at risk, Davis commented to confused conservative voters in 1984 that he did not believe conservativism could thrive without diversifying its constituent base.[71] MECLA in turn put its full weight behind Davis's campaign, donating the maximum amount allowable under its charter.

Coupled with the respectability politics of the city's neighborhoods of color, this backdrop to gay pride organizing explains why "the Dragons" were policed out of "gay" places like West Hollywood and Silver Lake into Skid Row. It also explains why Tony Castro's 1984 Skid Row exposé was careful to differentiate the homosexuality of its residents from the political projects being staked out in areas west of downtown. He wrote, "Although ['the Dragons'] are selling sex to other men, both police and gay rights activists hesitate to describe it as 'homosexual prostitution.'"[72] Although gay and lesbian activists continued to clash with the LAPD on other issues, this claim was significant because it signaled a general agreement between gay activists and the LAPD that the policing of "the Dragons" was somehow justified and appropriate. Here, it is clear how post-1960s gay rights campaigns primarily benefited white gay men at the expense of other homosexuals positioned as mentally disabled and troublesome, not for their sexual identity but for their primary association with a "permanent underclass."[73]

EXPLAINING THE RACE, SEX, AND PLACE OF THE PERMANENT UNDERCLASS

The creation of a "permanent underclass" suggests the arrival of a new way of viewing and thinking about race and sexuality in Los Angeles. The location of Black and Brown trans people in the concentrated space of Skid Row with the homeless, mentally disturbed, working poor, and the formerly incarcerated during and after the 1984 Olympics demonstrates the power of this new race-making process. Skid Row's multiracial poverty illustrates how Cannon and Hooker conceived of a new multicultural mainstream set apart from a "permanent underclass" that departed from a previous landscape divided between a white heterosexual mainstream and segregated ghettos. Here, both Cannon's and Hooker's affirmations of healthy Black and gay identities mirror the work of activists and sociologists, detailed in the work of Roderick Ferguson, who set out to define Black and gay communities as healthy "neighborhoods" rather than backward "ghettos" by purging queer figures from their communities.[74]

This process of disavowing the least normative members of marginalized communities illustrates how community mental health leaders in LA's neighborhoods of color and gay neighborhoods opened up new opportunities for others to provide new frames to explain the existence of those still deemed to be " severely mentally ill" by new multicultural community standards. Although Cannon's and Hooker's theories worked toward opposite outcomes to police "the Dragons" into Skid Row, the shared discursive belief that mental illness and criminality were manifestations of a thwarted developmental sequence began to appear in new social scientific ideas about how to police space by the 1980s.

Municipal leaders and everyday citizens in all different types of neighborhoods began passing legislation to target unwanted street activity as criminal, hoping to both prevent blight and spur economic development. Such ideas were popularized particularly after George Kelling and James Wilson coined the term *broken windows policing* to describe strategies to maintain order by directing police resources to patrol low-level street activity in an attempt to curb more dangerous forms of crime under the theory that "crime and disorder are inextricably linked, in a kind of developmental sequence."[75] Their strategy targeted so-called "disreputable or obstreperous or unpredictable people" such as "panhandlers, drunks, addicts, rowdy teenagers, prostitutes, loiterers, and the mentally disturbed" under a belief that this zero-tolerance approach prevented serious crimes such as drug trafficking, homicides, theft, and rioting.

Kelling and Wilson admitted that their theory rested on approaches first propagated "in the 1960s, when urban riots were a major problem" and when "social scientists began to explore carefully the order maintenance function of the police ... to reduce the incidence of mass violence." Similar to how community mental health activists defended their ideas as benign, Kelling and Wilson insisted that their theory constituted a new benevolent form of "community policing" because it directed police to enforce the will of "decent folks" in neighborhoods of color rather than that of racist police chiefs or aloof city halls. Their linking of new policing strategies with 1960s social science tied the birth of broken windows policing to the history of community mental health professionals like Cannon, Morales, and Hooker who worked at the intersection of psychiatry and social science to clarify who, in Black, Asian, and Gay neighborhoods, counted as "decent folks" and what constituted "community norms."

The public's desire for increased policing, prisons, and containment strategies like Skid Row was also underwritten by new racially and sexually liberal discourses of "color-" and "sex-blindness" in psychiatry. In 1969, UCLA undertook new steps to extend the scholarship of Hooker and Cannon by hiring Louis Jolyon "Jolly" West as the medical school's new chair of psychiatry and director of the Neuro-Psychiatric Institute. Like Cannon and Hooker, West shared research interests about questions of race and homosexuality as part of a larger field of abnormal psychology focused on "outcasts."

Even though Hooker and Cannon diverged from each other on who or what counted as "normal," West took seriously their arguments that race and homosexuality generally held no intrinsic value in explaining violent behavior.[76] West followed the logic of childhood development underlying explorations about race and homosexuality to focus his research on childhood trauma. In doing so, West unified the concerns of Black elites working in South Los Angeles with those of gay elites in West Los Angeles to propose what he would later term *epidemiology of violence theory*, a concept proposing that dysfunction witnessed as a child created a psycho-*biologic* basis for violent behavior as an adult.

West's theory arose out of joint psychiatric studies conducted by the University of Southern California and UCLA in which he and his research team analyzed the case histories of violent offenders "from all walks of life" who collectively could not be "distinguished by belonging to any particular groups."[77] His findings argued that a significant percentage of the study's violent offender subjects tended to share the same history of being "victims of violence in childhood themselves."[78] In other words, West not only incorporated the basic arguments of Cannon and Hooker but extended them by arguing that the childhood trauma that accounted for the development of a permanent underclass also produced them as violent.

In his writing and speeches, West tended to refer to his research subjects as "violent people" because he believed that it was a more useful category to understand mental illness than race and sexuality and because it helped mark his growing belief that "violent people" were biologically different from nonpathological individuals. During the 1970s and 1980s, West dedicated UCLA's resources to studying his hypothesis that childhood exposure to trauma biologically altered brain functioning in ways that left individuals predisposed to violent behavior in adulthood. To solidify his theories and link UCLA's research agenda with California's mental health and criminal justice system, West proposed the Center for the Study of Reduction of Violence (CSRV) in 1972, known more popularly as the "violence center." The CSRV prioritized investigations of the impact of violence on children through research topics such as violence against children, violent adolescents, the normalization of family violence, sexually violent males, and chromosomal factors to violence.

As Alondra Nelson relates, the Black Panther Party formed a community coalition that in 1973 killed the state's plan to fund the center.[79] Despite the CSRV proposal's relatively race-neutral language, the Panther coalition pointed to the center's proposed heavy use of incarcerated Black and Brown men and children and its rumored deployment of invasive psycho-surgeries to investigate violence as proof that the project was "racist, fascist, sexist, and dangerous to human rights."[80] Although activists were successful in withholding funds to build the center, West nonetheless boasted subsequently that the defeat did not stop researchers at UCLA "from asking questions" about the epidemiology of violence and from "studying it anyway."

By the late 1980s, the rise of broken windows policing and epidemiology of violence theory in mental health discourses revealed that the city's response to the sudden appearance of immigrant Mexican and Central American families living in Skid Row was guided by the threat of a new biological dimension to culture of poverty theory. By 1988, the city admitted that all its efforts to develop the real estate surrounding Skid Row by containing the city's homeless and mentally ill had had the unintentional effect of making Skid Row the most affordable housing district for recently arrived immigrants and asylum seekers. Since 1980, the city had unofficially tracked the number of families living in the neighborhood's SRO hotels by relying on the

Los Angeles Police Department to count heads. The city's census reports revealed that Skid Row's population not only had more "Hispanic" than Black residents but that most of its "Hispanic" residents also "had a higher rate of labor force participation than either whites or blacks."[81]

In 1983, *Los Angeles Times* reporter Dorothy Townsend used these census reports to help readers become more familiar with the new presence of at least three hundred working-poor families that she described as "illegals and refugees" living in SRO hotels.[82] Like many other reporters, Townsend relied on the testimony of Los Angeles police officer Robert Lamont to describe the neighborhood's demographic change. Whereas Lamont recalled that "there wasn't a family with children living on the row" when he first started patrolling in 1972, the neighborhood by 1983 felt "a little worse" because it not only played home to "transvestites," "prostitutes," "winos," "robbers," "dope dealers," and "crazies" but also "kids" whom Townsend described as "mostly tots and some teenagers, who live in seedy walk-up rooms in Skid Row hotels with their parents." With nearly half of the eight hundred children estimated to be living in Skid Row under the age of five, both Townsend and Lamont drew public attention to an alleged public health crisis caused by exposing children to violence. They claimed that violence seemed to "lurk" everywhere—in the neighborhood's doorways, alleys, and especially, in the "bathroom down the hall."

Recognizing that "the ill effects of homelessness on children have been well-documented and the continued homelessness of children contributes to the immediate and future social and psychological pathology," an official city report deemed Skid Row to be "no place for children."[83] To reinforce the identity of Skid Row as a place for unemployed, single, unattached adults, the city prohibited the construction of shelters to house "homeless families," discouraged Skid Row SROs from renting to families with children, and empowered social service workers to facilitate, coordinate, and maximize supportive services to allow families to "re-enter mainstream society in outlying communities."[84] In turn, to ensure that working-poor immigrant families could find housing elsewhere, the city promoted the construction of low-cost multiple-family housing units and developed special rent-subsidy programs and new rental-assistance programs (via loans and direct grants) to enable them to secure permanent housing outside Skid Row. The sum of these programs helped account for the growing identity of neighborhoods like Westlake–MacArthur Park, Pico-Union, and Hoover as Central American neighborhoods.

VIEWING THE LANDSCAPE OF MENTAL WELLNESS FROM KING-DREW

Looking at the landscape of increasing working poverty, homelessness, policing, and incarceration from the vantage point of Watts, Cannon could not help but feel disillusioned. In 1977, he expressed fear that the tide of the 1960s Black social revolution had receded and that the possibilities for seeing Black people as fully human had gone with it. Cannon soberly wrote that "the system is so brutal" that instead of the "rehabilitative experience" he had dreamed of and worked so hard to implement, it had become "a re-criminalizing one."[85] Testifying that "black males are being institutionalized at an alarming rate and are presently, as environmentalists might say, an endangered species," Cannon's account suggests that his critique of "the system" referred to the seamless enmeshment of criminal justice and mental health systems in locking up men of color in both prisons and state hospitals. Hoping to revive a Black social revolution from a distance in Africa, Cannon sent himself into exile to work for the newly formed government of Zimbabwe in 1983.[86]

As this chapter has shown, by the late 1970s and early 1980s municipal leaders and the public increasingly replaced their desire to fund community mental health programs with policing and new segregation patterns exemplified by Skid Row. Eroded by a growing belief within psychiatry that community mental health's psychoanalytic-based practices and methods were unscientific and too immeasurable to prove effective, psychiatry as a discipline progressively turned to revive biological approaches to explain mental illness and relied more deeply on lab-based pharmaceutical solutions to treat it. Such a trend benefited pharmaceutical companies by materially incentivizing physicians to treat mental illness as an individual problem solvable through medication.

These lab-based solutions to individual "race problems" contrast with and are connected to the "race problems" of locking up and keeping perceived troublesome citizens hidden away from sight. Indeed, as Sam Roberts Jr. argues, instead of including all Black people into citizenship as promised, these endeavors underwrite surveillance and policing in communities of color as a common good while reinforcing a liberal conceit within medicine that "health ultimately is purchasable" and "limited only by access to a level economic playing field."[87] Without access to housing and medical care, those abandoned by capital are at greater risk of being incarcerated as a solution.

Cannon's 1977 observations about the mental health system's tendency to recriminalize patients coincided with the passage of California's Uniform Determinate Sentencing Act, a legislative policy that reversed the state's previous commitment to use its criminal justice system to rehabilitate prisoners.[88] According to Ruth Wilson Gilmore, while the law "did not *forbid* rehabilitation," it "excised its central importance" such that the main "purpose of imprisonment for crime is punishment."[89] As a result, California's prison population grew from 16,500 inmates in 1967 to an astonishing 180,000 prisoners by 2018.[90] The scale of incarceration now makes criminal detention centers the largest purveyors of mental health services in the nation—a phenomenon Alisa Roth and others argue serves as strong evidence that the functions of state hospitals have been transferred to other institutions since "deinstitutionalization."[91]

The public's lost appetite for funding community mental health programs but growing taste for policing and incarceration helps explain the renewal of the use of state hospitals as places to cage people. Instead of abolishing them, California's deinstitutionalization movement resulted in a more highly securitized state hospital system to house those indicted as "criminally insane."[92] Instead of the welcoming, community-oriented mental health infrastructure that Cannon initially envisioned, national funding priorities for mental health clinics focused on treating patient populations with chronic illness (such as those afflicted with schizophrenia and drug and alcohol addiction) by requiring locked facilities and greater security measures. The loss of NIMH funding transformed even Cannon's and Morales's cherished youth programs by shifting their identities from being mental health programs towards city and county police-funded "delinquency" prevention programs. As Max Felker-Kantor has shown, these programs proliferated in the 1980s in ways that expanded policing while erasing their mental health origins.[93]

Whereas many community mental health leaders set out to normalize formerly excluded categories of belonging such as racial difference, the net effect of psychiatry's shared discourses of individual and community development produced a city where no "safe space" appeared to exist for the city's Black residents. Whether they lived in Skid Row or in the supposedly rebranded respectable working-class neighborhoods of color, Black residents seemed only to encounter violence—be it from the effects of working poverty or from being hyper-policed. However, as the next chapter shows, if working poverty and places like Skid Row could be made "productive" for the city's economy, so too could violence.

SIX

Profiting from Violence

IN THE FALL OF 1989, *Chicago Tribune* writer Mike Royko used his daily column to laud the Los Angeles County Board of Supervisors' recent decision to renew a military agreement using King-Drew's Trauma Unit and Emergency Medicine Department as a training ground for combat-bound Army surgeons. Since the rise of citizen-led tax revolts in the late 1970s, taxpayers increasingly viewed publicly supported emergency medical services in low-income neighborhoods as fiscally wasteful and ideologically misguided as other despised forms of what they considered welfare, including funding for housing, education, and hospital and clinic services. Royko, however, departed from most liberal progressives by arguing for emergency medicine's significance as a tool for public safety. According to him, public funding for emergency medicine was necessary to convert the number of gunshot wounds and stabbing victims in Watts into the raw clinical material to "prepare every Army doctor for, at the least, World War II 1/2."[1] "If and when the shooting starts," he declared, "the Army must have doctors who know how to treat bullet wounds."

In mounting such a defense, Royko helped illustrate how increased research and innovation within the field of emergency medicine since the 1960s had made it possible for American hospitals to build and sustain labor and technical arrangements previously seen only in US military field hospitals. King-Drew's emergency medicine infrastructure contributed to this history in a novel way by using the Black and Brown youth "who came out on the losing end of a disagreement between gang members" to make its emergency department "about as close to a genuine wartime medical situation as anything this side of Lebanon or Colombia." According to Royko, Watts provided clinicians with "the kinds of gaping, multiple wounds caused by automatic and semiautomatic gunfire" that Army surgeons could expect during war but "rarely" got to see while training in "peacetime" conditions. Royko urged readers, politicians, and other citizens in other large cities—such as New York, Chicago, Detroit, Washington, and Miami—to view the "gang mayhem" in their cities in a similar manner: as an untapped resource for military surgeons to "get a taste of real war, without the inconvenience of traveling abroad" and as an opportunity for taxpayers to "salute" the otherwise nameless young Black and Brown gang youth who unwittingly and unknowingly offered their maimed bodies "for their country."

As sobering of an outlook as Royko's commentary was, his plea actually represented the latest proposal by outside observers to marshal South Los Angeles's expected frequency of gunshot and stabbing wounds toward naturalizing military medicine as everyday medicine for all American citizens. In 1972, consultants for the Department of Health, Education and Welfare and the Commonwealth Foundation, who were reviewing King-Drew Medical Center's mission for its viability as an antipoverty machine, were the first in the nation to recommend extending emergency medicine's latest innovations around mobile treatment of heart attacks toward treating gunshot and stabbing wounds.[2] Together with recommendations around clinic care intended to deliberately concentrate working poverty in neighborhoods of color, King-Drew's emergency medical services helped demonstrate to others how signs of poverty and violence normally considered troublesome and backward could be made "productive" for global capitalism. As Stuart Schrader argues, these practices were not just about bringing America's wars home but also about exporting methods developed around urban policing and control to militarized sites overseas.[3]

Both the 1972 and 1989 recommendations stood in stark contrast to King-Drew's original aims for its health services. Its original master plan sought to combat neighborhood violence by marshaling President Lyndon B. Johnson's signature antipoverty and health initiatives to employ and educate all poor Black people through the new health system's hospital and clinic infrastructure. Rather than innovate emergency medicine, King-Drew's leaders strove to relieve the poor from reliance on emergency room care by giving them the same access as insured white patients to high-cost hospital services through personal family physicians in a public clinic. In this model, medical practitioners prescribed full employment and public access to comprehensive preventive and acute healthcare as antidotes to poverty and violence in a way that made gun and knife injuries preventable and provided precautionary measures against avoidable health conditions.

Growing evidence by 1972 that rates of poverty were likely to continue to worsen, however, pushed LA's city and county officials and opinion leaders to work together to reorient the area's public hospital and clinic infrastructure to help produce and expand the labor-capital relationships that regional business and municipal leaders needed within an emerging "global" economy. Rather than using public clinic and mental health services as vehicles to reverse economic development in neighborhoods of color, municipal officials used public health services as devices designed to keep and attract low-cost laborers that other municipalities were less interested in retaining. By managing rather than displacing or eradicating poverty, the local government's subsidization of health services for low-income residents allowed Los Angeles to attract the kinds of global financial firms needed to maintain economic growth in a period when most large cities experienced deep economic uncertainty.

This chapter traces how the renormalization of poverty and its biomedical effects throughout the 1970s proved productive in constituting emergency medical services as an entirely new biomedical infrastructure fitted to the interests of the nation's new "global" economy by the 1980s. King-Drew's leaders refocused their energies to make gun violence "productive" for new research in emergency medicine, as opposed to organizing employment for more Black breadwinners to better house and feed their families to prevent "the high incidence of homicides and accidents" in the neighborhood.[4] By the early 1980s, county leaders had transformed King-Drew's emergency "waiting room" into a full-fledged Emergency Medicine Department and Trauma Unit connected to a network of publicly and privately owned paramedic technicians, ambulances, helicopters, and base stations capable of addressing incidents in every corner of Southern California.

City and county leaders initially believed that investing in new labor arrangements and technology around treating gunshot wounds and stabbing victims could advance King-Drew's mission of producing healthy and normal citizens of color by expanding the number of employment opportunities for men of color. However, as scholars of sexuality have shown, public perceptions about racial manhood were increasingly influenced by new social scientific and medical research positing that men of color, particularly Black men, seemed incapable of obeying authority and were more prone to being violent. In many cases, scholars often used the discourses of racial and sexual liberalism found in the civil rights, Black Power, and gay liberation movements to portray Black men as somehow more pathological and violent than before the social movements of the 1960s. Psychiatrists and sexologists, for instance, not only used Black men's assertions of independence and power in the 1970s as grounds to diagnose them as schizophrenic but also used prevailing political discourses to portray Black men in prisons as predatory rapists and their supposedly unwilling white heterosexual sexual partners as unwitting "victims."[5]

The effect of these discourses produced a different meaning to research on the treatment of gunshot and stabbing wounds than was originally intended. Rather than being used to combat the problem of "absentee fathers" and "wild youth" through larger social service and job programs, by the early 1980s the rise of emergency medicine helped mobilize the city's mostly white electorate to support greater public funding for emergency medical services, prisons, and policing. Ruth Wilson Gilmore argues astutely that higher rates of violence, poverty, crime, and unemployment had everything to do with the nation's shift away from a manufacturing economy to an economy centered on global finance capital. Voters, by contrast, increasingly interpreted economic deterioration in putatively white rural and suburban neighborhoods as a problem of racial difference and deviance in the inner city (regardless of the actual presence of people of color or their proximity to urban neighborhoods).[6] Particularly after California voters approved a successful anti-tax measure known as Proposition 13 in 1978, politicians and citizens alike increasingly used the rhetoric of "smaller government" to defund public hospital and clinic services in order to fund the enlargement of a carceral state.

This pattern tended to center funding around ideas of public safety more than around ideas of public health. Gilmore observes that lowered property taxes for the wealthy resulted in cuts to a myriad of needed public and social services for all citizens including highway and street maintenance, sanitation, and public health and education. She argues that politicians and taxpayers then invested remaining public funds in the building of prisons and employment of prison guards as a means to recapitalize exurban areas made economically fallow by agricultural industrialization. Rather than result in less government spending, these processes simply represented a different kind of government spending.

White taxpayer desire for emergency medical services revealed a deep willingness to expand certain parts of the state associated with public safety (such as prisons, police, and the military) over other parts of the state associated with welfare (such as public hospitals, clinics, and housing) not out of economic rationality or government efficiency but because such state services constituted a "common good" that obfuscated what Daniel HoSang refers to as the privileges and preferences funneled to "political whiteness." HoSang defines political whiteness as "a formulation of political subjectivity, identity, and community in which whiteness functions as an absent referent within the putatively neutral and abstract terms of liberalism."[7] Politicians and voters, for instance, made "race-neutral appeals to political whiteness" by claiming that publicly funded emergency medicine—unlike locally situated and geographically bound public hospitals and clinics—served *everyone* for any ailment, at anytime, and anyplace. Such appeals, however, obfuscated how publicly funded emergency medical services expanded and guaranteed emergency medicine as a new service that complemented insured white people's access to private hospital and clinic services while increasingly limiting poor people of color's access to just one entry point for care—the emergency department.

The effect of "smaller government" discourses, by the mid-1980s, was thus less successful in producing a smaller state than in producing a landscape of relative health, safety, and security for mostly white citizens who used the ballot box to insulate themselves and their property from the normalization of gun violence and poverty produced by global economic restructuring in neighborhoods of color. Despite all efforts by politicians, physicians, and activists in the city's neighborhoods of color in the 1970s to demonstrate a shared commitment to health, normality, and sexual respectability, white suburban and rural voters in the 1980s empowered a new set of leaders at both local and national levels, such as conservative county supervisor Peter Schabarum and President Ronald Reagan, to carry out policies that literally and figuratively policed the boundaries between whiteness and race with larger police outfits. The cumulative effect of these relationships helped popularize and make profitable emergency medicine in the region's outlying white suburban hospitals while keeping the region's least profitable and sickest patients trapped in what most public health experts increasingly referred to as King-Drew's "safety net."

FROM WAR TO WATTS

Royko's column connected the United States' global military presence around the world to the everyday local dimensions of violence in Los Angeles. It sutured emergency medicine's contemporary and future uses to the history of military medicine that preceded it. Royko admitted that King-Drew's use as a training ground for combat military surgeons represented a "strange twist" in the history of military medicine because it reversed the historical direction of "research and development" around gunshot wounds.[8] According to Royko, the technology, knowledge, and labor arrangements to treat gunshot wounds did not originate in Watts but were developed, at first, by military surgeons empowered to perform "research and development" on soldiers wounded in the United States' military interventions in Asia and "sneak operations" in Africa, the Middle East, and Latin America since World War II. Instead of instantaneously adopting military medicine built for war for domestic uses, Royko intimated to readers that it took "several decades" of "government, industry and science" to pool their resources before everyday Americans came to enjoy the "fringe benefit" of military medicine adapted to peacetime.

What Royko failed to recognize is that King-Drew's role in the history of military medicine did not just connect Watts in time and place to Vietnam in the 1970s and Korea in the 1950s but also illuminated how these connections made it possible for LA's "global economy" to flourish by the 1980s. Highlighting the role of empire in reshaping the global economy after World War II illustrates how the United States began to transition from a manufacturing economy to one centered on transactions of global finance capital by reshaping the economies of newly independent nations in Asia, Africa, and Latin America through war. As US aid to Germany and Japan helped economies in Europe and East Asia rebound by the 1960s, US diplomats and businessmen tied the fates of newly independent nations along the Pacific Rim, the South Atlantic, and Caribbean waters to American cities like Los Angeles. The same economic context that normalized violence in the development of military medicine in these "developing" markets before the 1960s also normalized violence in American cities like Los Angeles that, in turn, regularized military medicine as emergency medicine by the 1980s.

Unlike the capitalist landscape dominated by European empires before 1945, the expansion of the United States' economy after World War II increasingly required US diplomats and businessmen to convince political, opinion, and business leaders and citizens in formerly colonized nations of the benefits of achieving economic and political independence as capitalist democracies. As many scholars of Cold War history have shown, US diplomats exploited the threat of communist invasion or internal revolt facing leaders of newly independent nations by offering US military protection to regimes in exchange for open trade with the United States. As the proliferation of US military bases and military exercises in "developing" nations (such as Mexico, South Korea, and the Philippines) and in US territories in the Pacific and the Caribbean (such as Hawai'i and Puerto Rico) shows, many international figures saw such arrangements as providing their otherwise vulnerable nations with security as they progressed toward modernity, economic maturity, and true political independence.[9] In other nations, however, such as Vietnam, Laos, Guatemala, the Congo, Chile, and Nicaragua, US diplomacy took a more aggressive and violent route by suppressing opposition to capitalist expansion through either direct military intervention or covert military support of leaders and paramilitary units allied with the United States.[10]

In many ways, the US efforts to expand capitalism and electoral democracy in newly independent nations took on approaches similar to domestic antipoverty efforts. They entailed recruiting and empowering indigenous actors by carrying out a shared vision of progress centered on capitalism and democracy. By the 1960s, US efforts to reflect the racial and ethnic composition of occupied territories in the faces of soldiers also increasingly reflected similar policies by American police departments to recruit more people of color.[11] By the 1960s, Asian American participation in the military had not only helped further entrench the US occupation of the Hawaiian Kingdom through American statehood but also helped bolster the willing participation of South Korean and Filipino soldiers in the United States' war on Vietnam. As Simeon Man argues, such operations advanced the interests of American empire in the region, while recruitment into the work of soldiering allowed Asian American and Asian soldiers alike to see their participation as forwarding an "Asia for Asians."[12]

Despite claims by a growing class of global elites of a more inclusive multiracial and multinational world stage, by the late 1960s the "stabilization" of new markets for trade through military intervention brought two opposing economic trends within the United States to bear on poor and working-class people in nations targeted by US business interests. First, agricultural innovations in technology and labor that had displaced workers of color in the rural South and West were also simultaneously applied to foreign markets targeted by US businesses for development.[13] As land reforms economically and spatially displaced workers in rural sectors, American businesses also used the military suppression of opposition to new economic policies as an opportunity to move manufacturing operations closer to consumer markets in Europe, Asia, and Latin America to better compete with German and

Japanese firms revived by US policy. Although politicians, bureaucrats, and diplomats rhetorically positioned the poor affected by US policies abroad as newly empowered "consumers" and as the intended beneficiaries of capitalist economic development, the reality of new economic development policies caused daily individual and intergenerational crises for the poor through displacement, violence, and underemployment and unemployment.

Although many Central and South Americans at the start of the 1960s were considered by power brokers to be both spatially and culturally distant from the Black Americans who had migrated to California since the 1940s, the tumult of widespread agricultural corporatization, industrialization abroad, and deindustrialization in the United States steadily pushed Central and Latin American migrants—with or without authorized entry—into the same South Los Angeles neighborhoods as Black Americans by the 1970s. American workers up until the 1960s understood their relative value and position within the US economy based on their proximity and relationship to manufacturing, but the combined result of all these processes newly subordinated employment in the United States to high-end "service" sector financial jobs geared toward transacting the capital needed to move manufacturing and goods from one market in a global economy to another. These shifts also led to a proliferation of low-wage producer and consumer service jobs.

While these processes further marginalized workers of color already made peripheral within a receding manufacturing economy, they also increasingly affected employment for white workers who had for some time felt secure in the nation's economy. Whereas following World War II white working-class men without college degrees could reliably count on achieving well-paying middle-class jobs by getting hired into unionized manufacturing plants, the emerging new global economy now required advanced college degrees in law, real estate, and finance to achieve the same level of job security.[14] For many white workers—especially those unable to quickly readjust, retool, and reeducate themselves in a rapidly deindustrializing economy—these shifting labor-capital relationships thrust their lives into economic precarity similar yet not identical to those of many newly arrived immigrants and people of color.

These shifting labor-capital arrangements between metropole and empire in the late 1960s and 1970s produced the conditions that made military medical techniques adaptable to civilian use through the conflict engendered by what economists term a "relative surplus population"—a population of laborers unable to be immediately absorbed by a given market because of their redundancy or lack of needed skills within a particular economic system. As

Ruth Wilson Gilmore argues, workers of all races and places took different approaches to cope with deindustrialization's patterns of worklessness and un- and underemployment, but many poor and working-class workers of color turned to "alternative modes of social production, given their utter abandonment by capital."[15] Instead of just waiting for the economy to change, she argues that urban residents turned to reproduce daily and intergenerational life through alternative kinship patterns such as single-headed households, multigenerational homes, and gangs.[16] The worsening economic conditions only exacerbated the preexisting "'concentration effects' of sociospatial apartheid" by increasing people of color's exposure to "high rates of intentional and accidental violence," "premature death from a wide range of causes," and "persistent but hostile interaction with state agencies, especially welfare, family services, courts, and the police."

Gilmore shows that voters turned to solve the problem of too many people chasing too few jobs, associated with deindustrialization and corporate agriculture, by incapacitating the labor of surplus populations through caging and deporting them with expanded prisons and policing. They rejected the alternative of enlarging the state's capacity to employ, feed, clothe, and care for every citizen. Politicians, bureaucrats, and activists from neighborhoods of color increasingly joined white voters in directing the police to target their own communities in order to distinguish hardworking and sexually respectable citizens from those considered violent and undesirable. In this way, militarized policing—by way of officers in the United States or soldiers in spaces of American empire—served as an important and necessary component in controlling populations abandoned by capital as economies were reengineered by racial elites toward unifying as many markets as possible into one "global" capitalist economy.

The overall effect of uninterrupted US military intervention in the Pacific and Latin America since World War II thus deepened by the early 1970s a crisis of unemployment for poor people of color in the United States while at the same time perfecting technology and techniques within combat military medicine to effectively address gunshot wounds, injuries, and other forms of somatic trauma. As early as the 1950s, advances in patient transport, evacuation, and surgical know-how were gathered and enhanced during the Korean War through what the US military referred to as "Mobile Army Surgical Hospitals," better known as MASH.[17] Yet, as the next section shows, the appetite and willingness to deploy military medicine for civilian use first required everyday Americans to normalize and naturalize gun violence as an expected and likely outcome of living in the metropole of empire. That is, voters remained unwilling to invest in emergency medicine until leaders made new compelling arguments as to why the government should invest in technology to save people from gunshot wounds rather than invest in programs designed to prevent them from getting shot in the first place.

THE PATH OF GOOD INTENTIONS

Although global economic restructuring eventually created the conditions that inspired politicians and taxpayers to fund military medicine for civilian use in the United States as emergency medicine, its adaptation did not immediately originate with a desire to naturalize gun violence or normalize policing and prisons as everyday expected facets of American life. In fact, the historical development of emergency medicine in Los Angeles was inspired by the 1965 Watts Uprisings, the very citizen revolt that precipitated the construction of King-Drew Medical Center. As the uprisings were widely interpreted as an illustration of how poor Black workers were already marginalized enough within the nation's manufacturing economy to protest it through revolt, the construction of King-Drew's public hospital and clinic system and the development of publicly funded emergency medical systems both illustrate how county leaders responded to a crisis, asking how to deliver healthcare to neighborhoods and regions that were too poor or too geographically isolated to sustain a private "community" hospital on their own.

Los Angeles County Supervisor Kenneth Hahn was particularly inspired to explore a new way to deliver healthcare to poor and distant neighborhoods after the County Board of Supervisors felt compelled to override the majority-white electorate's rejection of Proposition A in the spring of 1966, which would have built King-Drew Medical Center with taxpayer bonds. Throughout the campaign, many residents in other poor and rural areas of the county commented on their desire to have a publicly funded hospital in their neighborhoods. Although many voters attested in newspaper op-eds to their willingness to pass Proposition A so long as leaders also looked into passing a bond to build a new public hospital in their neighborhood, a quiet but discernible "Don't Reward Rioting" campaign picked up enough traction to cause the referendum to fail.[18] Some newspapers, such as the *Downey Leader*, for instance, wrote that "no one doubts the appalling need for a hospital in the Watts area," but contended that it was "the responsibility of county officials not to rest on their laurels once they have ensured help for Watts, but to maintain a vigilant eye on all of the county for service to all citizens—not just those in areas that have been brought to the public eye."[19]

Hahn interpreted the failure of Proposition A as evidence that taxpayers expected the government to continue funding healthcare services as a public good but were increasingly unwilling to raise new taxes to provide them. Fearing that Black citizens might renew rioting after the rejection of the referendum, Hahn moved to do two things. First, he rallied his fellow supervisors to explore using County General Funds (a large bank of unallocated funds in the county's budget) to fund the construction of the medical center without voter approval. Although the board eventually settled on funding King-Drew by entering into a "special districting" agreement with the City of Los Angeles to build it as a joint project, the existence of a general fund large enough to contemplate using it demonstrated how officials viewed approving new budget items as more or less a political and moral issue rather than as budget restraint due to lack of revenue.

Second, Hahn began to explore enhancing existing public and private services in his district to provide health services that did not require the costly expenditure of building new institutions. Knowing the difficulty of attracting private hospital investment in rural areas and in neighborhoods of color far from public hospitals, Hahn turned to the county forester and fire department warden, Chief K. E. Klinger, in September 1966 with a proposal to connect rural and poor regions to existing county hospitals through a new "paramedic program."[20] Hahn received early support from the American College of Surgeons' Committee on Trauma. He believed that the fire department's policy to have all employees obtain "Red Cross" training and its existing operation of rescue vehicles to address heart attacks, drownings, and emergencies could be extended to provide an "essential lifesaving service in certain areas where private ambulance companies fail to meet their responsibilities."[21]

Klinger and other fire officials, however, were hesitant to expand their services beyond firefighting until the assassination of New York Senator and presidential candidate Robert "Bobby" F. Kennedy illustrated the limitations of existing ambulance and emergency care. At 12:10 a.m. on June 8, 1968, Sirhan Sirhan famously assassinated Kennedy with two gunshot wounds to the head after Kennedy had just concluded his victory speech as the winner of the California Democratic presidential primary. The assassination set in motion a pair of ambulance "attendants" who—up until receiving a dispatch

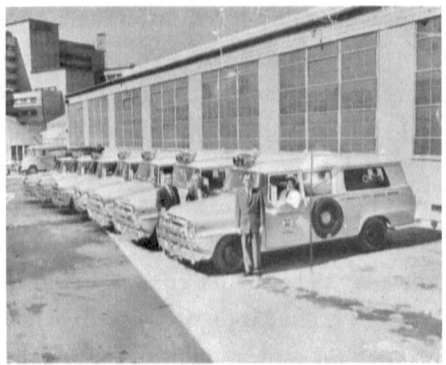

FIGURE 8. Ambulance services, 1958

These seven brand new ambulances, delivered to the County of Los Angeles in March of 1958, illustrate how ambulance design focused on transportation with little interest in technology or the application of medical expertise. Posing with Supervisor Hahn (center) are Leonard Beardslee, Walter Gross, and C. A. Ratliff. Source: "Ambulances for County General," HE Box 2078, Los Angeles Herald Examiner Collection (TESSA Digital Collections, Los Angeles Public Library).

describing an injured man who "had fell down in the Embassy Ballroom" of the Ambassador Hotel—had been "standing" around the Los Angeles Central Receiving Hospital, the city's designated "emergency hospital."[22] However, after successfully retrieving and transporting Kennedy from the hotel to Central Receiving's emergency room at 12:30 a.m., physicians were forced to transfer him four city blocks to Good Samaritan, yet another hospital, after realizing that they could not fully stabilize him without blood plasma and X-ray equipment. The doctors at Good Samaritan were equipped with the right tools but unprepared to immediately perform surgery. Kennedy was not wheeled into the ninth-floor surgical suite until physicians roused from their beds at home arrived at 2:45 a.m. After three hours and forty minutes of surgery, Kennedy was officially pronounced dead.

The missed opportunity to save Kennedy illustrated how emergency room systems prior to the late 1960s lacked the sophistication and coordination required to treat critically ill and injured patients. As Matthew Edwards has argued, "pre-hospital care" before the late 1960s "emphasized speedy and reliable 'transportation without treatment,'" and used hospital transporters in jobs that had "no formal requirements" and lacked "even basic first-aid training."[23] As the architecture of Good Samaritan's intensive care unit revealed, the few hospitals capable of addressing critically ill or injured patients before the 1970s often reserved the talent, labor, and resources to address them for insured patients scheduled for operations during the day. Most emergency rooms of the era were thus understood as services where working-class people without health insurance could access care after regular hours with physicians who picked up work to supplement wages they were unable to obtain through their regular work.[24]

The embarrassment over Kennedy's death renewed Hahn's appeal to innovate emergency medical services through existing public safety services. In 1969, county fire department chief Richard Houts joined Hahn in launching two pilot paramedic demonstration programs funded by the Department of Health, Education, and Welfare. According to Andrew Simpson, the federal government's grantee structure by the late 1960s did more than individually enrich program grantees with funds.[25] The iterative process of applying for grants and grant renewals also helped reconstitute technology and systems developed elsewhere and for other purposes into one coherent new purpose by forcing grantees to pay attention to each other's developments. In Los Angeles, the county's grant allowed officials to pull equipment formerly used in isolation toward new uses in mobile units. Hahn's "rescue vehicles," for instance, pulled defibrillators and electrocardiogram machines used in operating rooms for cardiac arrests; carried sirens, gurneys, and various medical splits used in fire rescue operations; and deployed two-way radios used in military operations into automobiles repurposed as modern ambulances.

The Department of Health, Education, and Welfare's paramedic grants to the county resulted in two different ambulance models to test whether maximizing a vehicle's technology or its speed produced better health outcomes. The experiments were each separately supervised by a different kind of agency, one private and one public, to check how portable and scalable each type of service could be for other locations. The first project, known the "heart ambulance" project, sought to maximize a vehicle's technology by reproducing the settings of an operating room on wheels. It was led by Dr. Walter Graf, president of the Los Angeles County Heart Association, and ran out of three private community hospitals and a private ambulance company to demonstrate how municipalities dependent on private providers could run a similar program.[26]

The second project, known as the "heart rescue vehicle" project, carried a modest amount of technology to prioritize speed. It was led by Dr. Michael Criley, director of cardiology at Harbor-UCLA, and involved Harbor-UCLA's emergency department and a local fire department station to illustrate how municipalities with larger budgets could run a program by re-training existing personnel and converting existing resources.[27] In the first year, the two programs trained eighteen county and eleven city firemen and two private ambulance attendants as some of the first paramedics in the United States.

Hahn was careful to make sure that residents in pilot demonstration neighborhoods understood that the new service was not like the "transport

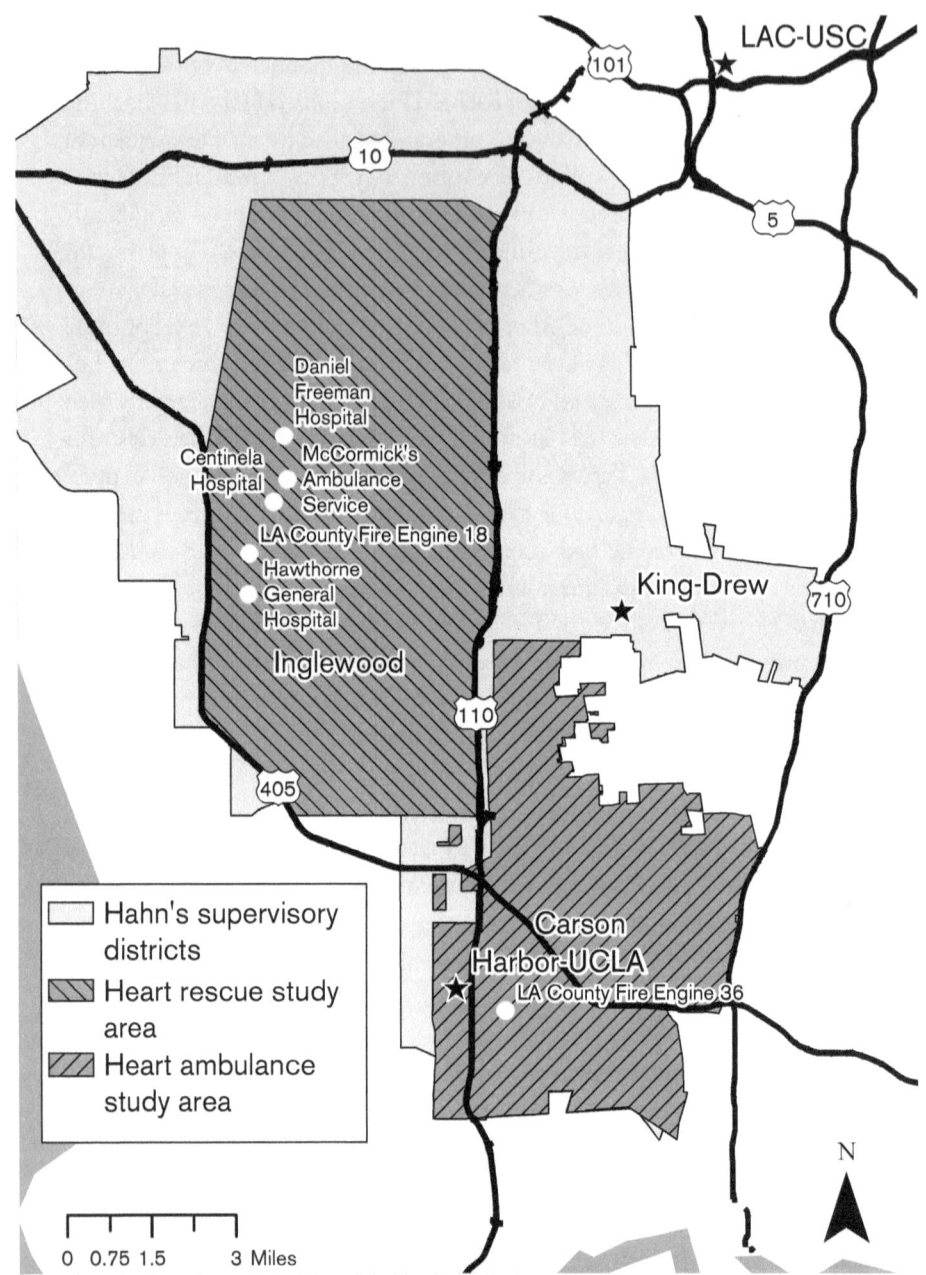

MAP 12. The county's paramedic demonstration projects

Hahn piloted two different paramedic demonstration projects in two suburban neighborhoods in his district. Each project was overseen by either a private or public agency in order to demonstrate the scalability and portability of paramedic programs to different kinds of municipalities. He hoped the success of these two projects would eventually be used at King-Drew. Map: Tyler Munn.

only" ambulance service they were accustomed to, highlighting that all the personnel associated with it were not "attendants" but newly specially trained "paramedics."[28] In a pre-recorded phone message to constituents in Carson, Hahn made sure residents knew the service was "not an ambulance" but "a highly skilled County Fire Rescue Team which will respond to calls from residents of the Carson area for cardiac and *other emergencies*" (emphasis mine). His mention of *other emergencies* reveal that, while the program was funded as a project addressing heart attacks, it was always understood as a program to address much more.

The new service was a far cry from private ambulance units driven by attendants with no first aid training. Hahn's message explained that instead of calling the hospital, having a physician diagnose a heart attack over the phone, and then dispatching a private ambulance service to pick up a nurse at the hospital before retrieving the patient experiencing a heart attack, its modernized rescue vehicles could be deployed "at the first sign of a heart attack" by either a fire or police department dispatcher "twenty-four hours per day, seven days per week." The critically ill or injured could expect "two Fire rescue personnel and a nurse" to use "portable equipment" to serve them "on-site" and "in-route" from the scene of an emergency to the hospital.

The use of two-way radios for simultaneous communication between paramedics in the field and staff at the hospital helped spur innovation that brought physician specialists once situated elsewhere in the hospital to the emergency room. In 1971, Los Angeles County General Hospital, with its affiliated medical school at the University of Southern California, became the first academic Emergency Medicine Department in the nation. Under the direction of an obstetrics and gynecology specialist, Dr. Gail V. Anderson, the program produced some of the first physicians ever trained specifically as emergency medicine doctors. The program's biggest innovation, however, was the assignment of a full complement of around-the-clock specialists (such as anesthesiologists, surgeons, surgical pediatricians, and orthopedic surgeons) who staffed the emergency room alongside emergency medicine doctors.

The simultaneous effect of increasing investment in the capital, labor, and knowledge of ambulance care and in emergency medicine departments helped account for the county's astonishing "perfect record" of receiving and saving 136 heart attack victims in the first six months of operation. The success and popularity of the program not only led to a series of city and county leaders inquiring about expanding the program to include their municipalities but helped convince conservative governor Ronald Reagan to support the expansion of emergency medical services. In 1971, Reagan helped Hahn pass a law authorizing paramedics to practice without the supervision of doctors or nurses and, in 1972, extended funding to expand paramedic training and enlarge the demonstration project's geography to encompass the entirety of Los Angeles County.

More important than establishing an entirely new publicly funded service was Hahn's innovation in funding emergency medical systems as a new municipal service. Despite the success of the pilot demonstration projects, Houts and his deputy Stanley Barlow feared new paramedic services would "dilute," drain, or take away from existing firefighting duties and budgets.[29] Rather than argue for continuing the service, they threatened to walk away from overseeing the project's expansion unless "funding [for new firefighting services] be provided from other sources."[30] As they pointed out, they believed that the budget to fund the twenty pairs of retrained firefighters and new ambulance units estimated to be needed to achieve full coverage for all of Los Angeles County would cost $3.5 to $4 million that the department did not have in its current budget.

Reluctant to raise taxes given the anti-tax posture voters took with Proposition A in 1966, and unwilling to bypass voters by creating a Special Tax District like the one used to build King-Drew, Hahn devised an entirely new funding scheme by contracting emergency medical services to independent municipalities willing to foot a portion of the county's total operating costs. By the end of 1972, the speculative belief that the county's emergency medical services would soon make profits from contracting its services with the nearly seventy-seven independent cities within Los Angeles County led the County Board of Supervisors to approve the opening of a second paramedic training program at Los Angeles County–USC Medical Center to complement its newly created academic emergency medicine department. By 1975, the scheme not only led to county contracts with thirty-seven cities but had also led twenty-six other cities to either fund their fire department units or contract with private ambulance companies who had raised their standards since 1969.[31] Hahn's efforts to create a solution to the problem of distributing health in response to voter rejection to Proposition A in 1966 led him to innovate emergency medicine by developing a system extending the reach of existing public and private hospitals while bringing the benefits of wartime medicine closer to home. More important, he also introduced a new way to govern by transforming government into a business catering to other municipalities.

NO GOOD DEED GOES UNPUNISHED

As well-intentioned as Hahn's actions were, his efforts to establish modern emergency medical systems eventually contributed to a budget crisis in the late 1970s that was only exacerbated by his simultaneous efforts to build clinics and expand preventative health services at King-Drew and in all of Los Angeles County's public hospital systems. In 1978, California voters revolted against such expenditures by passing new restrictive tax laws limiting the public expenditure of local and state governments; by the early 1980s they had also elected many conservative politicians who continued to slash government social welfare budgets on their behalf. The effect of these developments would pit proponents of public hospital and clinic services against proponents of emergency medical services in a series of budget crises that took place throughout the 1980s.

The irony of the anti-tax movements of the late 1970s and 1980s is that many voters failed to see how liberal politicians like Hahn, and the agents empowered by the county to carry out new government initiatives, such as the Drew Medical School's Black physician leaders, saw themselves as also working toward a "smaller" and more "efficient" government. Until fire department officials presented evidence of emergency medicine's true costs, Hahn initially framed his efforts around emergency medicine as a new efficient and cost-saving public service because it utilized "existing community resources" and did "not require additional personnel or vehicles."[32] Given that courses to retrain and outfit firemen and ambulance attendants as paramedics took only three months, he also naively believed that all agents involved in the enhancement of emergency medicine were already in the business of addressing emergencies—be they fire officials, ambulance company employees, or hospital staff.

Drawing on direct references to war and soldiering, Hahn also argued that the medical expertise perfected on the Vietnam War's battlefields could be marshaled toward fighting the War on Poverty, particularly around the nationwide physician and nursing shortage unleashed in the wake of Medicare and Medicaid. In this respect, Hahn preferred to refer to rescue workers as paramedics rather than the more increasingly popular term—emergency medicine technicians—because it helped citizens identify modern emergency medicine with military medicine rather than ambulance services once largely associated with funeral companies. If soldiers could "save men in the field of battle" as paramedics, he argued, they could "certainly save lives here" with the same title.[33]

Hahn's vision to redeploy Black veterans as paramedics brought the aim of Moynihan's culture of poverty thesis to masculinize Black men together with what William A. Williams calls an "empire way of life." In fact, according to Ellen Herman, the U.S. military's Project 100,000 directly recruited Moynihan's thesis into its program rationale.[34] The project sought to use military service as a social welfare program designed to recruit, in the words of Defense Secretary Robert McNamara, the "subterranean poor," and "cure" them of the "idleness, ignorance, and apathy" believed to be induced in Black men raised in female-headed households.[35] According to Williams, programs like Hahn's paramedic retraining asked Black veterans to extend the gendered logic of war well past the battleground to constitute an imperial "outlook" and "way of life" that informed their lives as everyday citizens.[36]

Hahn saw the success of the county's initial paramedic demonstration projects as a way to meaningfully transfer the education and skills that many Black veterans developed during the Vietnam War to employment opportunities they were normally ineligible to explore in the United States based on their class and educational backgrounds. Similar to other ambulance demonstration projects funded by the Department of Health, Education, and Welfare in the late 1960s, such as the Freedom House Ambulance Company in Pittsburgh, Hahn used subsequent paramedic training grants "to train discharged military medical corpsmen to become extensions of the physician."[37] Instead of the largely integrated "white" neighborhoods of Inglewood and Carson, Hahn organized representation on county paramedic advisory committees to situate new training programs and services to be based out of King-Drew's health service area under the hope that such programs would indirectly benefit taxpayers by reducing the number of welfare recipients in Black neighborhoods.[38]

However, despite Hahn's early promise to have paramedics "operating out of Martin Luther King Hospital when it opens," the Black physician leaders of King-Drew were more reticent about the place of emergency medicine in their vision for the hospital.[39] King-Drew's administrators, Dr. Mitchell Spellman and Dr. M. Alfred Haynes, like many of the National Medical Association's members, still regarded emergency room care as a sign of second-class citizenship because of its wide cultural association as the hospital's unofficial "back door." Instead of gaining access to hospital services through a private physician's referral and appointment, as most white patients were accustomed to, most poor patients and most people of color gained access to hospital services through the emergency waiting room, where wait times were often long, rooms were overcrowded, and care was brisk and impersonal.

Instead of the inferior treatment associated with emergency rooms, Spellman and Haynes's vision for modern healthcare aimed to acculturate poor Black people to mainstream medicine by emphasizing clinic services that would serve as the new "front door" to modern hospital services. Like Hahn, they framed clinic services as also ultimately serving the overriding interests of white taxpayers by creating "smaller" and more "efficient" government that reduced welfare rolls by using health services as a ploy to educate the poor on how to be more self-reliant and economically dependent. More important, it also sought to reduce commitments to public hospital care by mandating that Medicare- and Medicaid-eligible patients obtain a referral from a clinic physician before presenting themselves at the hospital. For all these reasons, King-Drew's decision-makers made sure that the hospital's emergency room was small and available only on weekends and at night.

By the time the hospital finally opened in early 1972, however, Black community health activists had come to believe that the medical center's emergency services would include the latest technological innovations because of Hahn's promises in September 1971 to locate a new paramedic base station and new training program for emergency medicine physician assistants at King-Drew.[40] When the hospital opened for operation, citizen activists registered their frustrations by protesting the perceived lack of emergency room services. For instance, an anonymous leaflet disseminated with the title "ATTENTION: The King Hospital is a Potential Death Trap" drew the public's attention to false claims by hospital leadership describing the hospital and its emergency services as "ready to open" and "fully equipped and adequately staffed with personnel, including bi-lingual employees."[41] Instead, the leaflet leaked information to community members that the hospital's "services were limited" and that its emergency room was "*not* accepting serious emergency cases!!"

The leaflet pointed to how local community members felt differently about emergency medical services than the hospital's leadership. Many savvy community activists, such as those involved with local welfare rights and antipoverty organizations, saw the medical center's referral policies as yet another ploy to deny and withhold lifesaving hospital and emergency services that welfare-eligible recipients were legally entitled to access as citizens. Many community members also saw the assumption that it was possible for poor and working-class people to make and maintain scheduled appointments as misguided and foolish, given that most worked for employers who did not make regular and predictable work shifts or lived lives where it was too difficult or

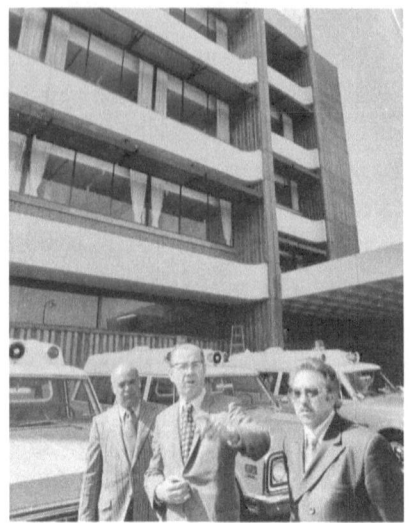

FIGURE 9. Bringing wartime medicine home

Hahn sought to use the opening of King-Drew as an occasion to showcase the county's latest emergency ambulances. These models illustrate the success of the more flexible and affordable "heart rescue" vehicles, which carried portable medical device kits and featured lights, sirens, two-way radios and other technology from police and military units. Standing with Hahn (center) are Carl Ballton and Dan Grindell. Source: "Hahn attends opening of new hospital," March 27, 1972, HE Box 1117, Los Angeles Herald Examiner Collection (TESSA Digital Collections, Los Angeles Public Library).

expensive to coordinate healthcare. Especially as the quality of emergency medical services made emergency rooms both popular and convenient in white neighborhoods and among paying patients, leaflets like the one distributed after the opening of King-Drew demonstrated how many poor Black residents no longer associated emergency medical care with stigma.

The consultants for the Department of Health, Education, and Welfare and the Commonwealth Foundation charged with reviewing King-Drew's mission and purpose in 1972 did not see emergency medicine in a negative light. Instead, they viewed the proliferation of discourses around emergency medicine as a sign of its significance within a larger consumer rights movement. The elevation of emergency medicine's technology, labor arrangements, and expertise was thus understood by experts to deliver healthcare on terms considered ideal for the "consumer." Under the banner of consumer rights, King-Drew's leaders were thus encouraged to implement programs to meet the consumer needs of those empowered by Medicare and Medicaid to seek care in its health system. To satisfy the projected health needs of women and children on welfare, for instance, King-Drew's administrators grouped various mother and baby services into program offices in its comprehensive health clinics. These services, in turn, complemented the pediatric, obstetrics, and gynecological services in the system's hospital.

The same rhetoric of consumer rights encouraged King-Drew's leaders to see a new opportunity to innovate emergency medicine's advancements around heart attacks to treat citizens affected by "homicides" and gun violence. To bolster the importance of treating gunshot and stabbing wounds, King-Drew's consultants used the rhetoric and methods of community medicine against itself by arguing that viewing violence as a social issue had led its leaders to overlook it as a medical issue. By 1972, Dr. M. Alfred Haynes, King-Drew's chair of community medicine, had prioritized the collection and ordering of a community's health data points to help community members direct resources and talent toward the community's "biggest killers." However, despite the fact that Haynes's data showed that gunshot and stabbing wounds were the fourth- and fifth-leading causes of death in the neighborhood, after cancer, heart disease, and stroke, Haynes and others continued to regard employment as the only appropriate answer to treating violence.[42]

Under the rhetoric that emergency medicine services were somehow more humane, sensitive, and relevant to the lives of poor people, after 1972 King-Drew expanded its emergency medicine infrastructure by immediately authorizing the construction of a new paramedic base station. By 1976, the hospital had expanded its emergency "waiting room" and built a separate trauma care area dedicated to treating gunshot wounds and car accidents. In 1978, the center formally transformed its emergency room into a full-fledged emergency department by launching a fully accredited emergency medicine residency program.[43] At the same time, the county built or repurposed infrastructure to operate nearly sixty comprehensive neighborhood health centers throughout the region to counterbalance emergency department usage at each of its public hospitals.

By the 1980s, the combined effect of the county's clinic and emergency medicine policies had helped make the economy of Los Angeles productive by attempting to manage poverty in unconventional ways. From the perspective of everyday poor citizens of color, the county's expansion of clinic, hospital, and emergency room services helped maintain California's reputation as an ideal destination for settlement because it provided poor workers of color with health services equal to those found in white neighborhoods and that were difficult to find in other big cities without having private health insurance. For city and county leaders, the ample number of poor and working-class workers of color made possible by publicly supported health services, in turn, helped attract and secure global financial firms looking to locate their headquarters in places where labor was cheap and healthcare coverage for low-income workers was not considered an "industry standard" needed for employers to hire and retain workers.

Rather than serve the interests of the poor, then, the true purpose of all the county's liberal "multicultural" health policies was to appease the interests of mostly white taxpayers through the city's renewed ability to address rising unemployment rates in white suburban neighborhoods through new "service sector" employment opportunities made possible by investments in poverty. Whereas workers of color increasingly found service-sector work that was infrequent and underpaid, white workers with the ability to retool their skills through education increasingly found stable and higher-paid work in expanded service-sector industries such as healthcare, government, law, and finance. In short, rather than regard the region's poverty as a negative or undesirable trend, the city's and county's investments in managing poverty through expanded hospital, clinic, and emergency room services throughout the 1970s helped insulate white workers and their neighborhoods from the most volatile effects of global capitalist restructuring.

However, despite the critical contributions of workers of color to the city's reinvention as a center for global finance, the region's mostly white taxpayers responded to the high rates of welfare and violence seen in neighborhoods of color by overwhelmingly passing Proposition 13 in 1978. Although the statewide measure formally amended California's constitution to limit the revenue that counties could generate from property taxes to just 1 percent of property value, citizens frequently referred to the referendum in political and everyday discourse as a "tax revolt" against "big government," welfare dependency, and the race-based antipoverty initiatives of the 1960s. Its architect and most public figure, Howard Jarvis, for instance, rallied supporters to view the initiative as an act affirming the rights of homeowners, "the most important people in this country," by reaffirming the principles of "life, liberty and property—not 'life, liberty and welfare or life, liberty and food stamps.'"[44]

Jarvis made it a point to use King-Drew's services as an example of reasons to roll back taxes. In fact, he developed early criticism of "big government" from observations of municipal leaders' more frequent use of bond mechanisms, like King-Drew's Joint Power Agreement authority, not requiring voter approval.[45] Although Joint Power Agreements made a whole host of services like running water, sanitation, and hospital services possible in white neighborhoods, King-Drew's close association with Black neighborhoods and welfare dependency made it an easy target for Jarvis. Just a month after King-Drew's opening, Jarvis took to the *Canyon Crier* to explain how voters were now on the hook for a reported $34.5 million hospital that was originally slated to only cost $12.5 million and that voters had "said 'No'" to in

1966. Jarvis called for Joint Power Agreement authority to be abolished or renamed "license to steal authority" because such arrangements bound taxpayers to "costs without limit."[46]

Proposition 13's effect did more than just give homeowners a massive tax break. It also indirectly subsidized large retail corporations and real estate companies through new sales tax zones and gated subdivisions. Denied the revenue generated by homeowners' property taxes, municipal leaders turned to generate revenue through the property taxes paid by "big box" retail stores. They also shifted towards developing special tax districts that essentially billed residents living in new high-end subdivisions to pay for roads, parks, and schools. The coupling of these phenomena led municipal officials to support exclusionary measures, like building gated communities and expanding police forces to protect both the property of retailers and homeowners. By weaving "financial cocoons around many suburban subdivisions," William Fulton argues Proposition 13 "forced [municipal leaders] to view the urban landscape not as a place where people live and work and die, but as a cash register."[47]

Although many liberal progressive Democratic leaders, such as Hahn, California's governor Ed "Jerry" Brown, and Los Angeles's mayor Tom Bradley, spent much of the late 1960s and 1970s sharing most voters' desires to reduce welfare dependency, the measure's success was politically interpreted as a boon for conservative Republicans at both local and national scales. The measure helped bolster the political influence of Schabarum, one of the only two supervisors to support the measure, and ex-governor Reagan, who heralded the measure's passage as proof that taxpayers wanted to end "excessive taxation, excessive spending and excessive government."[48] Both Schabarum, reelected as county supervisor in 1978, and Reagan, elected as US president in 1980, exploited the "tidal wave of protest" associated with Proposition 13's success to exert greater control over public resources as the leading voices for white suburban and rural voters in Los Angeles at the local and national levels.[49]

THE CALCULUS OF POLITICAL WHITENESS

The influences of Supervisor Schabarum and President Reagan by the early 1980s were critical because their elections empowered them to decide the distribution of public services after the fallout of Proposition 13. Although the proposition passed in 1978, California's legislature organized a statewide "bailout" that expended a statewide budget surplus on county and city services before fully confronting Proposition 13's budgetary constraints in 1981 and 1982. This "lag" in decision-making helped activists concerned about the distribution of public funding to health programs organize and mount arguments about how "essential" public health programs piloted during the early 1970s had become by the early 1980s. While defenders of publicly funded clinics and emergency medical services both drew on the importance of preventative healthcare and emergency healthcare as critical for modern public health, proponents of emergency medical services also increasingly drew upon its growing significance to ideas of public safety and policing.

The outcome of public health budget decisions in the wake of Proposition 13 demonstrates how the growth of emergency medicine increasingly took on greater meaning and significance for politicians and white voters in suburban and rural districts since its modern reinvention in the late 1960s. It was not long after the completion of Hahn's first paramedic demonstration program that advancements in emergency medicine began to capture the imagination of citizens well beyond the inner-city contexts that first inspired Hahn to explore innovating fire department rescue vehicles. In fact, Hahn's efforts to address the uneven distribution of healthcare helped launch the career of James O. Page, a fire chief who worked alongside Dr. Walter Graf in designing the first paramedic training program at Daniel Freeman Hospital in Inglewood. After retiring from the fire service in 1972, Page worked to innovate and replicate LA's emergency medical systems in mostly rural and suburban neighborhoods across the United States by serving first as a bureaucrat charged with building emergency medicine systems, and then as a lobbyist for the Advance Coronary Treatment Foundation, a special interest group dedicated to expanding emergency medicine.

Page did more than just design, build, and fund new emergency medical systems for municipalities across the United States as a bureaucrat and consultant; he also helped shape public opinion about it as a writer and consultant for *Emergency!*, the first television show to feature paramedics and emergency medical staff as central characters of a primetime drama series. After its premiere in early 1972, *Emergency!* was followed by the premiere of *M*A*S*H*, a television show that dramatized the military origins of emergency medicine in Korea. Along with growing newspaper coverage of advances in trauma medicine, both television shows brought modern emergency medicine into the living rooms of suburban and rural voters who, in turn, shaped Page into an advocate for an entirely new and profitable emergency medicine industry by the 1980s.

The show's popularity helped Page to shape a different future for emergency medicine than the one originally envisioned by Hahn. Whereas Hahn aimed to develop emergency medical services as a new publicly funded service to extend the reach of existing hospitals and employ more veterans of color, Page encouraged citizens to explore creating local emergency medical systems in the quickest and most efficient way possible. By 1976, Page argued to interested emergency medicine boosters that "the national experience" with emergency medicine had "clearly shown the reality that quality in an EMS system [did] not require uniformity of role throughout the nation."[50] He pointed out, for instance, that the Grand Rapids Police Department in Michigan and the Dallas and Houston Fire Departments in Texas ran their paramedic services just as well as "commercial ambulance" companies in Palm Springs, California.

Early on, Page also encouraged "activists" seeking to develop emergency medicine in their locations to be wary of affirmative action programs designed to benefit veterans and workers of color. He argued, for example, that state officials overseeing his role as North Carolina's EMS director hindered his ability to build an effective statewide emergency medical system because they were "overwhelmingly concerned for equity and equality in hiring."[51] He suggested that while "former military medics" might appear "on the basis of written statements of training and experience" to be ready to easily transfer their military skills to a "civilian atmosphere," he found that most veterans "failed to accomplish the transition" because they lacked the intellectual capacity to work "without day-to-day supervision" and follow "standard operating procedures." He argued instead that emergency medical service activists should focus on hiring employees who were "highly motivated, sensitive and socially acceptable professionals and technicians who see themselves as a team and who tend to exhibit a special form of pride and dedication to their work."

Page's efforts to discourage racial equity and equality in hiring policies were significant because he worked hard to institute new employment policies that preserved the historically white racial character of public safety occupations—especially since changes in the economy had made good-paying middle-class jobs less secure for white working-class men. Page's aim to end affirmative action was reinforced by new interpretations of civil rights law that protected and extended historical patterns of discrimination by abandoning the achievement of equal outcomes as the law's main objective. Kimberlé Crenshaw argues that new legal interpretations encouraged courts to balance and limit the interests of Black workers against the competing interests of white workers "even when those interests were actually created by the subordination of [Black people.]"[52]

Thus, in spite of the fact that the entire purpose of developing the paramedic industry initially rested on overcoming discriminatory employment and admission practices in fire departments and educational institutions, legal interpretations defending "equal opportunity" as the court's central objective protected the right of fire departments to exercise hiring preferences for white men. As opposed to relying on previously exclusionary language based on race, employers defended the hiring of white candidates by arguing they were, by mainstream educational and social standards, generally more "qualified" than Black candidates. Such legal reasoning enshrined racism using race neutral approaches to remedying inequality by eliding the fact that Black candidates continued to be excluded from gaining access to the kinds of education and resources needed to make themselves "qualified." The effect of Page's recommendations thus helped preserve hiring preferences for white employees in a turbulent economy.

As anti-tax sentiment around Proposition 13 increasingly threatened to undermine the budgets of fire and police departments across the nation, Page encouraged fire and police chiefs to consider defending public safety and fire protection funding by expanding their services to include some level of what he referred to as "advanced life-support" services. He did this by encouraging fire officials to do more than just support paramedic units within their departments. Pointing to exemplary firefighting units in Wichita, Kansas, and Santa Monica, California, Page advocated for every firefighter to be trained in "basic life support," a level of training below that of a paramedic but above that of basic first aid, and for every fire truck and "pumper" to be outfitted with paramedic gear.[53] Page explained that these initiatives transformed every firefighter and police officer into medical personnel he referred to as "first responders" because their spatial coverage and likely proximity to people in distress made their arrival before trained paramedics more likely. He was inspired to weave all firefighting and police units into a larger and more alert medical system after following a North Carolina paramedic unit to the house of a woman suffering from a heart attack, where "several over-fed firemen" sat, five houses down, "in wicker chairs . . . looking curiously at the ambulance that was coming and passing them."

Page was keen to blur the responsibilities between public safety officers and medical personnel because, as he put it, publicly funded fire departments could "no longer exist on smoke and water alone" and because "the ratio of life threatening emergencies in hospital departments" was "relatively small." According to his own estimates, while "only five percent of patients" who used emergency medical services turn out to be genuine medical emergencies and only "four percent of reported fires turn out to be working fires," Page argued that emergency medical systems came "to the fire service at a time when it [was] increasingly difficult to justify an expensive body of personnel for the occasional single function of fire protection." After the passage of Proposition 13, Page increasingly defended the utility of medically trained public safety officers by comparing the number of reported building fires (992) to the number of emergency medical incidents handled (23,775) by a single paid fire department within an unnamed "midwestern city."

The linking of public safety duties and emergency medical services was increasingly important because the cost of the latter was quickly growing. Although few calls to paramedic units and few visits to emergency departments constituted genuine medical emergencies in the eyes of medical professionals, Page's interactions with taxpaying citizens reveal an insatiable appetite for more and more expensive personnel and technology. Page's foundation regularly shared with interested politicians and bureaucrats just how expensive services were by parsing out the elements of Dallas's annual $1.8 million ambulance operation (notwithstanding the costs related to purchasing and retrofitting vehicles *and* staffing, operating, and equipping emergency departments in hospitals).[54] Despite such high costs, Page observed that many municipal officials continued to press him about the possibility of adding "helicopter and air evacuation"—a service he understood received a lot of "extravagant praise and drama" on television but felt obliged to admit was impractical given the "economics, geography, and weather" of many locations throughout the United States.[55]

By the early 1980s, a large part of the allure of emergency medicine drew upon the fact that it authenticated, in the eyes of insured patients, that the care they received in a particular hospital was modern, cutting-edge, and sophisticated. Speaking at a 1982 conference, Page recalled that "forty years ago, hospitals were trying to get rid of their ambulance services," but "needing a feeder mechanism to fill empty beds, and responding to the current hospital industry buzz word—'marketing'—it appears that hundreds of hospitals are getting back into the ambulance business."[56] Such observations about hospital "marketing" revealed how hospitals struggling to make profit from their traditional services believed that emergency medical services could revive their ailing businesses. However, as emergency medical services increasingly proved to be too costly for many hospitals by the early 1990s, many hospital owners, particularly those who considered themselves market leaders within a particular region, continued to operate high-level emergency departments and trauma centers because these facilities marked them as "luxury" medical centers.

The problem with emergency medicine's proliferation in Los Angeles by the early 1980s is that it caused patients to be sent to hospitals unequipped and unprepared to handle critically ill and injured patients despite being advertised as "emergency" hospitals. Although, for instance, the number of hospital owners who self-advertised their hospitals as having an emergency room grew to ninety-seven by 1982, the *Los Angeles Times* reported that only thirteen were fully equipped and staffed to handle critically ill and injured patients.[57] Los Angeles County General nurse Andrea Bourquin relayed the effect of such policies to readers by saying that she had "watched patients die" because local protocol required paramedics to take the critically ill or injured to "the nearest hospital with a 24-hour emergency room rather than the hospital best equipped to care for them."

The profit motive and costs associated with emergency medicine's spatial unevenness caused proponents of emergency medicine to be much more spatially aware of the physical location and quality of emergency medicine departments than of their profitability. As Page reminded proponents of emergency medicine in 1979, emergency medical systems only work "when multiple components (pre-hospital, in-hospital, and inter hospital) work together."[58] For Page and other proponents of emergency medicine, it was thus less important for proponents to regulate who advertised themselves as an "emergency hospital" and more important to direct public funding to sustain emergency departments in regions where it was well-known to be difficult to operate a hospital, let alone an emergency department.

The need to ensure that an emergency department remained operational in South Los Angeles, where only a handful of private hospitals existed, and even fewer were willing to provide emergency care for poor and indigent patients, pushed proponents of emergency medicine to increasingly focus their efforts on funding King-Drew's emergency department. Rather than see all the services offered at King-Drew as equally important for all citizens in Los Angeles, Page took a decidedly antagonistic position against the fur-

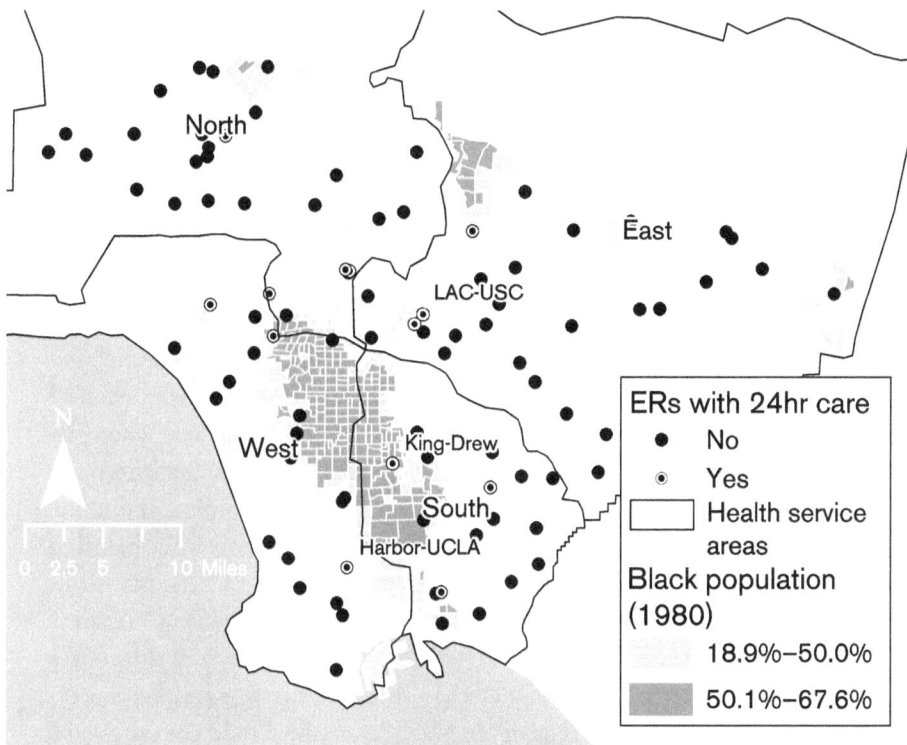

MAP 13. Race, false advertising, and emergency rooms, 1981

By 1981, a total of ninety-seven hospitals advertised themselves to consumers as having emergency room capabilities. A survey, however, revealed that only thirteen hospitals had staff on hand to handle around-the-clock emergency services. Except for King-Drew, the location of most emergency rooms in relation to Black census districts shows most providers sought to avoid opening an emergency room if surrounded by Black neighborhoods. Map: Tyler Munn.

ther funding of public hospital and clinic services he considered not essential to the operation of emergency medicine. Speaking to attendees of a Houston conference in the wake of nationwide budget cuts, Page encouraged emergency medicine proponents to see "health education, especially preventative health education" like that offered within King-Drew's health clinics, as "one of government's biggest failures."[59]

Drawing on well-worn racist beliefs that people of color were incapable of self-governance and hygiene, Page insisted that public funding would be better put to use to serve those he considered "responsible." Alluding to the now persistent belief that poor people of color lacked the proper motivation and willpower to lift themselves out of poverty, Page argued that "probably more than any other factor," health education's perceived failure in neighborhoods of color could be "traced to a lack of individual motivation" and, since "all learning is tied to motivation," that "people who are not motivated to accept personal responsibility for their own health are not likely to learn how."[60] As he put it, "The failure of our government to change life-styles, change personal habits, improve diet, while at the same time promising quality health care for all citizens, has resulted in an economic imbalance that could easily break our nation."

Page's strategically deployed comments amid nationwide deliberations over the distribution of tax revenues show how his decade-long career helping mostly white suburban and rural community leaders build emergency medical systems in their neighborhoods shaped his imagination about whom he believed emergency medicine's "true" constituents were. His statements putatively cast those who exclusively used publicly funded hospital and clinic services as immutably unhygienic and "irresponsible" citizens while painting putatively white voters and homeowners as beneficiaries of emergency medicine's lifesaving services. In suggesting that white homeowners or taxpayers were somehow more motivated and educated about how to keep themselves individually healthy, Page intimated that white citizens were entitled to services to treat medical "emergencies" and "accidents" they could not reasonably predict or prevent on their own. In Page's imagination, publicly funded emergency medical services seemed a particularly important entitlement for insured white patients who regularly traversed neighborhoods of color between home and work. Such observations made King-Drew's emergency medical services of paramount importance because without public funding, commuters faced being stranded in a region that few private hospitals even dared to serve.

A MEANING GREATER THAN THE SERVICE ITSELF

By the time Proposition 13's cuts hit Los Angeles County's budget in 1981, the vision to prioritize emergency medicine over other public health services manifested in the actions of Schabarum, who had become the de facto leader of the County Board of Supervisors' new conservative majority, and President Reagan, who greatly expanded military funding while severely diminishing federal funding to health and welfare programs beginning in 1980. Conservatives increasingly saw their support for emergency medical services as a way to either isolate liberals from their traditional constituencies or organize them under the aegis of the Republican Party. Their vision to consolidate political power in the aftermath of Proposition 13 conflated public clinic services with race and crime and portrayed emergency medical services as needed for law and order.

Initial efforts show that the county's conservative leaders sought at first to sustain public funding for emergency medical services by cutting budgets for public hospital and clinic care. The county supervisors received help in achieving this endeavor through a July 12, 1981, *Los Angeles Times* article that Black community leaders described as an "attack" designed to influence public opinion about the direction of public health budgets.[61] Described by the team of writers who wrote it as an investigatory piece exploring the growth of the "permanent underclass," "Marauders from Inner City Prey on L.A.'s Suburbs" described how, over the previous decade, LA's "ghettos and barrios" had become "staging areas for robbers, burglars and thieves who ride the freeways like magic carpets to hit homes and businesses" in the region's various white suburban enclaves. Rather than directly attribute the violence, criminality, and predatory nature of so-called marauders to their race, writers used computerized data sets from police departments to declare that nearly 41 percent of all "felons who stole money or property" in 1979 hailed from "the inner city," a figure that the newspaper claimed had doubled since 1969.

Black community activists, however, felt that the article exacerbated "an already tense racial situation" because it "literally depicted the residents of Watts as little more than gutter rats" shortly after the county supervisors proposed eliminating as many as eight public clinics and several key health services at King-Drew.[62] In response to the article, the proposed budget cuts, and the rate of violence and drug use in the neighborhood, a group of prominent Black political leaders, such as Reverend James Lawson, Avalon-Carver Community Center leader Mary Henry, and Assemblywoman Maxine Waters formed the Coalition for Economic Survival, an alliance that gathered community leaders and organizations from South Los Angeles "to persuade the conservative-dominated Board of Supervisors to reverse its decision" on cutting health services to Black and Brown neighborhoods.[63] The coalition's members felt compelled to act because of rumors since the passage of Proposition 13 of proposals to close some or all of the county's public hospitals, eliminate as many as thirty-two of its fifty-seven health centers, and lay off as many as 1900 county health employees.

The rhetoric that the coalition deployed in its public rallies to defend funding for public hospital and clinic services, however, tended to reinforce conservative opinions that the only services worth defending were those related to emergency medicine and public safety. Rather than organize voters around the idea that poor people of color deserved health care as a human right, the coalition mounted a series of "anti-PCP" street rallies, arguing that public health services, especially mental health services, were part of an arsenal of tools that responsible Black community leaders felt they needed to fight poverty, drug use, and violence in their neighborhoods.[64] Indeed, organizers made sure to feature the voices of several prominent Black law enforcement figures, such as Inglewood police chief Joseph Rouzan, LAPD deputy chief Jesse Brewer, and Celes King III, a local bail bondsman and a former president of the local NAACP chapter. King noted the article in the *Times* had ignored "some of the positive things and people who have come out of the Watts community," and that the cuts hindered them from "dealing with the root causes" of street crime and drug use.[65]

The implementation of budget cuts shows that the supervisors ultimately agreed with Black community leaders on the importance of public safety but did not agree that Black community leaders had effectively utilized public health services in the fight against crime. The county supervisors cut $75 million from the county health budget in 1981 and over $100 million in 1982. The cuts led to reduced hospital services at King-Drew and Harbor-UCLA not considered essential to the operation of emergency medical services and the closure of eight public clinics in predominantly low-income neighborhoods that included Pacoima, Compton, Bell Gardens, Culver City, Santa Fe Springs, and Norwalk.[66] County officials, for example, cut outpatient services attached to the ear, nose, and throat, orthopedic-gynecology, pediatric, and urology clinics at Harbor-UCLA's hospital and eliminated "follow up work on about 1,800 surgical patients a month" at King-Drew by forcing patients to seek private care after only one postsurgery follow-up. It also reduced King-Drew's family medicine program by 75 percent.

The county's 1981 and 1982 budget cuts were more striking because of what the supervisors did not cut or put up for debate. While the supervisors required all departments to reduce their budgets by 10 percent, they left the budgets related to police and fire protection intact. In contrast to their very public disagreements with Black community activists, county officials spent most of 1981 and 1982 working with private hospital owners to designate all county-run emergency departments as "trauma centers," a designation ensuring that patients with the "worst injuries—not the broken arm or the cut toe, but the life-threatening car accident, gunshot wound or knifing injury" were sent to emergency departments capable of treating them appropriately.[67] Although many hospital owners contested the designation because it unfairly directed paying patients away from their emergency rooms to the county's large teaching hospitals, many physicians throughout the county believed that the designations would save lives. In fact, one report shared that many off-duty physicians began to "carry cards in their wallets telling paramedics to take them to large teaching hospitals rather than to the nearest emergency room in the event of a serious accident."[68]

Public responses by citizens after the first budget cut revealed that voters increasingly associated conservatives with emergency medicine, law, and order, while they identified public clinics as "liberal" causes, regardless of how individuals using public clinics actually politically identified. J. Smith of Los Angeles, for instance, wrote a letter to the *Los Angeles Times* arguing that the budget cuts clearly targeted "the poor and minorities" who "cannot afford to pay for private doctors or hospitals."[69] Lynn McKibben of Long Beach agreed in another letter by stating that she ultimately believed the "decision to close certain neighborhood clinics was based primarily on political gain rather than use or needs of the communities." She warned readers, however, against treating health decisions along party lines. Pointing out that Norwalk's "very busy 1,500-patient-visit-a-month clinic" also served a "city full of legal and illegal aliens, Southeast Asian refugees, poor whites and Hispanics," she warned that the "profound effects" of its closure would mean that "we will all suffer the consequences" of spreading disease and poverty.

The belief that liberal political power was connected to the strength and reach of public clinics inspired conservatives to explore ways to undermine and reorganize that relationship to their benefit. Schabarum initially tried to sever these perceived relationships by attempting to implement a new policy in 1981 known as County Health Department Policy 516, which required any citizen seeking care to divulge evidence of either Medicare/Medicaid eligibility or immediate ability to pay for health services.[70] The policy not only would have made any undocumented immigrant ineligible for any health service but would have served as a way to identify and apprehend health seekers for eventual deportation. When courts ruled the policy unconstitutional, conservative leaders found new leadership on the issue from President Reagan.

In 1986, Reagan successfully undermined and reorganized the Democratic Party's perceived relationships between immigrant rights activists and public health clinics by proposing and securing passing of the Emergency Medical

Treatment and Labor Act (EMTALA) and the Simpson-Mazzoli Act (more commonly known as the Immigration Reform and Control Act or as Amnesty) in the same year. Although the latter preserved access to public hospital and clinic care for an estimated 2.9 million people by granting them citizenship, Reagan's signature emergency medicine law effectively empowered Los Angeles County officials to deny undocumented immigrants access to publicly funded preventative health services and follow-up care by compelling all hospitals to treat and stabilize any individual, regardless of citizenship status, who presented at an emergency department, emergency room, or trauma unit. Despite its benevolent appearance, the law forced immigrant rights activists and public health advocates to share common cause with conservatives in preserving emergency medical services as a new common good.

Although later regarded by Thomas Scully, former director of the Federal Centers for Medicare and Medicaid, as an unfunded and "backdoor way to get people universal access to at least emergency room 'care,'"[71] Reagan's law manipulated the policy landscape of large cities by forcing municipalities to prioritize emergency care over public hospital and clinic care by reorganizing the debt mandate that guided antipoverty efforts around preventative health under emergency medical services. Although in practice women and children on welfare and undocumented immigrants continued to seek healthcare in ways that did not differ from before 1986, the imagined policy outcomes of limiting clinic services to Black women and children on welfare and limiting undocumented immigrants to emergency medical services helped renew conservative talking points in the 1990s that portrayed each group as "welfare cheats" and fiscal "burdens."[72] The effect, in turn, only heightened citizen calls for more policing and prisons as a way to protect white suburban citizens from the normalization of gun violence in inner cities.

Ultimately, Reagan's "solution" to emergency medical services funding showed that he cared less about the actual costs or the health outcomes of the service and more about how his mandate helped preserve profits for private hospitals operating outside King-Drew's neighborhoods. By tipping health policy to favor public funding of emergency medical services over public clinic funding, private hospitals saw Reagan's policy as saving them from having to serve the patient populations they properly believed belonged to the county's public hospital system. For some, the law permitted hospital owners to insulate themselves from poor patient populations they believed were unprofitable by closing their emergency rooms. For others, who kept their emergency departments open to cater to middle-class clientele, the

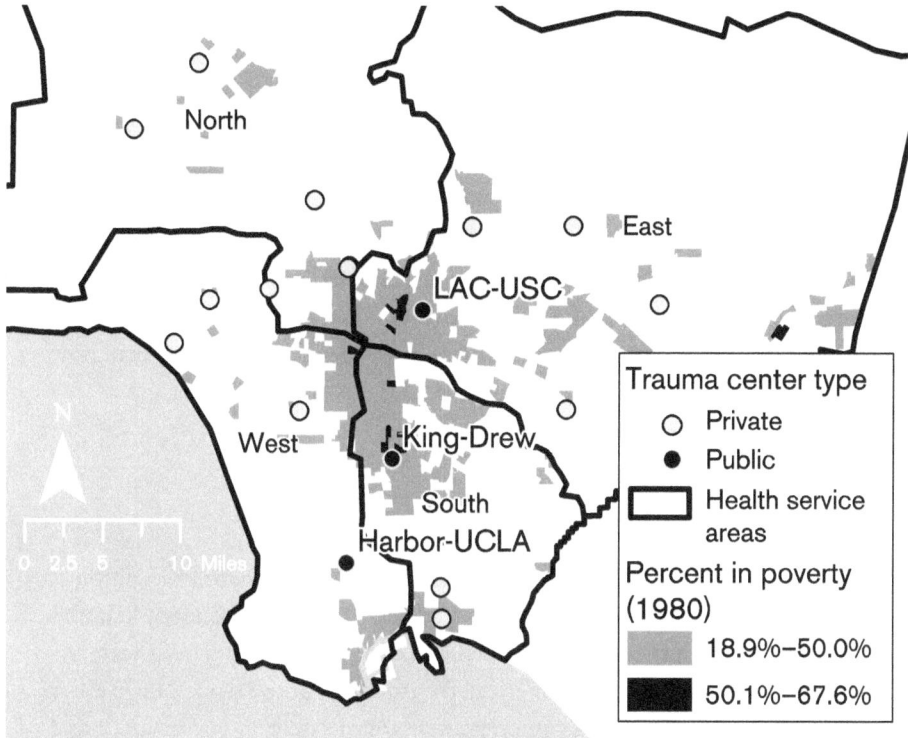

MAP 14. Safety net hospitals: patient dumping in Los Angeles

By 1986, hospital leaders created a trauma center designation that stabilized modern emergency medical systems. Trauma center designations are set by region and require hospitals to voluntarily opt in. Unlike privately-run trauma centers, the county's three trauma centers—LAC-USC, King-Drew, and Harbor-UCLA—are required by California's Pauper Act to accept any and all patients. The Pauper Act has subsidized the profitability of privately run hospitals by leaving the county's public hospitals to shoulder the county's poorest, sickest, and most expensive patients. Map: Tyler Munn.

existence of publicly funded emergency departments like King-Drew's offered a convenient place to transfer, or "dump," unprofitable patients who presented in their emergency rooms.

As Beatrix Hoffman has argued, by the late 1980s and early 1990s the total effect led public health experts to refer to the existence of publicly funded emergency rooms as a "safety net," a term that curiously denoted the perceived openness of emergency rooms relative to the otherwise near total exclusionary nature of America's healthcare system.[73] Such a skewed vision of funding priorities demonstrates how Reagan's policies banked on the belief that taxpayers would continue to tolerate certain kinds of debt and certain types of government growth not because the state outcomes were more financially sound or socially equitable but because such outcomes offered some citizens a meaning greater than the service itself. That is, in the case of emergency medicine, being a direct beneficiary of King-Drew's emergency services signified little to nothing compared with the meaning and profits it produced for those outside the city's neighborhoods of color. For many white suburban homeowners, for instance, it represented the safety of having a government willing to go to great lengths and into great debt to maintain a particular way of life; it increasingly signified, for many hospital owners, the ability to make profits in a landscape made otherwise risky by the greater acceptance of poverty and normalization of everyday violence.

TWO WORLDS IN ONE

The outcome of public health budget decisions in the wake of Proposition 13 reveals how the growth of emergency medicine since the late 1960s had dramatically undermined older approaches to evenly distributing healthcare. As opposed to caring for every American by situating a hospital or clinic in every *neighborhood* to provide a comprehensive complement of preventative and acute care services, emergency medical services introduced an alternative vision for distributing healthcare by prompting citizens to think of situating an emergency department in every *region* as serving a greater good than older approaches to distributing healthcare. Particularly as white citizens increasingly took on longer commutes between their homes and their places of work to sustain a living, support for publicly funded emergency medical services in rural and urban regions, where private funding for healthcare continued to be a problem, rose in importance over the funding of publicly funded hospitals and clinics in urban areas.

The resulting political whiteness of emergency medicine exposes how its meaning produced two contradictory but overlapping ways of seeing race by the 1980s. Looking at the city from King-Drew, liberal politicians such as Mayor Bradley and Supervisor Hahn viewed the city and the "global" economy they helped engineer as an exemplary landscape for a new multicultural society based on capitalist inclusion and sexual respectability. Looking at the city from the edges of its suburbs, however, conservative politicians such as Supervisor Schabarum and President Reagan saw the city as a dystopian landscape in need of rescuing through law and order.

Emergency medicine oddly served as both a meeting ground and a departure point for these two visions. Hahn's efforts to innovate emergency medicine to serve as a new vehicle for employment and racial inclusion ultimately had the opposite effect. Emergency medicine not only encouraged politicians to turn away from older policy approaches to achieving healthier citizens by situating a hospital in every neighborhood but replaced that political vision with emergency medical services designed, by their very nature, to stabilize rather than maximize life. This shifting political horizon made it more difficult for politicians and citizens alike to make claims on government to provide for a "good life" for every citizen if society, through emergency medicine's proliferation, helped normalize a "bare life" as a universal common good.[74]

In this regard, emergency medicine's popularization as a service did not negate a "good life" as an outcome but simply distributed its possibility to insured patients who enjoyed emergency services as part of a larger world of privately run hospital and clinic services. As this last chapter has shown, however, for a short time during the 1970s poor people of color enjoyed a city where leaders boldly dared to provide the same hospital, clinic, and emergency care in their neighborhoods as most white insured patients found in theirs. Still, as the entire book has shown, such "equality" hid deeper relationships of power that subordinated all workers in Los Angeles to the same forces of subordination facing workers in Asia, Africa, and Latin America.

And still, there are other worlds possible.

Epilogue

"A PESSIMIST, IF I AM NOT CAREFUL"

BE IT DEATH BY ARSON or slavery by "choice," the alternatives framed in Octavia Butler's 1993 novel *The Parable of the Sower* illustrate the consequences of what she believed would take place in Los Angeles if the electoral politics and economic phenomena of the late 1980s and 1990s continued. In her novel, by 2024 LA's economy and environment have grown so unstable that public services, such as police, firefighters, and first responders, are untrustworthy and corrupt. Homeowners rely on "smart pills" to manage their own healthcare and build walls and gates around their neighborhoods to keep the leagues of homeless and poor people throughout the region from enacting their resentment on the affluent by setting fire to their homes. For the homeless and poor unwilling to join those who resort to arson, crime, and drug use to cope in a deteriorating economy, the answer to attaining housing, healthcare, and food security has led them to exchange their labor for the safety of towns owned and policed by foreign corporations.

So powerful and viscerally real were her observations that Judith, a homeowner in the affluent city of Newport Beach in Orange County, called in to National Public Radio's *Talk of the Nation* in 2000 to ask for Butler's opinion on whether she thought it was feasible "to plant a vegetable garden" on the property of her gated neighborhood.[1] Judith explained that the novel felt so accurate that she had come to fear that the walls of the gated neighborhoods of the "middle-income housing projects" around her "weren't high enough." So frightened was Judith of the seeming inevitability of the chaos featured in *Parable* that she felt she needed a survival garden because she was "afraid to go to any stores." As she put it, "especially down here in Los Angeles in Octavia's story ... you can't get to Los Angeles without being killed mostly."

Butler responded by taking the time to politely explain that so many readers have mistakenly read *Parable* as "prophecy" when it instead ought to be understood as a "cautionary tale." Butler explained, "It's a book that says, 'If we keep doing what we're doing, here's what we might wind up with.'" "I've heard people call it prophecy, and I generally respond to that with horror because certainly I don't want it to be prophecy. I don't want to live in that world."

As a "cautionary tale," Butler expressed relief over Judith's confession that the novel haunted her, because she wrote *Parable* with the intention of showing people how social norms that citizens usually considered productive were actually dangerous. As this epilogue discusses, Butler hoped that amplifying the danger of American political and economic norms most were programmed to think of as benign, such as homeownership, respectable marriage and family life, and biomedicine, would prompt citizens to rethink the wisdom of distributing life's basic necessities according to free market capitalism. Across her body of work, Butler drew on and portrayed a city where pinning happiness and personal security on respectable homeownership neither conferred safety nor protected citizens from exposure to contagious disease, murder, police harassment, sexual violence, drug trafficking, and slavery. That Judith seemed to accept a future involving the need to plant a survival garden as inevitable, however, underlines how Butler urgently saw that the *true crisis* facing most Americans was less a crisis of capital than a crisis of the *imagination*.

By plunging *Parable*'s mixed-race protagonist Lauren Olamina into a predicament more akin to the daily crisis of survival facing queer, trans, and poor people of color in the 1980s and 1990s, Butler used her writing to force readers to experience a world of survival already taking shape in their own time and in their own city. In so doing, she used science fiction as a platform to criticize the rise of racial and sexual liberalism in Los Angeles and its shortcomings in addressing the ongoing legacies of white supremacy. She saw her writing as a way to help readers see how narratives of respectable sexuality and homeownership were so deeply entrenched in society as common sense that even when people "are aware" of its controlling forces, "they can still possess or control you because you're not necessarily aware of exactly what they're doing when they're doing it."[2]

In contrast to Los Angeles's Black middle-class elites like Mayor Tom Bradley, Congressman Augustus Hawkins, and King-Drew's physician founders and administrators, Butler was a native Californian with a working-class background. Born in 1947 in Pasadena to a mother who worked as a domestic and a father who worked as a shoe shiner before he passed away when she was seven, Butler spent part of her childhood living in the high desert between Victorville and Barstow on a chicken farm owned by her grandmother and her herbalist grandfather. She spent most of her life, however, in LA's "racially mixed" and "integrated" neighborhoods of Pasadena, Altadena, and Crenshaw. Even after winning $295,000 as part of being a 1995 recipient of the MacArthur "genius" Fellowship, Butler continued to labor for nearly a year as a hospital laundry worker, a job she described as "bad" but no less good than other jobs she held throughout her life like "washing dishes, sweeping floors, doing warehouse inventory, sorting potato chips."[3]

In addition to being a woman, Butler also differed from many of the city's Black middle-class elites in other distinctive ways. Although she did not positively identify as gay, she knew others around her interacted with her as if she were queer based on her appearance and on her deep voice. Despite ultimately choosing to identify as a "hermit" after several trips to explore her sexual identity at the Los Angeles Gay and Lesbian Community Services Center, she made it a point to "play around with ['gay sexuality']" in her imagination and in her work.[4] She additionally differed in perspective from other Black women activists, who at the time rejected the label "feminist" because they "assumed it was for white people."[5] Butler, in contrast, positively identified as a Black feminist because she felt it "was just as important to have equal rights for women as it was to have equal rights for Black people."

> "SOME OF THE THINGS THAT ARE REALLY HARD TO
> TALK ABOUT IN THE BLACK COMMUNITY I TALKED
> ABOUT IN *DAWN* AND IN *MIND OF MY MIND*"

The interviews Butler gave throughout her life reveal that she was as unsatisfied with the future proposed by proponents of racial and sexual liberalism in the 1960s and 1970s as she was with the world of white supremacy. She also felt that the labels of "fantasy" and "science fiction" used to describe her work diminished the criticisms she had of both. As a Black woman writing in genres dominated by white male authors who often wrote stories with virtually no people of color, Butler's writing gained attention for centering characters who frequently were not white, not men, and not straight. Although often read for the ways her writings challenged normative cultural narrations of American life where the "norm is white" and where men exist at the "top of the hierarchy," Butler also challenged the ascendance of new racially and sexual liberally discourses of power in city politics as it unfolded around her.[6]

In an interview in 1997, Butler revealed to readers that most of her writing—five novels published between 1976 and 1984 known as the *Patternist* series; *Kindred*, published in 1979; and *Dawn*, published in 1987—were written, as she phrased it, as a "comment" on "Black America."[7] Published three years after the election of Bradley in 1973, Butler's most striking criticism about the rise of racial and sexual liberalism in LA's politics appeared in *Mind of My Mind*, a novel about the ascendance of the Patternists, a race of humans gifted with a telepathic power once considered by others to be a sign of mental disability and exclusion. Similar to how Dr. J. Alfred Cannon's racial scientific narratives of racial normality sought to help Black people in Los Angeles see their race as a tool for power, rather than a disability, Butler's Patternists come to no longer see their telepathy as a disability by following the leadership of Mary, the biracial daughter of an ancient and immortal African man named Doro. As a "healer," Mary teaches the Patternists how to draw upon their disability as a source of power that they can control. As opposed to having a disability that controls them, the Patternists eventually use their telepathic powers to control their former oppressors. By the novel's end, the Patternists have not only transformed humans without telepathic power into their own unwitting servant and consumer class but have also colonized the best neighborhoods in the city as their own.

As a novel that essentially serves as a historical allegory for the 1960s and 1970s triumph over the social stigma of race and mental illness and the success of residential integration campaigns in Los Angeles by the city's professionals of color, Butler was not shy about indirectly criticizing their politics by calling the Patternists "people who think that they've won."[8] In the fictive universe of *Mind of My Mind* and in the real universe of 1960s Los Angeles, both groups attain their status as part of society's new ruling class by relying on the labor and patronage of the oppressed for their survival. Although relatively successful in comparison with their pasts, Butler sought to highlight in *Mind of My Mind* how the appropriation of and renewal of techniques of oppression, bounded spatially in the symbolism of homeownership, made the Patternists in *Mind of My Mind* and the middle-class professionals of color who abandoned their former neighbors in real life both "not very nice."

Butler did not just limit her criticism to middle-class professionals but also faulted Black nationalists who disparaged the masses of poor Black people for failing to murder, rebel against, and poison their enslavers at a rate and scale large enough to win Black freedom sooner. Butler recalled that she felt compelled to write *Kindred*, a novel about the journey of a modern-day Black woman sent back in time to navigate her odds as an enslaved person, as a "reaction to some of the things going on during the sixties when people were feeling ashamed of, or more strongly, angry with their parents for not having improved things faster."[9] Especially after a classmate expressed a desire to "kill off" all the "old people who have been holding [Black people] back for so long,"[10] Butler wrote *Kindred* as a way to imagine what it *felt* like to make choices in an era that so many Black history enthusiasts were quick to judge. For Butler, the experience helped underline the disconnect of some ideological approaches to Black nationalism that increasingly blamed poor Black people for a system that white patriarchs had designed to control them.

As she later revealed, the rise of the Patternists to positions of power allowed her to discuss other "things that are really hard to talk about in the black community."[11] It allowed her, for instance, to criticize the prevailing use of culture of poverty theory to make Black community development and race survival dependent on kinship patterns pinned to Black breadwinning manhood. It also allowed her to highlight the shortcomings of certain feminist and gay and lesbian inclusion narratives as women began to appear as leaders in the city's new financial district and as white gays and lesbians gained greater police protection for their status as taxpaying voters and homeowners in the 1970s.

All these criticisms come to a head in *Mind of My Mind*, where Doro's and Mary's social visions come into direct conflict. In *Mind of My Mind*, Butler indirectly criticized the eugenic, patriarchal, and sexist undertones of culture of poverty theory through the figure of Doro, Mary's father, who is set on his own quest of "breeding a master race" by using the authority and power he has over the women he marries, kidnaps, and fathers to keep all his "experiments" under control. Butler argued that the Patternists were "awful" because they had, as she put it, "a bad teacher" in Doro.[12] His willingness to kidnap, breed, and use women as he saw fit eventually accounts for his ill treatment at the hands of Mary and the Patternists she controls. According to Butler, Mary and the Patternists not only do "nasty things" to Doro but "also do nasty things to everybody else, because they've learned that's how you behave if you want to survive."[13]

Butler traced the renewal of oppressive practices and the deferral of true freedom in the "nasty things" she saw both radical feminists and mainstream feminists deploy in their respective quests for gender equality. She disagreed with radical feminists who advocated "completely getting rid of males" and was troubled by the emergence of a form of corporate feminism that advocated scrapping gender-based affirmative action programs as soon as women achieved positions of power.[14] She believed that feminist proposals that encouraged women to become men politically, to replace men, or to get rid of men obscured how patriarchy recruited more than just men to sustain its power. She understood that using the same methods of exclusion to produce gender equality just produced a world no different than the old.

Butler also strove to show the shortcomings of gay and lesbian movements in real life by portraying the Patternists as a society full of gays and lesbians who, despite their inclusion within the ruling class, continued to do "nasty things" to other people. Whereas the first half of *Mind of My Mind* uses Mary's critical eye of Doro's ruling practices as a narrative device to problematize culture of poverty theory and Black and multicultural forms of capitalism, Butler criticizes the renewal of capitalism in LA's gay and lesbian neighborhoods through the exclusionary spatial and labor practices of the Patternists. Unlike the heteropatriarchal kinship patterns that telepathically lock Doro's experiments into a patriarchal "pattern" pinned to his leadership, Mary's leadership permits those locked into her "pattern" to form queer kinships outside traditional heterosexual couplings. Although the Patternists are tolerant of nonnormative kinship patterns such as same-sex couples, polyamorous unions, and intergenerational households, they renew the ethical quandary of Doro's practices of coercion and entrapment by representing and reproducing capitalism under more than just heterosexual forms.

Given that so many of LA's urban planning policies had been underwritten by the latest advances in racial science, it should come as no surprise that Butler connected her criticisms of Southern California's electoral and economic trends to common assumptions of biological evolution shared across the disciplines of sociology, anthropology, sexology, criminology, and psychiatry in "sociobiology," a field that, according to Butler, "became popular and unpopular at the same time" in the late 1960s and early 1970s.[15] Her interest in sociobiology reveals that she understood that the renewal of oppression after the rise of civil rights, feminist, Black, gay, Chicano, and Asian pride movements relied on a basic evolutionary biologic principle that held that the gender distinctiveness and sexual complexity of individuals as men and women indicated their capacity for civilization and self-governance. As this book has shown, this basic principle undergirded the popularity of culture of poverty theory, epidemiology of violence theory, new discourses of racial and homosexual normality, and broken windows theory by deferring questions of evolutionary fitness once only associated with white heterosexual men and women in the mid-nineteenth century to ideas of gender and sexual stability associated with twentieth-century home and property ownership.

Rather than affirm the gender and sexual stability of Black individuals, Butler witnessed how well-intentioned efforts by Black physicians, psychiatrists, and politicians to stabilize society's opinion of Black people as heterosexual only deferred the conferral of racial modernity and independence on Black people. The translation of culture of poverty theory into antipoverty policies first designed to cement normative gender and sexual roles in Black communities through breadwinning manhood only fueled the criminalization of all Black women as "welfare queens" in political discourse by the 1970s. Likewise, by the 1980s efforts to push women on welfare into working motherhood not only marked the renewal of Black women's labor subordination within the economy but also resignified Black men as equally sexually aberrant for their status as "absent fathers" and "wild youth." Instead of validating the proposal of Black people as "modern," just as supposedly sexually evolved and stable as white people, these proposals ended up recriminalizing Black men and women as sexually "backward" and incapable of self-governance.

Despite being putatively "straight," popular discourses around "welfare queens" and "absent fathers" not only effectively denied Black men and women the same attributes of gender and sexual stability assigned to straight white men and women but also helped renew the pathologization of queer and trans people of color by denying them the same social acceptance conferred upon white gays and lesbians through normal homosexuality discourses. The elaboration of culture of poverty discourses within the realms of sexology and policing recast queer and trans people as biologically prone to violence and crime. Thus, whereas the sexuality of white gays and lesbians was increasingly described by scholars and historians in the 1980s and 1990s as the emergence of a "modern sexuality," the sexuality of all people of color, regardless of their stated sexuality or gender, continued to be discussed in common discourse as "atavistic," "backward," and "Black."

As a science fiction writer who relied on countering sociobiological texts that many understood were broadly eugenic in nature, Butler was consistently asked about her opinion on biological determinism. Butler was clear that she felt the development of biological traits as a response to survival was a normal, natural, and expected phenomenon. She argued, however, that while "behavior is controlled to some extent by biological forces," it was possible for people to, as she put it, "work around our programming if we understand it."[16] That is, she challenged the scientific assumption that "every behavior has a purpose important to survival" and argued against the use of "sociobiology" to advance social Darwinism.[17]

Butler argued for scientific uses of sociobiology that helped people "learn to work with" genetic traits and argued against using sociobiology as a way to uplift the voices of those "who see it as a good reason to let the poor be poor."[18] Moreover, the idea that poor people of color "must be poor because of their genes" was a "kind of foolishness" that was not helpful. She expressed this belief in the actions of some of her most famous characters, such as *Parable of the Sower*'s Lauren, who possesses a congenital trait that allows her to feel other people's physical pain as well as her own. Rather than reduce or define Lauren to her disability, Butler showcases how Lauren is able to make choices about her future based on what she knows about her own body—something that Butler referred to as "body knowledge." Thus, while some of Lauren's abilities are biologically determined, her life and social position are not.

THE FUTURE, IN PRESENT TENSE

Despite her own criticisms of the Patternists' alternative kinship patterns, Butler spent more time in her novels exploring queer kinship patterns because her observations about life at the end of the twentieth century and into the twenty-first demonstrated that the promises of prosperity, security, and homeownership once associated with the nuclear family home were either increasingly unattainable or outright meaningless. Indeed, although the nation's productivity generally increased after 1973, average expenses related to the costs of living rose while wages across all income brackets except the wealthiest remained stagnant or declined. Declining wages for low-wage workers meant that fewer and fewer families in the United States by the 1980s could afford to own a home based on the income of one wage earner. According to some estimates, whereas nearly half of US households in 1960 consisted of a nuclear family with a single breadwinner, that percentage dropped by half to only a quarter of US households.

As many of her interviews in the late 1980s and 1990s reveal, Butler felt inspired to write about the potential benefits of alternative family formations because, unlike most depictions of poor neighborhoods in Southern California, she had witnessed how successful poor families were in surviving in the city despite their relative political and economic abandonment. News reports of gangs and "broken homes" obfuscated how families used alternative kinship patterns, such as single-parent and multigenerational homes, communes made up of multiple families, and households of adopted kin to develop ways of reproducing life outside the official state-sanctioned unions found in single-family homes. Judith's perception that she needed a survival garden in her future belies the fact that Butler spent more time discussing the potential possibilities for successfully surviving a bleak future in *Parable* by looking to the lives of queer, trans, and poor people of color in her present.

By the late 1980s and 1990s, Butler was increasingly convinced that the need of California's homeowners and voters "to feel superior to make themselves feel better" increasingly led them to vote "against their own interests."[19] Her statements referenced the increasing frequency by which California's homeowners voted to erode the public health and social service benefits established as a public safety net for the poor since the New Deal by targeting undocumented immigrants. After passing referendums targeting "welfare queens" and Black communities in the 1970s and early 1980s, California's voters passed a series of laws in the late 1980s and early 1990s designed to exclude undocumented immigrants from public life, such as laws enforcing English as the state's official language and laws denying undocumented immigrants access to public healthcare, education, safety, and social service provisions. Together with ballot initiatives designed to end affirmative action and enhance sentencing for low-level crimes, the effect of California's postwar referenda sought to criminalize and incarcerate poor people of color in a growing number of prisons throughout the state.

Butler connected the impact of these laws to economic processes that she argued signaled the return of slavery and the emergence of what she called "throw-away" labor. Butler, for instance, traced the impact of Mayor Bradley's 1970s and 1980s efforts to secure cheap labor for global capital to the 1995 "discovery" of seventy-two undocumented Thai women held captive as garment workers in a makeshift residential home in El Monte, a neighborhood just outside downtown Los Angeles. In an interview published for the Black readers of the NAACP's *The Crisis*, Butler described the mostly poor and undocumented Asian and Latina women garment workers she saw being "held against their will and forced to work" in the city's sweatshops as no different than the Black migrants who had been "seduced" to Los Angeles "by lies about good salaries" several generations prior.[20] While she argued that the terms of labor for garment workers were not exactly the same as those enslaved under chattel slavery or Jim Crow sharecropping, she described the phenomena on similar terms by arguing that garment factory owners "work them and [do] not pay them" and "forbid them to leave"—"if they try, they're beaten or killed."

She also traced these local patterns in Los Angeles to the emergence of "throw-away" labor in maquiladora plants on the US-Mexico border, which were duty-free and tariff-free factories expanded and strengthened in 1992 under the North American Free Trade Agreement. As Butler explained, the irony of their existence was the fact that factory owners designed them to undercut the already low wage and work conditions in LA's garment industry by taking advantage of Mexico's even more lax labor and environmental standards to achieve even more competitive profit margins. Describing maquiladoras as "the opposite of slavery," Butler testified that employers provided employment for poor people but provided neither protections for worker safety nor wages high enough to sustain basic necessities such as food and housing. Forced to "live in horrible shacks" with "no plumbing, open sewers" and "not really enough money to sustain life," Butler argued most families resorted to putting their entire families to work. The cumulative effect "used up" women at such a young age that many thirty-five-year-old women were regularly "tossed aside for younger workers."[21]

Butler's *Parable of the Sower* illustrated what she thought would happen to the safety and sanctity of homeownership and the nuclear family if electoral trends continued on the same trajectory as those she observed in real life. The two opposing forces figuratively meet in the home of Lauren Olamina's parents in *Parable*. According to Butler, the walled cul-de-sac of Lauren's parents' home symbolized how unrealistic and foolish defending traditional kinship patterns and property ownership was in light of the complete dismantling of public services by voters and the deterioration of the economy at the hands of ruthless capitalist corporations. Despite the fact that "their way of life" was "going nowhere," Butler points out that Lauren's parents still desperately try to "hold on until the good-old-days come back."[22] It is here where Butler's statements about the "short-sighted behavior" of California's voters (in real life) are made apparent.[23] In Butler's opinion, California's homeowners had unwittingly exposed themselves to the unbridled ravages of capitalism already lurking in their midst by dismantling the social safety net of public services.

Readers of *Parable* sometimes responded to Butler's assertions that electoral trends and economic trends were "setting things up so that the poor will get a lot poorer and the middle-class will get a lot poorer too" with disbelief. Such a reaction was so common that Butler commented, "I don't think a lot of members of the middle-class have figured out yet [that they are destroying society]."[24] Others, as her interview with *The Crisis*'s Jerome Jackson revealed, did not think Black readers would understand why an economic crisis facing "Hispanics" mattered to Black folks. In both instances, Butler alluded to her earlier comments about slavery and throw-away labor: "If you only pay attention to what's happening to your own folk, by the time you notice, then it's creeping into your people too; and very well entrenched."[25] For those who continued to insist they could just not see "how we could possibly get from where we are to where they are in *Parable*," Butler responded with the thought, "You poor baby."[26]

Despite her bleak assessments of real-life electoral and economic phenomena, Butler saw promise for more equitable and fair societies in the way that most poor people of color responded to their marginalization within liberal democratic capitalist societies. Butler drew upon her own experience growing up working class with a complicated family life to encourage readers to recognize the value of distributing life's most basic necessities to individuals not based on their marriage and obedience to male breadwinners. According to her, "Growing up without a father influenced my life," and "my [difficult] childhood had something to do with the way I sometimes present parents as not being able to raise their own children."[27] Although marriage and blood relations did not do as much work for her as others, she argued that "other family"—"other adults, friends, people who simply came into the household and stayed"—constituted "our most important set of relationships" and "so much of what we are."[28]

Parable serves as the greatest illustration of these concepts through the motley band of people that joins Lauren on her journey to create a new society in Northern California. Unlike Lauren's parents, who remain "waiting for the times of plenty to come back," Butler claimed that it was "the kids" who picked up and carried on society because their present and future were unencumbered by the weight of respectable family and home life that defined the normative expectations of the past.[29] Despite a previous "deep-seated feeling that wanting power, seeking power, was evil," Butler wrote that

Lauren served as an experiment to show that a "Black woman could be convincing as not just a power-seeker but a power-holder over people who were not necessarily Black and not necessarily female."[30] In *Parable*, Lauren goes on to create a community founded on the belief that survival depended on respect for people's abilities and disabilities and on communal willingness to accept change.

Such assertions placed Butler's worldview closer in perspective to the Black welfare activists who contested the vision for organized employment offered by King-Drew's leaders with their own. Instead of using the functions of the state to achieve the distribution of income security, housing, education, and healthcare to women and children through universal employment of men, welfare rights activists demanded universal access to income security, housing, education, and healthcare as rights that allowed poor women of color to choose careers (be it as stay-at-home mothers or otherwise) free from the coercive powers of patriarchy, racism, and sexism. In short, their vision pushed the state to invest in the autonomy and self-determination of all citizens regardless of race, gender, or stated sexual identity. For Butler, achieving such a vision meant that women would have "no more" or no less "a special place in the future" than men because, as she put it, "the better a society is treating women, the better the society is likely to be."[31]

Although Butler believed that being a Black woman allowed Black women to perceive more humane alternatives for organizing employment and life, she did not believe that one's birth determined one's ideological or political outlook. She made sure that readers still understood the dangers of empowering people just on identity alone by arguing that "wisdom and power and money are all [just] tools . . . that can be used in any way you like. You can use them to tear things up. You can use them to build things up."[32] In this regard, she offered Lauren's leadership as more of a way to achieve a deeper analysis of power than as a prescription of who, by birth, could be expected to be "good." As she claimed, although "people are happier reading about good and evil," "I don't tend to give them that, because I find it boring. It's difficult to go out and find causes and find people who are 100 percent good or 100 percent evil."[33]

Thus, despite her willingness to *criticize* "Black America" and the manifestation of racial and sexual liberalism in history and in her work, she was adamantly unwilling to *condemn* those who sought to end white supremacy and its gendered and sexualized iterations, no matter how imperfect and faulty such attempts might have been. Like many scholars of postwar US history, she recognized that just because power worked in multiple directions did not mean that people in subordinated positions were powerless to create change. She argued that oppressed people "do what [they] have to do" by "mak[ing] the best use of whatever power [they] have."[34] Speaking in regard to her depiction of Black America's 1970s gender war in *Wild Seed*, Butler claimed that what she hoped to achieve in her work was "a series of shadings that correspond to the way concepts like 'good' and 'evil' enter into the real world—never absolute, always by degrees. In my novels, generally, everybody wins and loses something—*Wild Seed* is probably the best illustration of that—because as I see it, that's pretty much the way the world is."[35]

THE PARABLE OF THE HEALER

Like *Wild Seed*, this book I have written has attempted to write history as "a series of shadings that correspond to the way concepts like 'good' and 'evil' enter into the real world—never absolute, always by degrees." I also share Butler's description of herself as "a pessimist, if I am not careful."[36] For some readers, the history I have written might be interpreted only as a story of tragedy and failure. To do so, however, would miss how all the speculative visions for a more equitable society offered by Black people—King-Drew leaders' vision to universalize breadwinning manhood, welfare rights activists' vision for universal basic income, and even Tom Bradley's multicultural vision for capitalist inclusion—remain unfulfilled and incomplete. They are all, as the historian Robin D. G. Kelley would frame them, "freedom dreams" far more inventive and imaginative than many white voters and taxpayers came to understand them.

In this regard, it is indeed hard not to feel pessimistic about society when so much of what Butler has written about Los Angeles has come to pass. In 2005, my attempts to help unionized resident physicians stop the closure of King-Drew's obstetrical and gynecological services only inspired the Board of Supervisors to create special contracts with private hospitals to take some of King-Drew's patients so that they could achieve what they set out to do in closing the medical center's trauma and emergency medical services a year prior. In 2007, the Board of Supervisors officially closed King-Drew, a process that triggered the privatization or closure of most of its neighborhood health clinics.

Much like Medicare and Medicaid in the 1960s, the passage of President Barack Obama's Affordable Care Act in 2010 led to the rebirth of a new hospital in 2015: Martin Luther King Jr. Community Hospital, a small private hospital on the same premises as the previous public hospital. Unlike its public predecessor, MLK Community Hospital accepts only patients who can pay for their healthcare or have Medicare and Medicaid benefits to apply to their care. Patients who cannot pay or are ineligible for Medicare and Medicaid must, just like all indigent patients in Los Angeles, seek care at the remaining public hospitals in Los Angeles or go without healthcare. The closure and rebirth of King Hospital as a private hospital is distinctive because this transformation was overseen by the first Latina and Black woman supervisors elected to the County Board of Supervisors and by the first Black president ever elected to the highest political office of the United States.

Since then, the political backlash to the representation of racial diversity in political offices by way of the 2016 election and 2024 re-election of ultra-far-right President Donald Trump has only obscured how most queer, trans, and poor people of color have been left politically and economically behind by political leaders of all stripes. Butler's assessments of the future seem more urgent and timelier than ever. The widespread belief that police officers and prisons are unreliable, unnecessary, and costly manifested in the Black Lives Matter movement and the George Floyd protests; the deep recognition of unequal access to healthcare unearthed by COVID-19; and the rash of unionization by warehouse workers, graduate students, resident physicians, and coffee baristas—all serve as crisis points where the future can be remade in the present.

NOTES

INTRODUCTION

1. Bielensen hearing testimony submitted by Dr. Ramy Eskandar (2005), author's personal collection.

2. John McCone, "Violence in the City—An End or a Beginning? A Report by the Governor's Commission on the Los Angeles Riots," December 2, 1965, vol. 1, Los Angeles Riots Collection, University of Southern California Special Collections Library, Los Angeles, 1.

3. McCone, "Violence in the City," 7. McCone argued that anti-poverty measures like King-Drew were needed to avoid future rioting and larger police forces. He wrote, "If the city were to elect to stand aside [and not build projects like King-Drew], the walls of segregation would rise ever higher. The disadvantaged community would become more and more estranged and the risk of violence would increase. The cost of police protection would increase, and yet would never be adequate. Unemployment would climb; welfare costs would move apace. And the preachers of division and demagoguery would have a matchless opportunity to tear our nation asunder."

4. A global city is a city that serves as a primary node in a global economic network. The term comes from Saskia Sassen, *The Global City: New York, London, Tokyo* (Princeton University Press, 1991). For more on Los Angeles as a global city and California as a global economy, see Mike Davis, *City of Quartz: Excavating the Future in Los Angeles* (Vintage, 1992); and Ruth Wilson Gilmore, *Golden Gulag: Prisons, Surplus, Crisis, and Opposition in Globalizing California* (University of California Press, 2007).

5. The contradictions of racial liberalism I trace are indebted to many scholars. These include Mary Dudziak, *Cold War Civil Rights: Race and the Image of American Democracy* (Princeton University Press, 2000); Gary Gerstle, *American Crucible: Race and Nation in the Twentieth Century* (Princeton University Press, 2017); Daniel Martinez HoSang, *Racial Propositions: Ballot Initiatives and the Making of Postwar California* (University of California Press, 2010); Jodi Melamed, *Represent*

and Destroy: Rationalizing Violence in the New Racial Capitalism (University of Minnesota Press, 2011); Nikhil Pal Singh, *Black Is a Country: Race and the Unfinished Struggle for Democracy* (Harvard University Press, 2004); Michael Omi and Howard Winant, *Racial Formation in the United States: From the 1960s to the 1990s* (Routledge, 1994).

6. For a broad overview of these processes in medicine, see Nancy Tomes, *Remaking the American Patient: How Madison Avenue and Modern Medicine Turned Patients into Consumers* (University of North Carolina Press, 2016); Dorothy Roberts, *Fatal Invention: How Science, Politics, and Big Business Re-Create Race in the Twenty-First Century* (New Press, 2012). For its expression in racial liberal and radical terms, see John Dittmer, *The Good Doctors: The Medical Committee for Human Rights and the Struggle for Social Justice in Health Care* (University of Mississippi Press, 2009); Dennis A. Doyle, *Psychiatry and Racial Liberalism in Harlem, 1936–1968* (University of Rochester Press, 2016); Darlene Clark Hine, "Black Professionals and Race Consciousness: Origins of the Civil Rights Movement, 1890–1950," *The Journal of American History* 89, no. 4 (2003): 1279–94; Johanna Fernandez, *The Young Lords: A Radical History* (University of North Carolina Press, 2020); Jenna Loyd, *Health Rights Are Civil Rights: Peace and Justice Activism in Los Angeles, 1963–1978* (University of Minnesota Press, 2014); Alondra Nelson, *Body and Soul: The Black Panther Party and the Fight Against Medical Discrimination* (University of Minnesota Press, 2011); Dorothy Roberts, *Killing the Black Body: Race, Reproduction, and the Meaning of Liberty* (Vintage, 1998); David Barton Smith, *The Power to Heal: Civil Rights, Medicare, and the Struggle to Transform America's Health Care System* (Vanderbilt University Press, 2016). For its expression in sexual liberal and radical terms, see Jules Gill-Peterson, *Histories of the Transgender Child* (University of Minnesota Press, 2018); Regina Kunzel, *In the Shadow of Diagnosis: Psychiatric Power and Queer Life* (University of Chicago Press, 2024); A.J. Lewis, "We Are Certain of Our Own Insanity," *Journal of History of Sexuality* 25, no. 1 (2016): 83–113; Sandra Morgen, *Into Our Own Hands: The Women's Health Movement in the United States, 1969–1990* (Rutgers University Press, 2002).

7. See Margot Canaday, *Queer Career: Sexuality and Work in Modern America* (Princeton University Press, 2023); Allison Elias, *The Rise of Corporate Feminism: Women in the American Office, 1960–1990* (Columbia University Press, 2022); Clayton Howard, *The Closet and the Cul-De-Sac: The Politics of Sexual Privacy in Northern California* (University of Pennsylvania, 2019); Scott Kurashige, *The Shifting Grounds of Race: Black and Japanese Americans in the Making of Multiethnic Los Angeles* (Princeton University Press, 2008); Raphael Sonenshein, *Politics in Black and White: Race and Power in Los Angeles* (Princeton University Press, 1994); Daniel Widener, *Black Arts West: Culture and Struggle in Postwar Los Angeles* (Duke University Press, 2010).

8. George Aumoithe, "Dismantling the Safety-Net Hospital: The Construction of 'Underutilization' and Scarce Public Hospital Care," *Journal of Urban History* 49, no. 6 (2023): 1282–311; Mehrsa Baradaran, *The Color of Money: Black Banks and the Racial Wealth Gap* (Belknap Press of Harvard University Press, 2017); Laura Briggs,

How All Politics Became Reproductive Politics: From Welfare Reform to Foreclosure to Trump (University of California Press, 2018); Charlie Eaton, *Bankers in the Ivory Tower: The Troubling Rise of Financiers in US Higher Education* (University of Chicago Press, 2022); Beatrix Hoffman, *Health Care for Some: Rights and Rationing in the United States Since 1930* (University of Chicago Press, 2012); HoSang, *Racial Propositions*; Destin Jenkins, *The Bonds of Inequality: Debt and the Making of the American City* (University of Chicago Press, 2021); Mical Raz, *Abusive Polices: How the American Child Welfare System Lost Its Way* (University of North Carolina, 2020); Dorothy Roberts, *Torn Apart: How the Child Welfare System Destroys Black Families* (Basic, 2022); Keeanga-Yamahtta Taylor, *Race for Profit: How Banks and the Real Estate Industry Undermined Black Homeownership* (University of North Carolina Press, 2019); Elizabeth Todd-Breland, *A Political Education: Black Politics and Education Reform in Chicago Since the 1960s* (University of North Carolina, 2018); Tomes, *Remaking the American Patient*; Lawrence Vale, *Purging the Poorest: Public Housing and the Design Politics of Twice-Cleared Communities* (University of Chicago Press, 2013).

9. Christopher Lowen Agee, *The Streets of San Francisco: Policing and the Creation of a Cosmopolitan Liberal Politics, 1950–1972* (University of Chicago Press, 2014); Lisa Marie Cacho, *Social Death: Racialized Rightlessness and the Criminalization of the Unprotected* (New York University Press, 2012); Nathan B. Connolly, *A World More Concrete: Real Estate and the Remaking of Jim Crow South Florida* (University of Chicago Press, 2014); Max Felker-Kantor, *Policing Los Angeles: Race, Resistance, and the Rise of the LAPD* (University of North Carolina Press, 2018); Christina B. Hanhardt, *Safe Space: Gay Neighborhood History and the Politics of Violence* (Duke University Press, 2013); Mae Ngai, *Impossible Subjects: Illegal Aliens and the Making of Modern America* (Princeton University Press, 2004); Ana Minian, *Undocumented Lives: The Untold Story of Mexican Migration* (Harvard University Press, 2018); Chandan Reddy, *Freedom with Violence: Race, Sexuality, and the US State* (Duke University Press, 2011).

10. I use the term *underemployment* here to refer to workers underpaid and underworked in the formal waged labor market. I also use the term *worklessness* to refer to the lack of opportunities related to temporary work, day work, and contract work at the edges of the formal economy. The term *working poverty* thus signals regular consistent work and employment that pays under-poverty wages. All of these categories of labor point to work outside the formal economy. For more on policing and prisons, see Felker-Kantor, *Policing Los Angele*; Kelly Lytle Hernandez, *Migra! A History of the U.S. Border Patrol* (University of California Press, 2010); Kelly Lytle Hernandez, *City of Inmates: Conquest, Rebellion, and the Rise of Human Caging in Los Angeles* (University of North Carolina Press, 2017).

11. Derrick A. Bell, Jr. "Brown vs. Board of Education and the Interest-Convergence Dilemma," *Harvard Law Review* 93 (January 1980): 518–33.

12. Bell, "Brown vs. Board of Education," 522–23.

13. Bell, "Brown vs. Board of Education," 522.

14. Bell, "Brown vs. Board of Education," 523.

15. Bell, "Brown vs. Board of Education," 524.

16. Bell, "Brown vs. Board of Education,", 524.

17. Jefferson Cowie, *Stayin' Alive: The 1970s and the Last Days of the Working Class* (New Press, 2010).

18. Guian McKee, *Hospital City, Health Care Nation: Race, Capital, and the Costs of American Health Care* (University of Pennsylvania Press, 2023); Andrew T. Simpson, *The Medical Metropolis: Health Care and Economic Transformation in Pittsburgh and Houston* (University of Pennsylvania Press, 2019); Gabriel Winant, *The Next Shift: The Fall of Industry and the Rise of Health Care in Rust Belt America* (Harvard University Press, 2021).

19. Nell Irving Painter calls this period the "the enlargement of American whiteness." See Ira Katznelson, *When Affirmative Action Was White: An Untold History of Racial Inequality in Twentieth-Century America* (W. W. Norton, 2005); and Painter, *The History of White People* (W. W. Norton, 2010).

20. Robert B. Baker, "The American Medical Association and Race," *American Medical Association Journal of Ethics* 16, no. 6 (2014): 479–88; Douglas Melvin Haynes, "Policing the Social Boundaries of the American Medical Association, 1847–70," *Journal of History of Medicine and Allied Sciences* 60, no. 2 (2005): 170–95; Hine, "Black Professionals and Race Consciousness"; Vanessa Northington Gamble, "'Sisters of a Darker Race': African American Graduates of the Woman's Medical College of Pennsylvania, 1867–1925," *Bulletin of History of Medicine* 95 (2021): 169–97; Vanessa Northington Gamble, *Making a Place for Ourselves: The Black Hospital Movement, 1920–1945* (Oxford University Press, 1995); Gretchen Long, "I Studied and Practiced Medicine Without Molestation: African American Doctors in the First Years of Freedom," in *Precarious Prescriptions: Contested Histories of Race and Health in North America*, ed. Laurie B. Green, John McKiernan-Gonzalez, and Martin Summers (University of Minnesota Press, 2014); Thomas J. Ward, *Black Physicians in the Jim Crow South* (University of Arkansas Press, 2003); Lynn E. Miller and Richard M. Weiss, "Re-Visiting Black Medical School Extinctions in the Flexner Era," *Journal of History of Medicine and Allied Sciences* 67, no. 2 (2012): 217–43; Christopher D. E. Willoughby, *Masters of Health: Racial Science and Slavery in U.S. Medical Schools* (University of North Carolina Press, 2022).

21. Dan Georgakas and Marvin Surkin, *Detroit, I Do Mind Dying: A Study in Urban Revolution* (South End Press, 1998); David Goldberg and Trevor Griffey, *Black Power at Work: Community Control, Affirmative Action, and the Construction Industry* (Cornell University Press, 2010); David Goldberg, *Black Firefighters and the FDNY: The Struggle for Jobs, Justice, and Equity in New York City* (University of North Carolina Press, 2020); Robin D. G. Kelley, *Hammer and Hoe: Alabama Communists During the Great Depression* (University of North Carolina, 1990); Philip F. Rubio, *There's Always Work at the Post Office: African American Postal Workers and the Fight for Jobs, Justice, and Equality* (University of North Carolina Press, 2010); Joe Trotter, *Black Milwaukee: The Making of an Industrial Proletariat* (University of Illinois Press, 1985); Joe Trotter, *Coal, Class, and Color: Blacks in Southern West Virginia, 1915–1932* (University of Illinois Press, 1990); Joe Trotter,

Workers on Arrival: Black Labor in the Making of America (University of California Press, 2019).

22. On politics of respectability, see Evelyn Brooks Higginbotham, *Righteous Discontent: The Women's Movement in the Black Baptist Church, 1880–1920* (Harvard University Press, 1993). For excellent illustrations of the concept across class divides, see Kevin Gaines, *Uplifting the Race: Black Leadership, Politics, and Culture in the Twentieth Century* (University of North Carolina Press, 1996); Cheryl D. Hicks, *Talk with You Like A Woman: African American Women, Justice, and Reform in New York, 1890–1935* (University of North Carolina Press, 2010); Michele Mitchell, *Righteous Propagation: African Americans and the Politics of Racial Destiny After Reconstruction* (University of North Carolina Press, 2004); Mary Patillo, *Black Picket Fences: Privilege and Peril Among the Black Middle Class* (University of Chicago Press, 1999); Martin Summers, *Manliness and Its Discontents: The Black Middle Class and the Transformation of Masculinity, 1900–1930* (University of North Carolina Press, 2004). On linked fate, see Michael Dawson, *Behind the Mule: Race and Class in African-American Politics* (Princeton University Press, 1994).

23. Dawson, *Behind the Mule*, 48.

24. Patillo, *Black Picket Fences*, 17.

25. There are many different ideological interpretations for the term *Black capitalism*. To some, like Malcolm X, the term encouraged Black consumers to use and frequent Black-owned banks and businesses as a part of a larger political strategy to achieve eventual independence from white society; others, however, like President Richard Nixon and every other U.S. president after him (including Ronald Reagan and Barack Obama), saw it as a way to renew "white capitalism" under new representative signs. The framing I use is indebted to Baradaran, *The Color of Money*.

26. See Warwick Anderson, "Making Global Health History: The Postcolonial Worldliness of Biomedicine," *The Social History of Medicine* 27, no. 2 (2014): 372–84; Anne-Emanuelle Birn and Raul Necochea Lopez, *Peripheral Nerve: Health and Medicine in Cold War Latin America* (Duke University Press, 2020); Paul Farmer, *Pathologies of Power: Health, Human Rights, and the New War on the Poor* (University of California Press, 2005); Randall M. Packard, *A History of Global Health: Interventions into the Lives of Other Peoples* (Johns Hopkins University Press, 2016); Sebastian Gil-Raino, *The Remnants of Race Science: UNESCO and Economic Development in the Global South* (Columbia University Press, 2023).

27. Tomás Amalguer, *Racial Faultlines: The Historical Origins of White Supremacy in California* (University of California Press, 2009 [1994]); David Gutierrez, *Walls and Mirrors: Mexican Americans, Mexican Immigrants, and the Politics of Ethnicity* (University of California Press, 1995); Ngai, *Impossible Subjects*; Carey McWilliams, *California: The Great Exception* (University of California Press, 1999).

28. Isabel Wilkerson, *The Warmth of Other Suns: The Epic Story of America's Great Migration* (Vintage, 2010); Josh Sides, *L.A. City Limits: African American Los Angeles from the Great Depression to the Present* (University of California Press, 2003).

29. In addition to the works on migration by communities of color mentioned above, see Eric Avila, *Popular Culture in the Age of White Flight* (University of California Press, 2006); Laura Barraclough, *Making the San Fernando Valley: Rural Landscapes, Urban Development, and White Privilege* (University of Georgia Press, 2010); Lisa McGirr, *Suburban Warriors: The Origins of the New American Right* (Princeton University Press, 2001); Becky Nicolaides, *My Blue Heaven: Life and Politics in the Working-Class Suburbs of Los Angeles, 1920–1965* (University of Chicago Press, 2002).

30. On discrimination against homosexuals and suspected homosexuals in federal programs, see Margot Canaday, *The Straight State: Sexuality and Citizenship in Twentieth Century America* (Princeton University Press, 2009); Howard, *The Closet and the Cul-De-Sac*. For on residential segregation in Los Angeles, see Emily Hobson, "Policing Gay LA," in *The Rising Tide of Color*, ed. Moon-Ho Jung (University of Washington Press, 2014).

31. Kurashige, *The Shifting Grounds of Race*; Widener, *Black Arts West*.

32. Lyn Goldfarb and Alison Sotomayor, dirs., *Bridging the Divide: Tom Bradley and the Politics of Race* (Our L.A., 2016); Sonenshein, *Politics in Black and White*.

33. Josh Bloom and Waldo E. Martin Jr., *Black Against Empire: The History and Politics of the Black Panther Party* (University of California Press, 2016); Scot Brown, *Fighting for US: Maulana Karenga, the US Organization, and Black Cultural Nationalism* (New York University Press, 2003); Premilla Nadasen. *Welfare Warriors: The Welfare Rights Movement in the United States* (Routledge, 2005).

34. The conflict between Black nationalist groups, such as US and the Black Panthers, and the violent repression of Black activist groups by state actors such as the Los Angeles Police Department and the Federal Bureau of Investigation, in Los Angeles is well known. For more, see note 33.

35. Black scientists and physicians often used the terms of racial science to contest it. For the multiple contending versions of the Black Radical Tradition in science and medicine, see Britt Rusert, *Fugitive Science: Empiricism and Freedom in Early African American Culture* (New York University Press, 2017); Ayah Nuriddin. "Engineering Uplift: Black Eugenics as Black Liberation," in *Nature Remade: Engineering Life, Envisioning Worlds*, ed. Luis Campos et al. (University of Chicago Press, 2021), 186–201. Other scholars have argued that many white scientists and physicians also used racial science to argue for slavery's abolition, albeit for self-serving economic purposes or to preserve racism without slavery. See Wendy Gonaver, *The Peculiar Institution and the Making of Modern Psychiatry, 1840–1880* (University of North Carolina Press, 2018); Eric Herschthal. *The Science of Abolition: How Slaveholders Became the Enemies of Progress* (Yale University Press, 2021)

36. Merlin Chowkwanyun. *All Health Politics is Local: Community Battles for Medical Care and Environmental Health* (University of North Carolina Press, 2022); Nic John Ramos, "Pathologizing the Crisis: Psychiatry, Policing, and Racial Liberalism in the Long Community Mental Health Movement," *Journal of History of Medicine and Allied Sciences* 74, no. 1 (2019): 57–84; Martin Summers, "Psychia-

try, Mental Health Care, and the Black Freedom Struggle: Chicago's Woodlawn Mental Health Center," *Journal of American History* 110, no. 2 (September 2023): 282–307. There is a bounty of work on how Black clinical representation became increasingly important during and after the Black Power Movement. See Susan Reverby, *Examining Tuskegee: The Infamous Syphilis Study and its Legacy* (University of North Carolina Press, 2009); Nelson, *Body and Soul*.

37. Barbara Ehrenreich. *Nickel and Dimed: On (Not) Getting By in America* (Metropolitan Books, 2001).

38. Manning Marable. *How Capitalism Underdeveloped Black America: Problems in Race, Political Economy, and Society* (South End Press, 2000 [1983]), 2.

39. Kimberlé Crenshaw. "Race, Reform, and Retrenchment," *Harvard Law Review* 101, no. 7 (May 1988): 1331–87.

40. Crenshaw, "Race, Reform, and Retrenchment," 1331.

41. Ruth Wilson Gilmore, *Abolition Geography: Essays Towards Liberation* (Verso Press, 2022), 451.

42. Kimberlé Crenshaw, "Demarginalizing the Intersections of Race and Sex: A Black Feminist Critique of Antidiscrimination Doctrine, Feminist Theory and Antiracist Politics," *University of Chicago Legal Forum*, vol. 1989, no. 1, Article 8: 139–67.

43. Crenshaw, "Demarginalizing the Intersections of Race and Sex," 139–40.

44. Crenshaw, "Demarginalizing the Intersections of Race and Sex," 152.

45. Roderick A. Ferguson, *Aberrations in Black: Towards a Queer of Color Critique* (University of Minnesota Press, 2004).

46. Ferguson, *Aberrations in Black*, 6.

47. Patricia Hill Collins famously wrote, "What sense does it make to talk about 'Black People' as if all Black people are male when gender differences are so pronounced?" See *Black Sexual Politics: African Americans, Gender, and the New Racism* (Routledge, 2004), 5–6.

48. Cathy J. Cohen, "Punks, Bulldaggers, and Welfare Queens: The Radical Potential of Queer Politics?" *GLQ* 3: 438.

49. Audre Lorde, *Sister Outsider* (Freedom: Crossing Press, 1984), 61.

50. Lorde, *Sister Outsider*, 74.

51. Hortense Spillers. "Mama's Baby, Papa's Maybe: An American Grammar Book." *Diacritics* 17, no. 2 (1987): 64–81.

52. Cheryl I. Harris, "Whiteness as Property," *Harvard Law Review* 106, no. 8 (June 1993): 1715.

CHAPTER ONE

1. White was likely one of a handful of Black medical graduates accepted to USC's residency program before his arrival in 1954.

2. Simeon Booker, "Watts Report: Doctor with 10,000 Patients / Called 'Odd ball' Medic in Watts," *Jet Magazine*, April, 1966, 16.

3. For more on the concept of terra nullius, see Glenn Clouthard, *Red Skin, White Masks: Rejecting the Colonial Politics of Recognition* (University of Minnesota Press, 2014). A bevy of scholars working at the intersection of Black Studies and Indigenous Studies have shown that Western lands were not "empty" but full of Indigenous people and Black migrants. See Sarah E. K. Fong, "Racial-Settler Capitalism: Character Building and the Accumulation of Land and Labor in the Late Nineteenth Century," *American Indian Culture and Research Journal* 43, no. 2 (2019): 25–48; Tiffany Lethabo King, *The Black Shoals: Offshore Formulations of Black and Native Studies* (Duke University Press, 2019); Bayley Marquez, *Plantation Pedagogy: The Violence of Schooling Across Black and Indigenous Space* (University of California Press, 2024); Tiya Miles, *Ties That Bind: The Story of an Afro-Cherokee Family in Slavery and Freedom* (University of California Press, 2015); Alaina E. Roberts, *I've Been Here All the While: Black Freedom on Native Land* (University of Pennsylvania Press, 2021); Fay A. Yarbrough, *Race and the Cherokee Nation: Sovereignty in the Nineteenth Century* (University of Pennsylvania Press, 2008).

4. The terms here are words used by Drs. Oscar J. Jackson and Waldenese Nixon, two Black physicians practicing in Northern California, to describe, as they put it, "a group of physicians that the black community calls claim-jumpers and parasites" that "are usually non-black physicians who are somewhat self-seeking." See "Medicine in the Black Community," *The Western Journal of Medicine* 114, no. 4 (October, 1970): 58.

5. The full quotation is: "Considering himself as Watts' social worker-oriented physician, Dr. White strongly believes that Negro leadership must embrace segregation 'for a while' to solve problems in the ghettos." See Booker, "Watts Report," 20.

6. James Baldwin, *Another Country* (Vintage Books, 1993).

7. As Maria Josefina Saldaña-Portillo argues, "Development's discursive emergence was . . . paradoxically, *both* a liberatory strategy for decolonizing the world *and* a 'neutral' rearticulation of racialized colonized categories as national difference"; see *The Revolutionary Imagination in the Americas and the Age of Development* (Duke University Press, 2003), 23. For Alyosha Goldstein, this "foreign" and international dimension inspired US policy makers to approach urban and rural poor neighborhoods of color within the US in a similar fashion but towards more limited means. According to him, "US policymakers seized on the alignment of the foreign with underdevelopment when it could be cast as a transitional moment in the process of incorporation and assimilation, but when the conjunction threatened to seem a consequence of market or colonial relations, they considered it not only inassimilable but impermissible." See *Poverty in Common: The Politics of Community Action During the American Century* (Duke University Press, 2012), 78.

8. Gamble, *Making a Place for Ourselves*, 183–92.

9. Karen Kruse Thomas, *Deluxe Jim Crow: Civil Rights and American Health Policy, 1935–1954* (University of Georgia Press, 2011).

10. Hine, "Black Professionals and Race Consciousness."

11. W. Montague Cobb, "The Crushing Irony of De Luxe Jim Crow," *Journal of the National Medical Association* 44 (September 1952): 386–87.

12. For scholarship on successful desegregation efforts in medicine, see Dittmer, *The Good Doctors*; and D. Smith, *The Power to Heal*. For on the limits of such efforts, see Kevin McQueeney, "Health Care in the Era of Civil Rights and Resistance, 1950–1968," in *A City Without Care: 300 Years of Racism, Health Disparities, and Health Care Activism in New Orleans* (University of North Carolina Press, 2023); and T. Ward, *Black Physicians in the Jim Crow South*.

13. Dittmer, *The Good Doctors*; and D. Smith, *The Power to Heal*.

14. McQueeney, *A City Without Care*.

15. According to Martha Derthick, the NMA essentially "represented the medical professional" between 1963 and 1965, since the AMA was "implacably hostile to government health insurance." See *Policy Making for Social Security* (Brookings Institute, 1979), 96.

16. John Dittmer observes that many NMA activists, particularly those in Alabama and Mississippi, resented mainstream media's portrayal of the MCHR as the "medical wing of the civil rights movement" (*The Good Doctors*, 61–84).

17. Booker, "Watts Report," 16–21.

18. Booker, "Watts Report," 20.

19. Booker, "Watts Report," 16.

20. Charles Briggs, *Incommunicable: Towards Communicative Justice in Health and Medicine* (Duke University Press, 2024).

21. Gary Okihiro claims that "the power to know and the disciplining of space-time" associated with Western medicine's discourses "are imperial projects insofar as they claim the mastery over selves over others and of humans over other life-forms and their habitats." See *Third World Studies: Theorizing Liberation*, 2nd ed. (Duke University Press, 2024), 70.

22. Sharla Fett, *Working Cures: Healing, Health, and Power on Southern Slave Plantations* (University of North Carolina Press, 2002); Pablo F. Gómez, *The Experiential Caribbean: Creating Knowledge and Healing in the Early Modern Atlantic* (University of North Carolina Press, 2017); Pablo F. Gómez and Diego Armus, eds., *The Gray Zones of Medicine: Healers and History in Latin America* (University of Pittsburgh Press, 2021); Kalle Kananoja, *Healing Knowledge in Atlantic Africa: Medical Encounters, 1500–1850* (Cambridge University Press, 2021); Long, "I Studied and Practiced Medicine Without Molestation"; Kathleen Murphy, "Translating the Vernacular: Indigenous and African Knowledge in the Eighteenth-Century British Atlantic," *Atlantic Studies* 8, no. 1 (2011): 29–48; Carolyn Roberts, "To Heal and to Harm: Medicine, Knowledge, and Power in the Atlantic Slave Trade" (PhD diss., Harvard University, 2017); Todd Savitt, *Medicine and Slavery: The Disease and Care of Blacks in Antebellum Virginia* (University of Illinois Press, 1978); Sean Morey Smith and Christopher D. E. Willoughby, *Medicine and Healing in the Age of Slavery* (Louisiana State University Press, 2021); James Sweet, *Domingos Alvarez, African Healing, and the Intellectual History of the Atlantic World* (University of North Carolina Press, 2011); Harriet Washington, *Medical Apartheid: The Dark History of Medical Experimentation on Black Americans from Colonial Times to Present* (Anchor Books, 2006); Marli Weiner with Mazie Hough, *Sex, Sickness, and Slavery:*

Illness in the Antebellum South (University of Illinois Press, 2014); Karol K. Weaver, *Medical Revolutionaries: The Enslaved Healers of Eighteenth-Century Saint Domingue* (University of Illinois Press, 2006).

23. Pablo F. Gómez, "The Circulation of Bodily Knowledge in the Seventeenth-Century Black Spanish Caribbean," *Social History of Medicine* 26, no. 3 (2013): 386.

24. Fett, *Working Cure*.

25. Deirdre Cooper Owens. *Medical Bondage: Race, Gender, and the Origins of American Gynecology* (University of Georgia Press, 2017); Rana Hogarth, *Medicalizing Blackness: Making Racial Difference in the Atlantic World, 1780–1840* (University of North Carolina Press, 2017); Willoughby, *Masters of Health*.

26. In addition to Willoughby, see Daina Ramey Berry, *The Price for Their Pound of Flesh: The Value of the Enslaved, from Womb to Grave, in the Building of a Nation* (Beacon Press, 2017); Andrew S. Curran, *The Anatomy of Blackness. Science and Slavery in an Age of Enlightenment* (Johns Hopkins University Press, 2011).

27. Willoughby, *Masters of Health*.

28. In addition to Willoughby, see Hogarth, *Medicalizing Blackness*; Siobhan Somerville. *Queering the Color Line: Race and the Invention of Homosexuality in American Culture* (Duke University Press, 2000).

29. Jonathan M. Metzl, *The Protest Psychosis: How Schizophrenia Became a Black Disease* (Beacon Press, 2009).

30. Scholars Lundy Braun and Rana Hogarth have debated the importance of Cartwright in the development of American medicine. Braun argues that Cartwright "was not a fringe thinker at midcentury" because he was apprenticed by the United States's leading physician, Benjamin Rush, was educated in Maryland, Pennsylvania, and Europe, and was published in several prominent medical journals; see *Breathing Race into the Machine: The Surprising Career of the Spirometer from Plantation to Genetics* (University of Minnesota, 2014), 28. Hogarth asserts that several white physicians during his time took issue with the fact that his "suppositions on the black race were too heavily influenced by his political stance on slavery" in medical journals; see *Medicalizing Blackness*, 198n22. Despite this disagreement, both argue Cartwright's writings contributed to a long line of racial science physicians, such as Josiah Nott, Marli F. Weiner, and John Stainback Wilson, who legitimated and normalized racism in scientific and medical thought and practice.

31. Somerville, *Queering the Color Line*.

32. Long, "I Studied and Practiced Medicine Without Molestation."

33. D. Haynes, "Policing the Social Boundaries of the American Medical Association, 1847–70."

34. D. Haynes, "Policing the Social Boundaries of the American Medical Association, 1847–70."

35. Miller and Weiss, "Re-Visiting Black Medical School Extinctions in the Flexner Era."

36. T. Ward, *Black Physicians in the Jim Crow South*.

37. T. Ward, *Black Physicians in the Jim Crow South*.

38. Kevin Starr, *Inventing the Dream: California Through the Progressive Era* (Oxford University Press, 1985), 91.

39. Widney saw the "dull" Indigenous Tongva and Chumash people and the "sleepy" and "lazy" mixed-race Mexican *Indio* as degenerating racial groups whose neglect had left Southern California's land barren. He saw the climatically hearty "Aryan" as being the only race capable of awakening the "sleeping beauty" of Southern California's landscapes. Notably, Widney believed white settlers had a chance to correct the dangerous imbalance of industry and nature that (he claimed) not only had once caused the "race life" degeneration of once-great civilizations in the American Southwest, the Americas, Asia, and Southern Europe, but also was threatening to degenerate the "Engle" (Anglo) in the Eastern United States. He thus saw Los Angeles as being the center for the new development of new superior white societies to be located in the Western United States, Australia, and New Zealand. For more, see Joseph Pomeroy Widney. *Civilizations and their Diseases and Rebuilding a Wrecked World Civilization* (Pacific Publishing Company, 1937); *Race Life and Race Religions* (Pacific Publishing Company, 1936); *The Three Americas: Their Racial Past and the Dominant Racial Factors of Their Future* (Publishing Company, 1935). Kevin Starr's *Inventing the Dream* also has a compelling description of Widney's writings (91–98).

40. Charles Rosenberg, *The Care of Strangers: The Rise of America's Hospital System* (Johns Hopkins University Press, 1987); Paul Starr, *The Social Transformation of American Medicine: The Rise of a Sovereign Profession and the Making of a Vast Industry* (Basic, 1982); Rosemary A. Stevens, *In Sickness and in Wealth: American Hospitals in the Twentieth Century* (Basic Books, 1989)

41. The Pauper Act caused the Los Angeles County Board of Supervisors to give its first contract to the Daughters of Charity, who arrived in California in the wake of the Gold Rush to tend to the "new problems" caused by the "population increase" of white settlers. See Daughters of Charity, "Our Heritage," accessed December 12, 2012, http://www.daughtersofcharity.com/who/OurHeritage/Pages/default.aspx.

42. Deborah Reidy Kelch, *Caring for Medically Indigent Adults in California: A History* (California Healthcare Foundation, June 2005), 5.

43. Kevin Waite, *West of Slavery: The Southern Drum of a Transcontinental Empire* (University of North Carolina Press, 2021).

44. Du Bois noted the difference between the free wage labor of the "white worker" and the enslaved and free wage labor of the "Black worker" as primarily a difference in their spatial and economic mobility. In *Black Reconstruction* he wrote, "No matter how degraded the factory hand, he is not real estate." See *Black Reconstruction in America, 1860–1880* (Harcourt, Bruce and Company, 1935; repr., The Free Press, 1998), 7. Du Bois insisted on this term even after his publisher suggested his use of the word was a mistake or accident. Du Bois insisted the legal status of enslaved people was real estate, not personal property, writing that the publisher's desire to change "real estate" to "property" throughout the manuscript was done "without knowing the facts." For more, see Zach Sell, *Trouble of the World: Slavery and Empire in the Age of Capital* (University of North Carolina Press, 2021), 15–17.

45. Michael Magliari, "'A Species of Slavery': The Compromise of 1850, Popular Sovereignty, and the Expansion of Unfree Indian Labor in the American West," *The Journal of American History* 109, no. 3 (2022): 518–47.

46. A series of laws, including the Alien Land Law, impacted a wide range of Chinese, Japanese, Filipino, and South Asian immigrants. For more, see Rick Baldoz, *The Third Asiatic Invasion: Empire and Migration in Filipino America, 1898–1946* (New York University Press, 2011); Manu Karuka, *Empire's Tracks: Indigenous Nations, Chinese Workers, and the Transcontinental Railroad* (University of California Press, 2019); Susan Koshy, *Sexual Naturalization: Asian Americans and Miscegenation* (Stanford University Press, 2004); Erika Lee, *At America's Gates: Chinese Immigration During the Exclusion Era, 1882–1943* (University of North Carolina Press, 2003); Robert Lee, *Orientals: Asian Americans in Popular Culture* (Temple University Press, 1999); Beth Lew-Williams, *The Chinese Must Go: Violence, Exclusion, and the Making of the Alien in America* (Harvard University Press, 2021); Karen Leonard, *Making Ethnic Choices: California's Punjabi Mexican Americans* (Temple University Press, 1992); Lisa Lowe, *Immigrant Acts: On Asian American Cultural Politics* (Duke University Press, 1996); Ngai, *Impossible Subjects;* Gary Y. Okihiro, *Margins and Mainstreams: Asians in American History and Culture* (University of Washington Press, 1994); Nayan Shah, *Contagious Divides: Epidemics and Race in San Francisco's Chinatown* (University of California Press, 2001); Nayan Shah, *Stranger Intimacy: Contesting Race, Sexuality, and the Law in the North American West* (University of California Press, 2011); Isabel Wallace, *Not Fit to Stay: Public Health Panics and South Asian Exclusion* (University of Washington Press, 2017)

47. William Deverell, *Whitewashed Adobe: The Rise of Los Angeles and the Re-Making of its Mexican Past* (University of California Press, 2004); Miroslava Chávez-García, *States of Delinquency: Race and Science in the Making of California's Juvenile Justice System* (University of California Press, 2012); John McKiernan-González, *Fevered Measures: Public Health and Race at the Texas-Mexico Border, 1848–1942* (Duke University Press, 2012); Elena Gutierrez, *Fertile Matters: The Politics of Mexican-Origin Women's Reproduction* (University of Texas Press, 2014); Natalie Lira, *Laboratory of Deficiency: Sterilization and Confinement in California, 1900–1950s* (University of California Press, 2022); Natalia Molina, *Fit to Be Citizens?: Public Health and Race in Los Angeles, 1879–1939* (University of California Press, 2006); Lina-Maria Murillo, "Birth Control, Border Control: The Movement for Contraception in El Paso, Texas, 1936–1940," *Pacific Historical Review* 90, no. 3 (2021): 314–44; George Sanchez, *Becoming Mexican American: Ethnicity, Culture and Identity in Chicano Los Angeles, 1900–1945* (Oxford University Press, 1993); Alexandra Minna Stern, "Building Boundaries and Blood: Medicalization and Nation-Building on the U.S.-Mexico Border, 1910–1930," *Hispanic American Historical Review* 79, no. 1 (1999): 41–81; Alexandra Minna Stern, *Eugenic Nation: Faults and Frontiers of Better Breeding in Modern America* (University of California Press, 2005).

48. According to Tomas Amalguer, Black laborers were particularly "unwelcome" to the state because their "presence, or threatened presence" engendered labor

conflict with potential white working class laborers and because "their association with a slave system" was considered to be "antithetical to the society being created in California." See *Racial Faultlines*, 5; Ngai, *Impossible Subject*, 13.

49. Douglas Flamming, *Bound for Freedom: Black Los Angeles in Jim Crow America* (University of California Press, 2006); Sanchez, *Becoming Mexican American*; Molina, *Fit to Be Citizens?*

50. Sanchez, *Becoming Mexican American*.

51. Deverell, *Whitewashed Adobe*.

52. Deverell, *Whitewashed Adobe*, 10.

53. From 1915 to 1919, Los Angeles County monitored birthrates using the racial categories of "white," "Japanese," "Mexican," and "other," to "indicate where Japanese births outnumbered white births." After the 1921 and 1924 Immigration Acts and California Alien Land Law acts made the Japanese "no longer a visible threat," Natalia Molina argues the county introduced the word "alien" in hospital record-keeping practices to track Mexican birthrates. See *Fit to Be Citizens?*, 56–57, 129–31.

54. By 1915, county officials began reporting on the wide number of racial and ethnic groups receiving care at Los Angeles County General Hospital. By 1924, the swelling numbers of patients led county officials to campaign to relieve overcrowding through a bond measure by inviting reporters to witness the number of patients being placed "on the porches, verandas and even basement," the close quarters of tubercular patients, and the nearly three hundred patients it estimated were turned away daily. Although newspaper reports scrubbed the race and ethnicity of county patients, Emily K. Abel argues tuberculosis was widely associated in the cultural imagination with Mexican and Filipino workers and their neighborhoods. See "Many Sick Aliens: Figures Show Nearly Half of Patients Applying at County Hospital are Foreigners," *Los Angeles Times*, November 22, 1915, II2.; "Chamber Approves Bonds—County Issue for $7,000,000 for Finance Hospitals and Other Institutions Urged on People," *Los Angeles Times*, April 1, 1923; "County Bonds Called Saving," *Los Angeles Times*, April 22, 1923, II3; Emily K. Abel, "'Only the Best Class of Immigration:' Public Health Policy Toward Mexicans and Filipinos in Los Angeles, 1910–1940," *American Journal of Public Health* 94, no. 6 (2004): 932–39.

55. Mrs. M. M. James, "Letters to the Times," *Los Angeles Times*, April 19, 1923, I-10.

56. Margaret Gorsuch Morden and Richard Bigger, "Studies in Local Government, No. 11: Cooperative Health Administration in Metropolitan Los Angeles," Bureau of Governmental Research (University of California Los Angeles: June, 1949), 19.

57. *Goodall vs. Bright*, 11 California Court of Appeals, Second District 540 (1936), 541–54.

58. County Counsel to John Anson Ford re: *Goodall v Brite*, April 28, 1938, John Anson Ford Papers, Huntington Library.

59. County Counsel to John Anson Ford re: *Goodall v Brite*, April 28, 1938, John Anson Ford Papers, Huntington Library; *Goodall vs. Bright*, 11 California Court of Appeals, Second District 540 (1936), 549.

60. Most historians of medicine mark the 1920s as the birth of the modern hospital. See Rosenberg, *The Care of Strangers;* P. Starr, *The Social Transformation of American Medicine*; and Stevens, *In Sickness and in Wealth.*

61. This concept has long history in the American West. See Richard White, *The Middle Ground: Indians, Empires, and Republics in the Great Lakes Region, 1650–1815* (Cambridge University Press, 2010); Shah, *Stranger Intimacy*; Peter Boag, *Same-Sex Affairs: Constructing and Controlling Homosexuality in the Pacific Northwest* (University of California Press, 2003); Susan Lee Johnson, *Roaring Camp: The Social World of the California Gold Rush* (W. W. Norton, 2001).

62. *Goodall vs. Bright,* 11 California Court of Appeals, Second District 540 (1936), 549.

63. Regina Kunzel, *Criminal Intimacy: Prison and the Uneven History of Modern American Sexuality* (University of Chicago, 2008); Shah, *Stranger Intimacy*; Howard, *The Closet and the Cul-De-Sac.*

64. Canaday, *The Straight State.*

65. Gary Gerstle, Nelson Lichtenstein, and Alice O'Connor, eds., *Beyond the New Deal Order: US Politics from the Great Depression to the Great Recession* (University of Pennsylvania Press, 2019).

66. Canaday, *The Straight State*, 95–103.

67. Winant, *The Next Shift.*

68. Howard, *The Closet and the Cul-de-Sac.*

69. Canaday, *The Straight State;* Katznelson, *When Affirmative Action was White.*

70. Canaday, *The Straight State.*

71. Howard, *The Closet and the Cul-De-Sac.*

72. Local Hospital District Law section 32000 et. seq. of California Health and Safety Code.

73. According to the Desert Healthcare District and Foundation, "Prior to 1948, desert residents and visitors [of the West Coachella Valley] requiring hospitalization were transported to healthcare facilities in Indio, Loma Linda, Redlands, San Bernardino, and Riverside." In response, "Desert Healthcare District was created in 1948 to serve residents within a 458-mile-square-area of the Coachella Valley." See Desert Healthcare District and Foundation, "Our History," https://www.dhcd.org/Our-History, accessed August 25, 2022; "Hospital Board Elects President," *Los Angeles Times*, December 31, 1956, B9.

74. Rosemary A. Stevens, "Medical Specialization as American Health Policy: Interweaving Public and Private Roles," in *History and Health Policy in the United States: Putting the Past Back In*, ed. Rosemary Stevens, Charles Rosenberg, and Lawton Burns (Rutgers University Press, 2006); Kenneth Ludmerer, *Learning to Heal: The Development of American Medical Education* (Johns Hopkins University Press, 1985).

75. Harry Nelson, "Overhaul of Hospital Funds Rules Proposed," *Los Angeles Times*, December 7, 1962, A9.

76. "Hospital Beds Pose Problems: West Side Paradox: Too Many Here and Too Few There," *Los Angeles Times*, January 3, 1965, WS1; "Application for New Hospital Turned Down," *Los Angeles Times*, August 11, 1964, A8.

77. The phrase "invisible hand of the market" is generally attributed to Adam Smith's eighteenth-century writings on laissez-faire economics popularized in *The Theory of Moral Sentiments* (1759) and *The Wealth of Nations* (1776). It usually refers to the idea that trade and market exchange automatically channel self-interest toward socially desirable ends. See Adam Smith, *The Theory of Moral Sentiments*, ed. Knud Haakonssen (Cambridge University Press, 2002); Adam Smith, *The Wealth of Nations*, ed. Edwin Cannan (Modern Library, 1994).

78. Arnold Hirsch, *Making the Second Ghetto: Race and Housing in Chicago, 1940–1960* (University of Chicago Press, 2021, repr.).

79. The roots of these trends date back to farm policies initiated in the 1930s; see David Hamilton, *From New Day to New Deal: American Farm Policy from Hoover to Roosevelt* (University of North Carolina Press, 1991). For its impact on migrations, see Gutierrez, *Walls and Mirrors*; Matt Garcia, *A World of Its Own: Race, Labor, and Citrus in the Making of Greater Los Angeles, 1900–1970* (University of North Carolina Press, 2002); Christian Paiz, *The Strikers of Coachella Valley: A Rank-and-File History of the UFW Movement* (University of North Carolina Press, 2022); Sides, *L.A. City Limits*.

80. Wesley R. Brazier, Testimony Before the Governor's Commission on the Los Angeles Riots, October 14, 1965, Vol. IV Governor's Commission on the Los Angeles Riots, Los Angeles Riots Collection, Special Collections Library University of Southern California, 10.

81. Wesley R. Brazier, Testimony Before the Governor's Commission on the Los Angeles Riots, October 14, 1965, Vol. IV Governor's Commission on the Los Angeles Riots, Los Angeles Riots Collection, Special Collections Library University of Southern California, 23.

82. Guichard Parris and Sherwood Ross, Transcripts of Testimony, National Urban League Press Release, November 16, 1964, Vol. IV Governor's Commission on the Los Angeles Riots, Los Angeles Riots Collection, Special Collections Library University of Southern California, 2.

83. Willie F. Brown, Testimony Before the Governor's Commission on the Los Angeles Riots, November 4, 1965, Vol. IV Governor's Commission on the Los Angeles Riots, Los Angeles Riots Collection, Special Collections Library University of Southern California, 4.

84. Winston Slaughter, Testimony Before the Governor's Commission on the Los Angeles Riots, November 4, 1965, Vol. XIII Governor's Commission on the Los Angeles Riots, Los Angeles Riots Collection, Special Collections Library University of Southern California, 24.

85. Wendell Collins, Testimony Before the Governor's Commission on the Los Angeles Riots, November 4, 1965, Vol. V Governor's Commission on the Los Angeles Riots, Los Angeles Riots Collection, Special Collections Library University of Southern California, 18.

86. Louis Fleming, "Space Lack Prompts Hospital Bond Issue: More Room Needed for Bed and Clinic Patients, Doctors, Interns and Nurses," *Los Angeles Times*, May 20, 1960, B1. Under the article subsection titled "Training Stressed,"

Fleming quoted Dr. Thomas, the director of the hospital: "The part of the story that is hard to tell is the effect on our training program of inadequate facilities. This can seriously handicap the learning of medicine."

87. Lester Breslow, "New Partnerships in the Delivery of Services—A Public Health View of Need," *The American Journal of Public Health* 57, no. 7. (July 1967): 1095.

88. Breslow, "New Partnership in the Delivery of Services," 1095.

89. Taylor, *Race for Profit* (University of North Carolina Press, 2019).

90. See Fleming, "Space Lack Prompts Hospital Bond Issue."

91. "'Tokenism' Held Rap at Negro MDs," *Los Angeles Times*, August 11, 1963, G7.

92. Kurashige, *The Shifting Grounds of Race*.

93. Flamming, *Bound for Freedom*; Sides, *L.A. City Limits*.

94. George Sanchez, "'What's Good for Boyle Heights is Good for the Jews: Creating Multiracialism on the Eastside During the 1950s," *American Quarterly* 56, no. 3 (2004): 633–61.

95. John Buggs, Testimony Before the Governor's Commission on the Los Angeles Riots, Pre-submitted Testimony, September 28, 1965, Vol. V Governor's Commission on the Los Angeles Riots, Los Angeles Riots Collection, Special Collections Library University of Southern California, 5.

96. George Sanchez, *Boyle Heights: How a Los Angeles Neighborhood Became the Future of American Democracy* (University of California Press, 2022).

97. Thomas Roy Peyton, "The Negro Specialist and the Negro General Practitioner," *Journal of the National Medical Association* 55, no. 3 (May 1963): 248–50.

98. M. Alfred Haynes, "The Distribution of Black Physicians in the United States, 1967," *Journal of the National Medical Association* 61, no. 6 (November 1969): 470–73.

99. Peyton, "The Negro Specialist and the Negro General Practitioner," 248.

100. Peyton, "The Negro Specialist and the Negro General Practitioner," 249.

101. Avila, *Popular Culture in the Age of White Flight*.

102. Jean Gregg, Testimony Before the Governor's Commission on the Los Angeles Riots, Pre-submitted Testimony, October 21, 1965, Vol. VII Governor's Commission on the Los Angeles Riots, Los Angeles Riots Collection, Special Collections Library University of Southern California, 18.

103. Jean Gregg, Testimony Before the Governor's Commission on the Los Angeles Riots, Pre-submitted Testimony, October 21, 1965, Vol. VII Governor's Commission on the Los Angeles Riots, Los Angeles Riots Collection, Special Collections Library University of Southern California, 9.

104. John Buggs, Testimony Before the Governor's Commission on the Los Angeles Riots, Pre-submitted Testimony, September 28, 1965, Vol. V Governor's Commission on the Los Angeles Riots, Los Angeles Riots Collection, Special Collections Library University of Southern California, 2.

105. John Buggs, Testimony Before the Governor's Commission on the Los Angeles Riots, Pre-submitted Testimony, September 28, 1965, Vol. V Governor's

Commission on the Los Angeles Riots, Los Angeles Riots Collection, Special Collections Library University of Southern California, 2.

106. Daniel Martinez HoSang, "'Get Back Your Rights!' Fair Housing and the Right to Discriminate, 1960–1972," in *Racial Propositions*, 52–81.

107. H. H. Brookins, Testimony Before the Governor's Commission on the Los Angeles Riots, September 29, 1965, Vol. IV Governor's Commission on the Los Angeles Riots, Los Angeles Riots Collection, Special Collections Library University of Southern California, 27.

108. Arthur J. Viseltear, Arnold Kirsch, and Milton Roemer, *Medical Care Administration—Case Study No. 5: The Watts Hospital: Pilot Study US DHEW Public Health Service*, September 18, 1969, Series 18, Box 895 Charles R. Drew Postgraduate Medical School Papers, Commonwealth Fund Collection, Rockefeller Archives Center.

109. Booker, "Watts Report," 21.

110. John Buggs, Testimony Before the Governor's Commission on the Los Angeles Riots, Pre-submitted Testimony, September 28, 1965, Vol. V Governor's Commission on the Los Angeles Riots, Los Angeles Riots Collection, Special Collections Library University of Southern California, 18–19.

111. For more, see Chowkwanyun, *All Health Politics is Local*.

112. California State Hospital Advisory Council, Agenda and Minutes, December 13–14, 1965, Martin Luther King, Jr. Hospital 1965–1990, Kenneth Hahn Papers, Huntington Library, 13–14.

113. California State Hospital Advisory Council, Agenda and Minutes, December 13–14, 1965, Martin Luther King, Jr. Hospital 1965–1990, Kenneth Hahn Papers, Huntington Library, 13.

114. Wendell Collins, Testimony Before the Governor's Commission on the Los Angeles Riots, November 4, 1965, Vol. V Governor's Commission on the Los Angeles Riots, Los Angeles Riots Collection, Special Collections Library University of Southern California, 25.

115. Booker, "Watts Report," 21.

116. The idea that interracial fraternity could hasten national development is not new. See Ada Ferrer, *Insurgent Cuba: Race, Nation, and Revolution, 1868–1898* (University of North Carolina Press, 1999).

117. Viseltear, Kirsch, and Roemer, *Medical Care Administration*.

118. Viseltear, Kirsch, and Roemer, *Medical Care Administration*.

119. California State Advisory Hospital Council, "Agenda Minutes, December 13–14, 1965," Martin Luther King, Jr. Hospital 1965 Papers, Kenneth Hahn Papers, Huntington Library, 13.

CHAPTER TWO

1. Jeanne Theoharis, *A More Beautiful and Terrible History: The Uses and Misuses of Civil Rights History* (Beacon Press, 2018), 62–82.

2. John McCone, *Violence in the City—An End or a Beginning? A Report by the Governor's Commission on the Los Angeles Riots*, December 2, 1965, Vol. 1 Governor's Commission on the Los Angeles Riots, Los Angeles Riots Collection, Special Collections Library University of Southern California, 74.

3. Shah, *Contagious Divides*.

4. Neil Smith, *Uneven Development: Nature, Capital, and the Production of Space* (University of Georgia Press, 1984).

5. Smith, *Uneven Development*, 174.

6. Spillers, "Mama's Baby, Papa's Maybe."

7. Cohen, "Punks, Bulldaggers, and Welfare Queens," 452.

8. Hicks, *Talk with You Like A Woman*.

9. Higginbotham, *Righteous Discontent*.

10. Robert B. Baker, Harriet A. Washington, Ololade Olakanmi, Todd L. Savitt, Elizabeth A. Jacobs, Eddie Hoover, and Matthew K. Wynia, "African American Physicians and Organized Medicine, 1846–1968: Origins of a Racial Divide," *Journal of the American Medical Association* 300, no. 3 (2008): 306–13.

11. Gamble, "Sisters of a Darker Race," 186.

12. Miller and Weiss, "Re-Visiting Black Medical School Extinctions in the Flexner Era."

13. T. Ward, *Black Physicians in the Jim Crow South*, 31–57.

14. Vanessa Northington Gamble, "Black Autonomy versus White Control: Black Hospitals and the Dilemmas of White Philanthropy, 1920–1940," *Minerva* 35, no. 3 (October 1997): 247.

15. M. Alfred Haynes. "Problems Facing the Negro in Medicine Today," *The Journal of the American Medical Association* 209, no. 7 (August 18, 1969): 1069.

16. Gamble, "Sisters of a Darker Race."

17. Kelly O'Donnell, "Labors of Love and Marriage," *Journal of History of Medicine and Allied Sciences* (forthcoming).

18. "The Woman's Auxiliary of the NMA," *The Journal of the National Medical Association* 33, no. 6 (November 1941): 273.

19. Mrs. Marcus O. Tucker, "The Role of the Women's Auxiliary to the National Medical Association in the Talent Recruitment Program," *The Journal of the National Medical Association* 57, no. 6 (November 1965): 453–54.

20. McCone, *Violence in the City*, 72, 6.

21. Oral history transcript, John A. McCone, interview 1 (I), 8/19/1970, by Joe B. Frantz, LBJ Library Oral Histories, LBJ Presidential Library, https://www.discoverlbj.org/item/oh-mcconej-19700819-1-74-150.

22. For more on Oscar Lewis, see Laura Briggs, *Reproducing Empire: Race, Sex, Science, and US Imperialism in Puerto Rico* (University of California Press, 2003). The most noteworthy of popular social science studies depicting Black neighborhoods and their problems as isolated, detached, and separate from "mainstream" white society is Gunnar Myrdal's *An American Dilemma: The Negro Problem and Modern Democracy* (Harper and Brothers, 1944). Myrdal's work, however, followed upon the formation of sociology as a discipline under Robert E. Park's "Chicago

School," which included Ernest Burgess, William Thomas, George Herbert Mead, and Louis Wirth at the University of Chicago. These scholars produced new spatial imaginaries over immigrant and African American neighborhoods under the rubric of the study of "social problems." Although less well known, Emory Bogardus at the University of Southern California also played a role in propagating similar discourses by studying Mexican American neighborhoods in the American Southwest. By midcentury, debates about the relationship of "the ghetto" to mainstream society had produced a bevy of Black sociologists such as St. Clair Drake, Horace Cayton, E. Franklin Frazier, and W. E. B. DuBois.

23. Davis, *City of Quartz*, 128.

24. For more on this mayor rebellion, see: Richard M. Flanagan, *Mayors and the Challenge of Urban Leadership* (University Press of America, 2004), 116–17; "Sept 18, 196 Memo from Charles Schultze to President Johnson," Lyndon B. Johnson Collection Welfare 9 Box 26 Folder 8/1/65-9/21/65 (National Archives and Record Administration, Lyndon B. Johnson Library).

25. H. H. Brookins, Testimony Before the Governor's Commission on the Los Angeles Riots, September 29, 1965, Vol. IV Governor's Commission on the Los Angeles Riots, Los Angeles Riots Collection, Special Collections Library University of Southern California, 16.

26. Thomas Bradley, Testimony Before the Governor's Commission on the Los Angeles Riots, September 30, 1965, Vol. III Governor's Commission on the Los Angeles Riots, Los Angeles Riots Collection, Special Collections Library University of Southern California, 13.

27. James Baldwin, *No Name in the Street* (Knopf Doubleday Publishing, 1972), 129.

28. The full quote from Brookins: "First of all, the Negro male, for many years, was not given fair treatment and was not given equal job opportunity and was not able to hold a job and so, when he got to that frustrated point of inability to support his family, there was nothing for him to do but get out and get from it, because his wife was better off through the welfare programs and agencies of this country with him not being present than they were with him being present." H. H. Brookins, Testimony Before the Governor's Commission on the Los Angeles Riots, September 29, 1965, Vol. IV Governor's Commission on the Los Angeles Riots, Los Angeles Riots Collection, Special Collections Library University of Southern California, 46.

29. Mervyn M. Dymally, Testimony Before the Governor's Commission on the Los Angeles Riots, October 13, 1965, Vol. VI Governor's Commission on the Los Angeles Riots, Los Angeles Riots Collection, Special Collections Library University of Southern California, 19.

30. Augustus F. Hawkins, Testimony Before the Governor's Commission on the Los Angeles Riots, September 20, 1965, Vol. VIII Governor's Commission on the Los Angeles Riots, Los Angeles Riots Collection, Special Collections Library University of Southern California, 54.

31. H. H. Brookins, Testimony Before the Governor's Commission on the Los Angeles Riots, September 29, 1965, Vol. IV Governor's Commission on the Los

Angeles Riots, Los Angeles Riots Collection, Special Collections Library University of Southern California, 16.

32. Buggs reminded McCone that he knew of "no well integrated community anywhere in the United States in which a riot began." John Buggs, Testimony Before the Governor's Commission on the Los Angeles Riots, Pre-submitted Testimony, September 28, 1965, Vol. V Governor's Commission on the Los Angeles Riots, Los Angeles Riots Collection, Special Collections Library University of Southern California, 7, 18–19.

33. Simeon Man, *Soldiering Through Empire: Race and the Making of the Decolonizing Pacific* (University of California Press, 2018).

34. Augustus F. Hawkins, Testimony Before the Governor's Commission on the Los Angeles Riots, September 20, 1965, Vol. VIII Governor's Commission on the Los Angeles Riots, Los Angeles Riots Collection, Special Collections Library University of Southern California, 52.

35. McCone, *Violence in the City*, 72.

36. McCone, *Violence in the City*, 7.

37. McCone, *Violence in the City*, 74.

38. Lettergram from Harry Marlow to Kenneth Hahn, December 16, 1965, Martin Luther King, Jr. Hospital 1965–1990, Kenneth Hahn Papers, Huntington Library.

39. Harry Marlow's Notes from Dr. Arnold Sweeney Discussion, January 12, 1966, Martin Luther King, Jr. Hospital 1965–1990, Kenneth Hahn Papers, Huntington Library.

40. Robert Tranquada, "Racial Tensions in Health: 50 Years Since the Watts Riots," roundtable, November 20, 2015, Levan Institute for the Humanities and Ethics and Sidney Harman Academy for Polymathic Study ZYGO Lunchtime Series, University of Southern California, Los Angeles, CA.

41. Chowkwanyun, *All Health Politics is Local*, 118–19.

42. Julius W. Hill, "The Golden State Medical Association," *California Medicine* III, no. 1 (July 1969): 46–49.

43. White was emphatic that the Golden State Medical Society "were a bunch of Uncle Toms." See Daniel Simon, "The Creation of the King-Drew Medical Complex and the Politics of Public Memory" (PhD diss., University of Hawai'i at Manoa, 2014), 65.

44. State Advisory Hospital Council Meeting Minutes, February 10, 1965, Martin Luther King, Jr. Hospital 1965–1990, Kenneth Hahn Papers, Huntington Library. By 1960 standards, Watts had a population comparable to Long Beach, CA (344,168); Birmingham, AL (340,887); Oklahoma City, OK (324,253); and Rochester, NY (318,611).

45. Milton Roemer, November 1, 1965, "Health Services in the Los Angeles Riot Area," November 1, 1965, Vol. XVIII Reports of Consultants Papers, Governor's Commission on the Los Angeles Riots, Los Angeles Riots Collection, Special Collections Library University of Southern California.

46. Timothy Mitchell, "Origins and Limits of the Modern Idea of the Economy," paper presented at the Workshop on Positivism and Post-Positivism, University of Chicago, October 2001, 18–19.

47. T. Mitchell, "Origins and Limits of the Modern Idea of the Economy." See also Timothy Mitchell, *Rule of Experts: Egypt, Techno-Politics, Modernity* (University of California Press, 2002).

48. Breslow, "New Partnerships in the Delivery of Services," 1096.

49. "Peak Years and Decline (November 1970 to November 1974)," The Regional Medical Programs Collection, United States National Library of Medicine, Bethesda, MD, https://profiles.nlm.nih.gov/ps/retrieve/Narrative/RM/p-nid/99.

50. "School, Hospital in Watts-Willowbrook May Become a Prototype for Ghetto Care," *Medical Tribune and Medical News*, August 14, 1969, Box 3, Folder 15, Charles R Drew Postgraduate Medical School, John and Mary Markle Foundation Papers, Rockefeller Archives Center.

51. According to California Director of Public Health Lester Breslow, "To equalize the [health landscape], the legislature also provided that counties could henceforth open their hospitals to any patients, not just the indigent. Hence, the way is now clear to the conversion of county hospitals in California into general hospitals for all persons and the establishment of a single network of hospitals servicing every segment of the community equally." See Lester Breslow, "Medical Care and Public Health in California," *The Journal of the American Medical Association* 198, no. 10 (1966): 1080.

52. Harry Nelson, "Doctor Calls Healthcare for Poor Disgraceful," *The Los Angeles Times*, April 19, 1968, A6.

53. Letter from Reverend Roy L. Thompson, Chair of the Board of Directors of the South Central Area Welfare Planning Council, to Burton Chace, Chair of Board of Supervisors, January 11, 1966; News Release, "Community Organizations in Watts Unite for County Hospital," January 30, 1966; and Letter to Elmer Anderson from J. Alfred Cannon, Chairman of People in Community Action, February 18, 1966, Martin Luther King, Jr. Hospital 1965–1990, Kenneth Hahn Papers, Huntington Library.

54. The official ballot language read as follows: "Shall the County of Los Angeles incur a bonded indebtedness and issue bonds in the sum of twelve million, three hundred thousand dollars ($12,300,000) for the purpose of providing funds for the construction of hospital facilities in the southwest part of Los Angeles County consisting of hospital buildings for medical care of children and adults, surgeries, laboratories, post-graduate medical training, and related facilities and for uses incidental thereto, including the purchase of furniture and equipment from any funds remaining after construction and related costs have been paid?"

55. By 1975, the counties of Butte, Colusa, Imperial, Kings, Madera, Nevada, Santa Cruz, and Solano had closed their public hospitals. According to Elinor Blake and Thomas Bodenheimer, four counties (Humboldt, Placer, San Mateo, Yolo, and Yuba) came close to closing that same year, while eight counties (Tulare, Mendocino,

Santa Barbara, Sutter, Tehama, Sonoma, Santa Clara, and San Francisco) had open discussions about closing their public hospitals. Five counties contracted their indigent care services to private corporations, including El Dorado (Universal Medical Systems) and Siskiyou (Siskiyou Hospital, Inc.). Monterey County also held discussions about transferring their responsibilities to for-profit corporations. See "Closing the Door on the Poor: The Dismantling of California's Public Hospitals," *Health Policy Advisory Center Report* 16 (1975): 64–66.

56. See Robert Tranquada and Robert Maronde, "The Hospital Within A Hospital: An Empirical Experiment in Healthcare in a Major Metropolitan Hospital," *Bulletin of the New York Academy of Medicine* 48, no. 3 (March 1972): 560–61; and Blake and Bodenheimer, "Closing the Door on the Poor," 224–30.

57. Tony Cimurusti, "Reasons Hospital is Needed," *Monrovia Daily News Post*, May 19, 1966, Martin Luther King, Jr. Hospital 1965–1990, Kenneth Hahn Papers, Huntington Library.

58. Discussion of racial blackmail began to appear as early as late April. Enough discussion had taken place to prompt some newspapers, such as the *South Bay Daily Breeze*, to comment on it in order to defuse it. "Filling this need is not submitting to 'blackmail,' a charge leveled at some of the panicky moves to aid the area. Nor does it remove the area's responsibility to strive for law and order, or lessen the resolve of enforcement agencies to maintain it." See "This Hospital is Needed," *South Bay Daily Breeze*, April 24, 1966, Martin Luther King, Jr. Hospital 1965–1990, Kenneth Hahn Papers, Huntington Library, E6.

59. "Projects Included in Failing Bond Proposals Which Were Subsequently Constructed By Other Means 1947–1965," Martin Luther King, Jr. Hospital 1965–1990, Kenneth Hahn Papers, Huntington Library.

60. Jenkins, *The Bonds of Inequality*.

61. Haynes, "The Distribution of Black Physicians in the United States, 1967"; Haynes, "Problems Facing the Negro in Medicine Today."

62. Haynes, "Problems Facing the Negro in Medicine Today," 1069.

63. W. Montague Cobb, "Numa P.G. Adams, 1885–1940," *Journal of the National Medical Association* 43, no. 1 (January 1951): 42–54.

64. Mitchell Spellman Individual Grant, Subseries 2, Box 41, Folder 500 Commonwealth Fund Collection, Rockefeller Archives Center.

65. These diseases were identified as targets for the school at its opening. See Dr. Paul B. Cornely, "The Role of Health Care Institutions In an Era of Community Challenge" (January, 1970), 1 Subseries 2 Box 3 Folder 15, Charles R Drew Postgraduate Medical School, John and Mary Markle Fund Series, Rockefeller Archives Center.

66. M. Alfred Haynes, "Drew Postgraduate Medical School," *California Medicine/The Western Journal of Medicine* 118, no. 4 (April 1973): 81.

67. Harry Nelson, "South LA Medical School Sets Individual Care as Major Goal: Drew Facility, Teaching Arm of King Hospital, Hopes to Provide Quality Health Services for 400,000 in Area," *Los Angeles Times*, April 5, 1971.

68. See M. Alfred Haynes, "Additional Notes on Professional Experience," Commonwealth Fund MSS, 1. Haynes and his family preserved information regard-

ing each of these experiences in a personal website; for more, see, for example, M. Alfred Haynes, "Life with Native Americans," The Haynes Project, http://www.malfredhaynes.info/index.php?p = 1_12_Life-with-Native-Americans.

69. M. Alfred Haynes, "An Approach to the Teaching of Family Care," *Journal of the American Medical Association* 173, no. 3 (July 1960): 1340.
70. Haynes, "An Approach to the Teaching of Family Care."
71. Haynes, "An Approach to the Teaching of Family Care."
72. Haynes, "An Approach to the Teaching of Family Care."
73. Haynes, "An Approach to the Teaching of Family Care.".
74. M. Alfred Haynes, "Professionals and the Community Confront Change," *American Journal of Public Health* 60, no. 3 (March 1970): 519.
75. Haynes, "Drew Postgraduate Medical School," 80.
76. Haynes, "Professionals and the Community Confront Change."

CHAPTER THREE

1. Jack Jones, "The View from Watts Today: Political Fighting Slows Up Health Programs," *Los Angeles Times*, July 19, 1967, A1.
2. On community clinics see Chowkwanyun, *All Health Politics is Local*; Dittmer, *The Good Doctors*; Jack H. Geiger. "The First Community Health Center in Mississippi: Communities Empowering Themselves," *The American Journal of Public Health* 106, no. 10 (2016): 11,738–11,740; Molina, *Fit to Be Citizens?*; Bonnie Lefkowitz. *Community Health Centers: A Movement and the People Who Made It Happen* (Rutgers University Press, 2007); Stern, *Eugenic Nation*. On community mental health clinics see Phil Brown, ed., *Mental Health Care and Social Policy* (Routledge, 1985); Doyle, *Psychiatry and Racial Liberalism*; Gerald Grob, *From Asylum to Community: Mental Health Policy in Modern America* (Princeton University Press, 1991); Donald G. Langsley, "The Community Mental Health Center: Does It Treat Patients?," *Hospital and Community Psychiatry* 31 (1980): 815–19; Gerald Markowitz and David Rosner, *Children, Race, and Power: Kenneth and Mamie Clark's Northside Center* (Routledge, 1996); Gabriel Mendes, *Under the Strain of Color: Harlem's Lafargue Clinic and the Promise of an Anti-Racist Psychiatry* (Cornell University Press, 2015); Mical Raz, *What's Wrong with the Poor? Psychiatry, Race, and the War on Poverty* (University of North Carolina Press, 2013); Ramos, "Pathologizing the Crisis"; Nic John Ramos. "Poor Influences and Criminal Locations: Los Angeles' Skid Row, Multicultural Identities, and Normal Homosexuality," *American Quarterly* 72, no. 2 (2019): 541–67; Matthew Smith, *The First Resort: The History of Social Psychiatry in the United States* (Columbia University Press, 2023); Summers, "Psychiatry, Mental Health Care, and the Black Freedom Struggle."
3. Shah, *Contagious Divides*.
4. Shah, *Contagious Divides*, 8.
5. Shah, *Contagious Divides*, 8.

6. According to George Lipsitz, reliance on institutional programs often hides how activists have used them for what he calls "oppositional cultures" that forward social justice visions not tied to the stated bureaucratic aims of institutions. See "Shattering Silences: Dictions, Contradictions, and Ethnic Studies at the Crossroads" in *Kalfou* 7, no. 2 (Fall 2020): 222–48.

7. George Lipsitz, *A Life in the Struggle: Ivory Perry and the Culture of Opposition* (Temple University Press, 1995); Donna Murch, *Living for the City: Migration, Education, and the Rise of the Black Panther Party in Oakland* (University of North Carolina Press, 2010); Kofi-Charu Nat Turner, *Caffie Greene and Black Women Activists: Unsung Women of the Black Liberation* (Routledge, 2021).

8. Nancy Tomes, *Remaking the American Patient: How Madison Avenue and Modern Medicine Turned Patients into Consumers* (University of North Carolina Press, 2016), 11.

9. Alice O'Connor, *Poverty Knowledge: Social Science, Social Policy, and the Poor in Twentieth Century U.S. History* (Princeton University Press, 2001).

10. It is important to note that "design" and "use" of funds are two different aspects of anti-poverty programming funds. My earlier mention of Turner's, Lipsitz's, and Murch's scholarship shows that many antipoverty grantees stretched federal guidelines to meet their own vision of what alleviating poverty signified.

11. Goldstein, *Poverty in Common*, 16.

12. Crenshaw, "Race, Reform, and Retrenchment," 1335.

13. Hahn Press Release, "Palm Lanes Housing," October 11, 1966; Hahn Press Release, "Memo to the Press," October 20, 1966; Hahn Press Release to *Los Angeles Sentinel*, "Officially beginning the demolition ...," October 21, 1966, Martin Luther King, Jr. Hospital 1965–1990, Kenneth Hahn Papers, Huntington Library.

14. Hahn Press Release, "A 300-acre plot of ground ...," September 12, 1966, Martin Luther King, Jr. Hospital 1965–1990, Kenneth Hahn Papers, Huntington Library.

15. Bill Boyarski, "Far More Than Just a Hospital," *The Los Angeles Times*, February 18, 1996, B1.

16. Hahn Press Release, "A 300-acre plot of ground ...," September 12, 1966, Martin Luther King, Jr. Hospital 1965–1990, Kenneth Hahn Papers, Huntington Library, 2.

17. "Hospital Beds Pose Problems: West Side Paradox: Too Many Here and Too Few There," *Los Angeles Times*, January 3, 1965, WS1; "Application for New Hospital Turned Down," *Los Angeles Times*, August 11, 1964, A8.

18. Tomes, *Remaking the American Patient*; see also Nancy Tomes, "Patients or Health-Care Consumers? Why the History of Contested Terms Matters," in *History and Health Policy in the United States: Putting the Past Back In*, ed. Rosemary Stevens, Charles Rosenberg, and Lawton Burns (Rutgers University Press, 2006), 83–112.

19. Tomes, *Remaking the American Patient*, 7.

20. Grob describes the rise and fall of the mental hygiene movement over the course of two books: *Mental Illness and American Society, 1875–1940* (Princeton University Press, 1983) and *From Asylum to Community*. For an excellent overview of how state hospitals were impacted by Black migration and deinstitutionalization,

see Martin Summers, *Madness in the City of Magnificent Intentions: A History of Race and Mental Illness in the Nation's Capital* (Oxford University Press, 2019).

21. Ramos, "Poor Influences and Criminal Locations."

22. *Major Milestones: 43 Years of Care and Treatment of the Mentally Ill* (California Legislative Analyst's Office, 2000), http://lao.ca.gov/2000/030200_mental_illness/030200_mental_illness.html; Grob, *From Asylum to Community*, 90.

23. Dittmer, The Good Doctors; Geiger, "The First Community Health Center in Mississippi"; Lefkowitz, *Community Health Centers*.

24. "Nation's No. 1 Health Officer: Dr. Egeberg Strong Advocate of More Aid for Needy," *Fort Lauderdale News and Sun-Sentinel*, June 29, 1969, 12A.

25. "Doctors: Miracle in Charcoal Alley," *Time*, November 17, 1967.

26. "Construction Plans Unveiled for Watts Health Center," *The Los Angeles Sentinel*, August 11, 1966, D7.

27. *Office of Economic Opportunity: The Neighborhood Health Center*, US Government Printing Office, 1967, Box 93, South Central Multipurpose Health Center, Augustus Hawkins Papers, Charles Young Special Collections Library, University of California at Los Angeles, 10.

28. Harry Nelson, "New Watts Clinic Fights to Survive Many Problems," *Los Angeles Times*, July 8, 1968, A6.

29. Roger Egeberg, Robert Tranquada, and Elsie Giorgi, Office of Economic Opportunity Notice of Training or Demonstration or Research Project—Neighborhood Family Health Service Center Grant Application, 1965, Box 93, South Central Multipurpose Health Center, Augustus Hawkins Papers, Charles Young Special Collections Library, University of California at Los Angeles. For more on the rise of the family as a growing site of pathologization, see Debbie Weinstein, *The Pathological Family: Postwar America and the Rise of Family Therapy* (Cornell University Press, 2013).

30. Nelson, "New Watts Clinic Fights to Survive Many Problems."

31. Opal Gilliam, "Introducing: A New Health Service for Watts," South Central Multipurpose Health Services Center Brochure, 1967, Box 93, South Central Multipurpose Health Center, Augustus Hawkins Papers, Charles Young Special Collections Library, University of California at Los Angeles, 1.

32. Roger Egeberg, Robert Tranquada, and Elsie Giorgi, Office of Economic Opportunity Notice of Training or Demonstration or Research Project—Neighborhood Family Health Service Center Grant Application, 1965, Box 93, South Central Multipurpose Health Center, Augustus Hawkins Papers, Charles Young Special Collections Library, University of California at Los Angeles, 1–2.

33. Richmond's scholarly writing on the total health concept were directly quoted in USC's grant application to the OEO; see Roger Egeberg, Robert Tranquada, and Elsie Giorgi, Office of Economic Opportunity Notice of Training or Demonstration or Research Project—Neighborhood Family Health Service Center Grant Application, 1965, Box 93, South Central Multipurpose Health Center, Augustus Hawkins Papers, Charles Young Special Collections Library, University of California at Los Angeles, 1.

34. Raz, *What's Wrong with the Poor?*

35. Roger Egeberg, Robert Tranquada, and Elsie Giorgi, Office of Economic Opportunity Notice of Training or Demonstration or Research Project—Neighborhood Family Health Service Center Grant Application, 1965, Box 93, South Central Multipurpose Health Center, Augustus Hawkins Papers, Charles Young Special Collections Library, University of California at Los Angeles.

36. Chowkwanyun, *All Health Politics is Local.*

37. John Kendall, "Health Center in Watts Visited by Senator Percy," *Los Angeles Times*, July 19, 1968, 22.

38. "Dentist Cries 'Foul' in Poverty Practice," *Los Angeles Sentinel*, November 22, 1967, D2.

39. Nelson, "New Watts Clinic Fights to Survive Many Problems."

40. Unsigned Report to Augustus Hawkins, October 1968, Box 93, South Central Multipurpose Health Center, Augustus Hawkins Papers, Charles Young Special Collections Library, University of California at Los Angeles, 1.

41. Chowkwanyun, *All Health Politics is Local*, 120.

42. Thomas was also a close associate of Cannon; Cannon and Ron Karenga famously unsuccessfully campaigned for Thomas to win selection as the Director of UCLA's Black Student Center. Debate over Thomas's potential hire exacerbated growing tensions between students aligned with Karenga and those aligned with the Black Panther Party.

43. Milton S. Davis and R. Tranquada, "A Sociological Evaluation of the Watts Neighborhood Health Center," *Medical Care* 7, no. 2 (March-April, 1969): 105–17, quotations from 107, 108, and 115.

44. Study on Inpatients, Box 2, Folder 9, Los Angeles County Department of Mental Health Records, California Social Welfare Archives, Special Collections Library, University of Southern California.

45. In most cases in the United States, the imperative to maximize labor extraction from Black laborers (enslaved and free) in the antebellum period partly accounts for asylum policies that included refusing to admit Black patients into state care or treating them with inferior care in segregated wards and institutions; see Grob, *Mental Institutions in America*, 249–52. Other Atlantic World slave societies, such as Jamaica, created segregated asylums. For example see Hogarth, *Medicalizing Blackness*, 133–58. The great exception in the US context is Virginia's Eastern State. See Gonaver, *The Peculiar Institution and the Making of Modern Psychiatry, 1840–1880*.

46. Jim Downs, *Sick from Freedom* (Oxford University Press, 2012); Sarah Haley, *No Mercy Here: Gender, Punishment, and the Making of Jim Crow Modernity* (University of North Carolina Press, 2016); Talitha L. LeFlouria, *Chained in Silence: Black Women and Convict Labor in the New South* (University of North Carolina Press, 2016).

47. Mab Segrest, "Exalted on the Ward: 'Mary Roberts,' The Georgia State Sanitarium, and the Psychiatry 'Specialty' of Race," *American Quarterly* 66, no. 1: 69–94.

48. Gerald Grob, *Mental Illness and American Society, 1875–1940* (Princeton University Press, 1983), 144.
49. Gonaver, *The Peculiar Institution and the Making of Modern Psychiatry*.
50. Grob, *Mental Illness and American Society, 1875–1940*, 145.
51. Chávez-García, *States of Delinquency*; Hicks, *Talk with You Like a Woman*.
52. Grob, *Mental Illness and American Society, 1875–1940*, 144.
53. Somerville, *Queering the Color Line*.
54. Benjamin Kahan, *The Book of Minor Perverts: Sexology, Etiology, and the Emergences of Sexuality* (University of Chicago Press, 2019).
55. Gill-Peterson, *Histories of the Transgender Child*.
56. Warwick Anderson, *Colonial Pathologies: American Tropical Medicine, Race, and Hygiene in the Philippines* (Duke University Press, 2006); Gill-Peterson, *Histories of the Transgender Child*; Emmett Harsin Drager, "Early Gender Clinics, Transsexual Etiology, and the Racialized Family," *GLQ* 29, no. 1 (January 2023): 13–26; Nic John Ramos and Alex Burnett, "'One Out Gay Cop': Gay Moderates, Proposition 64, and Policing in Early AIDS-Crisis Los Angeles, 1969–1992," *Journal of History of Sexuality* 31, no. 3 (2022): 362–93.
57. Doyle, *Psychiatry and Racial Liberalism*; Kevin Mumford, "Untangling Pathology: The Moynihan Report and Homosexual Damage, 1965–1975," *Journal of Policy History* 24, no. 1 (2012): 53–73; Ramos, "Poor Influences and Criminal Locations."
58. Doyle, *Psychiatry and Racial Liberalism*, 101.
59. Mendes, *Under the Strain of Color*, 80.
60. The conceptual framework I use here is known as "Black Gender" and is drawn from Spillers, "Mama's Baby, Papa's Maybe." See also Haley, *No Mercy Here*; C. Riley Snorton, *Black on Both Sides: A Racial History of Trans Identity* (University of Minnesota Press, 2017).
61. I use the term "heterosexuals on the (out)side of heterosexuality" as Cathy Cohen does in "Punks, Bulldaggers, and Welfare Queens." See Doyle, *Psychiatry and Racial Liberalism*; Markowitz and Rosner, *Children, Race, and Power*; and Mumford, "Untangling Pathology."
62. J. Alfred Cannon, "The Psycho-Social Aspects of Segregation," *Journal of the National Medication Association* 56, no. 2 (1964): 160–63, quotations from 161–62.
63. Abram Kardiner and Lionel Ovesey, *The Mark of Oppression* (W. W. Norton, 1951).
64. Kardiner and Ovesey, *The Mark of Oppression*, 3.
65. Cannon, "The Psycho-Social Aspects of Segregation," 162.
66. J. Alfred Cannon, "Re-Africanization: The Last Alternative for Black America," *Phylon* 38, no. 2 (1977): 203–10.
67. Cannon, "Re-Africanization," 208.
68. "Down-to-Earth Psychiatry Helps in Los Angeles Slums," *Austin American Statesman*, October 10, 1968, B1.
69. "Down-to-Earth Psychiatry Helps in Los Angeles Slums."
70. "Down-to-Earth Psychiatry Helps in Los Angeles Slums."

71. Harry R. Brickman, M.D., PhD, interviewed by Frances Lomas Feldman in Dr. Brickman's Office, July 9, 1999, Oral History Transcripts, Special Collections Library University of Southern California, 7.

72. Cannon, "Re-Africanization," 208.

73. Here, I deploy the term as used by W. E. B DuBois to describe and criticize the ideological and economic project proposed by Booker T. Washington, which he accused of intensifying the "race-feeling" that separated white people from the "Negro race" through his economic development proposals. See *The Souls of Black Folk*, introduction by Patricia H. Hinchey (Myers Education Press, 2018), 43.

74. Cannon, "Re-Africanization," 209.

75. Du Bois, *Black Reconstruction in America*, 700.

76. Cannon, "Re-Africanization," 207.

77. Cannon, "Re-Africanization," 208.

78. David Colker and Marc Lacey, "From Watts Riot Ashes," *Los Angeles Times*, May 10, 1992, http://articles.latimes.com/1992-05-10/news/mn-2508_1_watts-riots.

79. This listing appears in an article advertising a fundraiser for the center: "Stars Plan Gala Night to Benefit Mafundi," *Los Angeles Sentinel*, December 25, 1969, C2.

80. E. Franklin Frazier, *The Black Bourgeoisie: The Rise of a New Middle Class in the United States* (Collier, 1962); Nathan Hare, *The Black Anglo-Saxons* (Collier-MacMillan, 1965).

81. Cannon, "The Psycho-Social Aspects of Segregation," 162.

82. Cannon, "The Psycho-Social Aspects of Segregation," 162.

83. J. Alfred Cannon, "Bama Will Never Be The Same," *Los Angeles Sentinel*, April 1, 1965, D1.

84. Cannon, "Re-Africanization," 204.

85. Martha Biondi. *The Black Revolution on Campus* (University of California Press, 2012); Bloom and Martin, *Black Against Empire*; Jared Leighton. "'All of Us are Unapprehended Felons': Gay Liberation, the Black Panther Party, and Intercommunal Efforts Against Police Brutality in the Bay Area," *The Journal of Social History* (2018): 1–26; Murch, *Living for the City*; Widener, *Black Arts West*.

86. Nelson, *Body and Soul*, 1.

87. Leighton, "All of Us Are Unapprehended Felons"; A. J. Lewis, "'We Are Certain of Our Own Insanity': Antipsychiatry and the Gay Liberation Movement, 1968–1980," *Journal of the History of Sexuality* 25, no. 1: 83–113.

88. Ashley D. Farmer, *Remaking Black Power: How Black Women Transformed an Era* (University of North Carolina Press, 2017), 78–79.

89. Leighton, "All of Us Are Unapprehended Felons."

90. Audre Lorde, *Sister Outsider*, 73.

91. Frantz Fanon, *Black Skin, White Masks*, trans. Richard Philcox, foreword by Kwame Anthony Appiah (Grove Press, 2008).

92. Ray Rogers, "Slayings Spotlight Split: Black Power in Turmoil," *Los Angeles Times*, February 16, 1969, B1, B2, B3.

93. Brown, *Fighting for US*; Bloom and Martin, *Black Against Empire*.

94. Letter from Congressman Hawkins to Charles Hall, March 21, 1968, Box 93, Community Development IMPAC Ujima 1968–1969, Augustus Hawkins Papers, Charles Young Special Collections Library, University of California at Los Angeles.

95. Letter from Congressman Hawkins to Charles Hall, March 21, 1968, Box 93, Community Development IMPAC Ujima 1968–1969, Augustus Hawkins Papers, Charles Young Special Collections Library, University of California at Los Angeles.

96. "Ujima Village Project to Open," *Los Angeles Sentinel*, October 23, 1969, C7.

97. "Drew Wins $500,000 In New Funds," *Los Angeles Sentinel*, September 27, 1973, C14.

98. "Drew Wins $500,000 In New Funds."

99. The other well-known Panther clinic to include mental health services is the Lincoln Hospital detoxification treatment center in New York City run in coalition with the Young Lords. For more, see Fernandez, *The Young Lords*, 302–3. As David Mechanic and Gerald Grob have argued, however, addiction and chemical dependency were not yet widely considered mental illnesses by psychiatrists until the end of the 1970s. See "The Plight of the Mentally Ill in America," in *History and Health Policy in the United States: Putting the Past Back In*, ed. Rosemary Stevens, Charles Rosenberg, and Lawton Burns (Rutgers University Press, 2006), 240–43.

100. Bloom and Martin, *Black Against Empire*.

101. Baradaran, *The Color of Money*.

102. At a meeting of the American Hospital Association in Anaheim, CA, Veneman "singled out the USC Multipurpose Health Center in Watts as an example of a 'one door' health service," which as a project "seems to hold bright promise" by "provid[ing] the kind of care in the community which will avoid more expensive care later." See Harry Nelson, "Prevention of Disease Called Best Curb on Hospital Costs," *Los Angeles Times*, April 29, 1969, C1.

103. Turner, *Caffie Greene and Black Women Activists*.

104. Historians of sexuality argue that class distinctions, gender presentations, and jobs played important roles in helping white citizens evade detection as homosexuals or non-normative heterosexuals. See Canaday, *The Straight State*; Julio Capo, Jr., *Welcome to Fairyland: Queer Miami before 1940* (University of North Carolina Press, 2017); George Chauncey, *Gay New York: Gender, Urban Culture, and the Makings of the Gay Male World, 1890–1940* (Basic Books, 1994); Howard, *The Closet and the Cul-De-Sac*; Jenn Manion, *Female Husbands: A Trans History* (Cambridge University Press, 2020).

105. See Ramos and Burnett, "One Out Gay Cop."

106. Letter from J. Alfred Cannon to Lilian Mobley, June 25, 1971, Martin Luther King, Jr. Hospital 1965–1990, Kenneth Hahn Papers, Huntington Library.

CHAPTER FOUR

1. Diana Pearce, "The Feminization of Poverty: Women, Work, and Welfare," *The Urban and Social Change Review* 11 (1978): 28–36. For more, see Pierrette

Hondagneu-Sotelo, *Domestica: Immigrant Workers Cleaning and Caring in the Shadows of Affluence* (University of California Press, 2001); Pierrette Hondagneu-Sotelo, *Gendered Transitions: Mexican Experiences of Immigration* (University of California Press, 1994); Pierrette Hondagneu-Sotelo, *Paradise Transplanted: Migration and the Making of California Gardens* (University of California Press, 2014); Ruth Milkman, *L.A. Story: Immigrant Workers and the Future of the U.S. Labor Movement* (Russell Sage Foundation, 2006); Rhacel Salazar Parrenas, *Servants of Globalization: Migration and Domestic Work* (Stanford University Press, 2015).

2. Clyde Adrian Woods, *Development Arrested: Race, Power and the Blues in the Mississippi Delta* (Haymarket, 1998), 2.

3. Louis R. Harlan, ed., *The Booker T. Washington Papers* (University of Illinois Press, 1974), 3:583–87.

4. Cowie, *Stayin' Alive*, 12.

5. For more on the political and cultural importance of this approach, see Benjamin Looker, *A Nation of Neighborhoods: Imagining Cities, Communities, and Democracy in Postwar America* (University of Chicago Press, 2015).

6. Davis, *City of Quartz*, 230.

7. Competitive Area Profile and On-Going Research, Development Research Associates, July 1969, Box 11, Folder 9, Bunker Hill Redevelopment Papers, Special Collections Library, University of Southern California.

8. "Sprawling Los Angeles Gets A New Skyline," *Business Weekly*, 1970, Box 12, Folder 51, Bunker Hill Redevelopment Papers, Special Collections Library, University of Southern California.

9. Davis, *City of Quartz*, 221–64.

10. "Sprawling Los Angeles Gets A New Skyline."

11. Section 6 of the Master Plan Vol. II. (Evaluation), The Master Plan Report, Box 981, Folder 891, Commonwealth Fund Series 18: Grants, Rockefeller Archives Center, 6-3.

12. Nadasen, *Welfare Warriors*.

13. Canaday, *The Straight State*, 126 and 130.

14. Annelise Orelick, *Storming Caesars Palace: How Black Mothers Fought Their Own War on Poverty* (Beacon, 2005), 14–15.

15. Haley, *No Mercy Here*.

16. Frances Fox Piven and Richard Cloward, "The Weight of the Poor: A Strategy to End Poverty," originally published in *The Nation*, May 2, 1966, reprinted in *New Political Science* 33, no. 3 (September 2011): 272–84.

17. For more on the importance of the professionalization of community organizers, see Saul Alinsky with Marion K. Sanders, *The Professional Radical: Conversations with Saul Alinsky* (Harper and Row, 1970); Barbara Ransby, *Ella Baker and the Black Freedom Movement: A Radical Democratic Vision* (University of North Carolina Press, 2003). For criticisms of the effects of professionalization, see Myrl Beam, *Gay, Inc.: The Nonprofitization of Queer Politics* (University of Minnesota Press, 2018). For a list of contributors to the NWRO, see Individual Contributions and

Foundations Boxes 10–12, National Welfare Rights Organization, George A. Wiley Papers, Wisconsin Historical Society.

18. "Ohio Adequate Welfare News," Newsletter, November, 27, 1968, Ohio Steering Committee for Adequate Welfare, Whitaker Papers, Box 1, Folder 17, Ohio Historical Society.

19. Nadasen, *Welfare Warriors*, 172.

20. Interview with Johnnie Tillmon, July 30, 1974, Box 11, Guida West Papers, Sophia Smith Collection of Women's History. Others, such as Barbara Ransby, have named this approach "Democratic Humanism"(see *Ella Baker and the Black Freedom Movement*.) In addition to Ransby, see note XXX on Saul Alinsky. A strong contemporary proponent of this approach is Jane McAlevey; see her books *No Shortcuts: Organizing for Power in the New Gilded Age* (Oxford University Press, 2016); *Rules to Win By: Power and Participation in Union Negotiations* (Oxford University Press, 2023); *Raising Expectations (and Raising Hell): My Decade Fighting for the Labor Movement* (Verso, 2012).

21. Interview with Johnnie Tillmon, July 30, 1974, Box 11, Guida West Papers, Sophia Smith Collection of Women's History.

22. Nadasen, *Welfare Warriors*.

23. Orleck, *Storming Caesars Palace*; Rosie Bermudez. "La Causa de los Pobres: Alicia Escalante's Lived Experience of Poverty" in *Chicana Movidas: New Narratives of Activism and Feminism in the Movement Era*, ed. Dionne Espinoza, Maria Eugenia Cotera, and Maylei Blackwell (University of Texas Press, 2018), 123–37; Alejandra Marchevsky, "Forging a Brown-Black Movement: Chicana and African American Women Organizing for Welfare Rights in Los Angeles" in Espinoza, Cotera, and Blackwell, *Chicana Movidas*, 227–44.

24. Interview with Catherine Jermany (n.d.), Box 11, Guida West Papers, Sophia Smith Collection of Women's History.

25. Tillmon recounted that control over the direction of the welfare rights movement between paid staff and women on welfare, and between different chapters for control of regional, state, and national leadership, had always characterized the organization. In 1974 she recounted how she rebuffed early efforts by paid staffers Tim Sampson and Arthur Jones in 1966 to create a "county-wide" welfare rights organization that would not have leadership represented from ANC Mothers Anonymous. When it finally formed, the county organization was led by Catherine Jermany, someone who organized alongside Tillmon. Interview with Johnnie Tillmon, July 30, 1974, Box 11, Guida West Papers, Sophia Smith Collection of Women's History.

26. Interview with Johnnie Tillmon, July 30, 1974, Box 11, Guida West Papers, Sophia Smith Collection of Women's History.

27. Hicks, *Talk with You Like A Woman*; LaShawn Harris, *Sex Workers, Psychics, and Number Runners: Black Women in New York City's Underground* (University of Illinois Press, 2016); Saidiya Hartman, *Wayward Lives, Beautiful Experiments: Intimate Histories of Riotous Black Girls, Troublesome Women, and Queer Radicals* (W. W. Norton, 2019).

28. Catherine Jermany described Governor Reagan's programs to place able-bodied recipients of welfare in public service jobs as a "slavery project." As she put it, "It's not productive work and they don't get any real training. These are dead-end jobs where they really don't learn any skills. We want to see recipients get off the rolls and get into jobs. But they need real training, not some Mickey Mouse training." See Jack Jones, "County Welfare: Many Recipients Work For It," *Los Angeles Times*, May 2, 1971, B1.

29. See Stevens, *In Sickness and in Wealth*, particularly "Pragmatism in the Marketplace: 1965–1980," 284–320.

30. HoSang, *Racial Propositions*, 16–19.

31. Interview with Johnnie Tillmon, July 30, 1974, Box 11, Guida West Papers, Sophia Smith Collection of Women's History.

32. Interview with Catherine Jermany (n.d.), Box 11, Guida West Papers, Sophia Smith Collection of Women's History.

33. Johnnie Tillmon's, Dee Johnson's and Catherine Jermany's interviews with Guida West all mention the deep personal and organizational connections welfare rights activists in Los Angeles maintained with Black political figures and organizations of all stripes. Tillmon had personal relationships with the Black Panther Party's leaders given her relationship with her sister Caffie Greene and was present for the Black Panther Party's launch of their first free clinic; see Nelson, *Body and Soul*.

34. Interview with Catherine Jermany (n.d.), Box 11, Guida West Papers, Sophia Smith Collection of Women's History.

35. Healthcare and child care remained consistent topics at every conference but were particularly emphasized in every conference after 1971. See "Welfare not Warfare," National Welfare Rights Organization Conference Program, Providence, RI, July 1, 1971; and "People Before Politics," National Welfare Rights Organization Conference Program, Miami Beach, FL, 1972, Box 26, Guida West Papers, Sophia Smith Collection of Women's History.

36. Interview with Johnnie Tillmon and M. Hayes, June 17, 1983, Box 11, Guida West Papers, Sophia Smith Collection of Women's History.

37. Johnnie Tillmon, "Profile of a Welfare Fighter," in *NWRO Welfare Fighter* newsletter, August 11, 1971, Box 11, Guida West Papers, Sophia Smith Collection of Women's History, 3.

38. Davis, *City of Quartz*, 128.

39. "Sprawling Los Angeles Gets A New Skyline."

40. The city officially first used the term in 1980 to describe "where growth occurs in stages." Planners claimed efforts since 1976 had strengthened "the existing character" of the neighborhoods targeted for redevelopment. See Community Redevelopment Agency of the City of Los Angeles. Progress Report 1976–1980, 1980, Box 12, Folder 21 Bunker Hill Redevelopment Papers, Special Collections Library, University of Southern California.

41. Milkman, *LA Story*; Ruth Milkman, *Organizing Immigrants: The Challenge for Unions in Contemporary California* (ILR Press, 2000).

42. Edna Bonacich and Richard Appelbaum, *Behind the Label: Inequality in the Los Angeles Apparel Industry* (University of California Press, 2000).

43. Edna Bonacich, Lucie Cheng, and Paul Ong, eds., *The New Asian Immigration in Los Angeles and Global Restructuring* (Temple University Press, 1994); Edna Bonacich, Lucie Cheng, Norma Chinchilla, Nora Hamilton, and Paul Ong, eds. *Global Production: The Apparel Industry in the Pacific Rim* (Temple University Press, 1994).

44. The study team published three volumes: "Volume I is a summary; Volume II comprises the text of the Master Plan; Volume III contains the appendices." See Grants, Box 981, Folder 891, Commonwealth Fund Series 18, Rockefeller Archives Center.

45. Section I of the Master Plan Vol. II. (Historical Context), The Master Plan Report, Grants, Box 981, Folder 891, Commonwealth Fund Series 18, Rockefeller Archives Center, p. I-7.

46. Section 1 of the Master Plan Vol. I. (Findings and Recommendations—Mission and Role), The Master Plan Report, Grants, Box 981, Folder 891, Commonwealth Fund Series 18, Rockefeller Archives Center, 4.

47. Service Area of the Los Angeles County-Martin Luther King, Jr. General Hospital Series 2, No. 1, 1971, Department of Community Medicine Background Information, Grants, Box 98, Folder 890 Charles R. Drew Postgraduate Medical School, Commonwealth Fund Series 18, Rockefeller Archives Center.

48. "The most recent [statistics on school dropout rates] (1965–1966) show that LA District High Schools located in the Hospital Service Area have experienced notably higher dropout rates than the average in the City School District. The estimate of dropouts in all senior high schools in the District was 21.5%. The equivalent figures for three of the senior high schools in the Service Area were 34.9% at Fremont, 42.4% at Jordan, and 43.6% at Jefferson." See Education, Department of Community Medicine Background Information, Series 2, No. 1, 1971, Grants, Box 98, Folder 890 Charles R. Drew Postgraduate Medical School, Commonwealth Fund Series 18, Rockefeller Archives Center, 36.

49. Adeljiza Sosa Riddell, "Chicanas and El Movimiento," *Atzlan* 5, no. 1–2 (1974): 155–65.

50. bell hooks, *We Real Cool* (Routledge, 2004).

51. Section 2 of the Master Plan Vol. II. (Mission and Strategies—The Mission), The Master Plan Study, Master Plan Report, Grants, Box 98, Folder 890 Charles R. Drew Postgraduate Medical School, Commonwealth Fund Series 18, Rockefeller Archives Center, 2-2.

52. Section I of the Master Plan Vol. II. (Historical Context—Drew's Community), The Master Plan Study, Master Plan Report, Grants, Box 98, Folder 890 Charles R. Drew Postgraduate Medical School, Commonwealth Fund Series 18, Rockefeller Archives Center, I-6.

53. Julilly Kohler-Hausmann, *Getting Tough: Welfare and Imprisonment in 1970s America* (Princeton University Press, 2017); Felicia Kornbluh and Gwendolyn Mink, *Ensuring Poverty: Welfare Reform in Feminist Perspective* (University of Pennsylvania Press, 2018); Alejandra Marchevsky and Jeanne Theoharis, *Not Working: Latina Immigrants, Low-Wage Jobs, and the Failure of Welfare Reform* (New

York University Press, 2006); Karen Tani, *States of Dependency: Welfare, Rights, and American Governance, 1935–1972* (Cambridge University Press, 2016).

54. Section I of the Master Plan Vol. II. (An Overview: Accomplishments and Problems), The Master Plan Study, Master Plan Report, Grants, Box 98, Folder 890 Charles R. Drew Postgraduate Medical School, Commonwealth Fund Series 18, Rockefeller Archives Center, 1-11.

55. "The ten leading causes of death in the community are, in order of importance, (1) heart disease, (2) cancer, (3) stroke, (4) accidents, (5) homicides, (6) cirrhosis of the liver, (7) influenza and pneumonia, (8) disease of early infancy, (9) diabetes, and (10) circulatory diseases. The high incidence of accidents and homicides is particularly notable." Section I of the Master Plan Vol. II. (Historical Context—Drew's Community), The Master Plan Study, Master Plan Report, Grants, Box 98, Folder 890 Charles R. Drew Postgraduate Medical School, Commonwealth Fund Series 18, Rockefeller Archives Center, I-6.

56. Section II of the Master Plan Vol. II. (Mission and Strategies), The Master Plan Study, Master Plan Report, Grants, Box 98, Folder 890 Charles R. Drew Postgraduate Medical School, Commonwealth Fund Series 18, Rockefeller Archives Center, 2-2.

57. Section I of the Master Plan Vol. II. (Historical Context—Drew's Community), The Master Plan Study, Master Plan Report, Grants, Box 98, Folder 890 Charles R. Drew Postgraduate Medical School, Commonwealth Fund Series 18, Rockefeller Archives Center, I-2.

58. Jonathan Engel, *Poor People's Medicine: Medicaid and American Charity Care since 1965* (Duke University, 2006); McQueeney, *A City Without Care*; Fernandez, *The Young Lords*.

59. Moving People in Los Angeles, Community Redevelopment Agency of the City of Los Angeles, June 1977, Box 22, Folder 1, Bunker Hill Redevelopment Papers, Special Collections Library, University of Southern California, 5.

60. Progress Report 1976–1980, 1980, Box 12, Folder 21 Bunker Hill Redevelopment Papers, Special Collections Library, University of Southern California, 8–13.

61. Thomas Bradley, Testimony Before the Governor's Commission on the Los Angeles Riots, September 30, 1965, Vol. III Governor's Commission on the Los Angeles Riots, Los Angeles Riots Collection, Special Collections Library, University of Southern California, 14.

62. "Neighborhood Health Centers" was the programmatic title given to clinics built and overseen by the Office of Equal Opportunity and Citizen Participation Programs from 1965 to 1972. Comprehensive Health Centers and Ambulatory Care Centers, although similar to the shape and character of OEO clinics, were administered and overseen directly by the Secretary of Health. For more on the history of Neighborhood Health Centers, see Geiger, "The First Community Health Center in Mississippi."

63. Memo from Dan Grindell, Deputy, to Philip M. Smith, MD, Acting Regional Director Florence-Firestone Educational Project, January 20, 1975, Martin Luther King, Jr. Hospital 1965–1990, Kenneth Hahn Papers, Huntington Library.

64. Sterilization has a well-known history in the American Southwest. For more on Madrigal vs. Quilligan see Gutierrez, *Fertile Matters*; Renee Tajima-Pena, dir., *No Mas Bebes* (PBS, 2015). For other scholarship on sterilization in the American Southwest, see Chávez-García, *States of Delinquency;* Lira, *Laboratory of Deficiency*; Molina, *Fit to Be Citizens?*; Murillo, "Birth Control, Border Control"; Stern, *Eugenic Nation*.

65. Section II of the Master Plan Vol. III (Reports of the Task Group on Maternal and Child Health Development), The Master Plan Study, Appendix, Grants, Box 981, Folder 891, Commonwealth Fund Series 18, Rockefeller Archives Center, 1-3.

66. "Ground Broken for Big Health Center," *Los Angeles Times*, March 31, 1974, G23.

67. "Program Stresses County Health Care," *Los Angeles Sentinel*, March 6, 1975, A3.

68. Carl Coates, "Child Care Center Opens," *Los Angeles Sentinel*, November 7, 1974, A8.

69. Progress Report 1976–1980, 1980, Box 12, Folder 21 Bunker Hill Redevelopment Papers, Special Collections Library, University of Southern California, 14.

70. Progress Report 1976–1980, 1980, Box 12, Folder 21 Bunker Hill Redevelopment Papers, Special Collections Library, University of Southern California, 2 and 5.

71. Richard K. Meyer, "The Impact of a Redevelopment Project on Downtown Los Angeles," June 1978, Box 12, Folder 23 Bunker Hill Redevelopment Papers, Special Collections Library, University of Southern California, 34.

72. Austin Scott, "Powerful Decision Makers," in *Downtown Los Angeles* from the *Los Angeles Times*, reprinted articles from April 25 through April 28, 1982, Box 13, Folder 31, Bunker Hill Redevelopment Papers, Special Collections Library, University of Southern California.

73. An Overview of Federally Assisted Projects in Downtown Los Angeles: Implemented Projects and Future Opportunities, Community Redevelopment Agency of the City of Los Angeles, December 1977, Box 12, Folder 24, Bunker Hill Redevelopment Papers, Special Collections Library, University of Southern California, 22.

74. Doris Byron, "Downtown L.A. High-Priced Boom Molds New Skyline," in *Downtown Los Angeles* from the *Los Angeles Times*, reprinted articles from April 25 through April 28, 1982, Box 13, Folder 31, Bunker Hill Redevelopment Papers, Special Collections Library University of Southern California.

75. Preliminary General Development Plan: Central City Los Angeles 1972/1990, 1972, Box 22, Bunker Hill Redevelopment Papers, Special Collections Library, University of Southern California, 22.

76. "Central City is a key element of the Regional Core—physically and commercially the center of the Western United States. It is unique and one-of-a-kind in nature. As the heart of the Region, its health reflects the Region's health—the two are tied irrefutably, one to the other—April, 1972." See Preliminary General Development Plan, 22.

77. As planners explained it: "Downtown's potential future reflects the Region's future; attitudes about what Downtown should be reflect Regional attitudes about land, open space, transportation, and social structure, among a multitude of additional factors." See Preliminary General Development Plan, 31.

78. "As planners are fond of pointing out, the Los Angeles region is rapidly converting itself into a Southern California megalopolis, stretching from Santa Barbara on the north, to San Diego to the south" ("Sprawling Los Angeles Gets A New Skyline").

79. Letter in reply to Francisca Flores's letter in *Regeneracion* Vol. II, No. 3, 1973, Box 23, Folder 17, La Causa de los Pobres correspondence, Alicia Escalante Papers, Special Collections Library, University of California at Santa Barbara.

80. Ehrenreich, *Nickel and Dimed*.

81. NWRO Press Release, August 6, 1977, Box 27, Folder 11, Guida West Papers, Sophia Smith Collection of Women's History.

82. NWRO Press Release, August 6, 1977, Box 27, Folder 11, Guida West Papers, Sophia Smith Collection of Women's History.

83. "She is troubled by this younger generation of welfare recipients, the unskilled, unwed mothers, women with far more obstacles than she faced and, she suspects, less grit." See John L. Mitchell, "A Dreamer and Her Dream Lose Ground," *The Los Angeles Times*, July 9, 1995, E1.

CHAPTER FIVE

1. Avila, *Popular Culture in the Age of White Flight*; Davis, *City of Quartz*; Deverell, *Whitewashed Adobe*; Widener, *Black Arts West*.

2. Official maps, Box 1355, Folder 20 and Box 1447, Folder 1, Los Angeles Olympic Organizing Committee Collection, Charles Young Special Collections Library, University of California at Los Angeles; Damron's Address Book, 1984, ONE Archives, University of Southern California, 32.

3. Max Felker-Kantor, "The 1984 Olympics Fueled LA's War on Crime," *Washington Post*, August 8, 2017, https://www.washingtonpost.com/news/made-by-history/wp/2017/08/06/the-1984-olympics-fueled-l-a-s-war-on-crime-will-the-2028-games-do-the-same; Dave Zirin, "Want to Understand the 1992 LA Riots?," The Nation, April 30, 2012, https://www.thenation.com/article/want-understand-1992-la-riots-start-1984-la-olympics.

4. Michael Dear and Jennifer Wolch, *Landscapes of Despair: From Deinstitutionalization to Homelessness* (Princeton University Press, 1987), 142–51.

5. Tony Castro, "Prostitutes Take Refuge in the Shadows of Skid Row," *Los Angeles Herald Examiner*, July 22, 1984, Box 6, Folder 1, Bunker Hill Redevelopment Papers, Special Collections Library, University of Southern California, 2-3.

6. Gilmore, *Golden Gulag*, 70–78.

7. Cathy Cohen, *Boundaries of Blackness: AIDS and the Breakdown of Black Politics* (University of Chicago Press, 1999), 13–16.

8. Davis, *City of Quartz*, 221–322; Christina Hanhardt, "Broken Windows at Blue's," in *Policing the Planet: Why the Policing Crisis Led to Black Lives Matter*, ed. Jordan T. Camp and Christina Heatherton (Verso, 2016), 41–62.

9. Robert McRuer, "Compulsory Able-Bodiedness and Queer/Disabled Existence," in *The Disability Studies Reader*, ed. Lennard Davis (Routledge, 2006), 91; Robert McRuer, *Crip Theory* (New York University Press, 2006); Jasbir Puar, "Bodies with New Organs," *Social Text* 33, no. 3 (2015): 48–51.

10. Grob, *From Asylum to Community*, 254.

11. Gerald Grob, *The Mad Among Us* (Free Press, 1994); Grob, *From Asylum to Community*; Dear and Wolch, *Landscapes of Despair*; Craig Willse, *The Value of Homelessness: Managing Surplus Life in the United States* (University of Minnesota Press, 2015); Joseph Morrissey, Howard Goldman, and Lorraine Klerman, "Cycles of Institutional Reform," in *Mental Health Care and Social Policy*, ed. Phil Brown (Routledge, 1985), 70–98.

12. Grob, *From Asylum to Community*, 257.

13. Chavez-Garcia, *States of Delinquency*; Doyle, *Psychiatry and Racial Liberalism in Harlem*; Hicks, *Talk with You like a Woman*; Kunzel, *Criminal Intimacy*.

14. William Fulton, *Reluctant Metropolis: The Politics of Urban Growth in Los Angeles* (Johns Hopkins University Press, 2001).

15. "Social Impact Evaluation," 1978, Box 5, Folder 16, Bunker Hill Redevelopment Papers, Special Collections Library, University of Southern California.

16. These reports include: "Social Impact Evaluation of Central City East" (1978); "Central City East" (1987); "The Changing Face of Misery" (1988); "To Build a Community" (1988); "Economic and Financial Situation of Los Angeles Single Room Occupancy Hotels" (1989); "Workshop on Homelessness" (1990); "Briefing Report: Central City East" (1991), all in Box 5, Bunker Hill Redevelopment Papers, Special Collections Library, University of Southern California.

17. This idea was evidently developed from reports conducted in 1969 by sociologist Robert Vander Koi, who noted the rise of the neighborhood's black men: see "Social Impact Evaluation," 1978, Box 5, Folder 16, Bunker Hill Redevelopment Papers, Special Collections Library, University of Southern California, 5-7.

18. Los Angeles Community Action Network (LA CAN), "All Show and No Substance: Proposition HHH First Year Performance Assessment" (November, 2017).

19. Rishi Manchanda, "Taming the Perfect Storm: Addressing the Impact of Public Health, Housing, and Law Enforcement Policies on Homelessness and Health in South Los Angeles," St. John's Well Child and Family Center, Esperanza Community Housing Corporation, Los Angeles Community Action Network, Strategic Actions for a Just Economy, and Southside Coalition of Community Health Centers (July, 2008).

20. "Changing Face of Misery," 51.

21. "Social Impact Evaluation" (1978), 6–11.

22. Eric Tang, "Cambodian Refugees in the NYC Hyperghetto," Organization of American Historians Process Blog, March 15, 2016, processhistory.org. For more

on the hyperghetto, see Eric Tang, *Unsettled: Cambodian Refugees in the NYC Hyperghetto* (Temple University Press, 2015); Loïc J. D. Wacquant, "Deadly Symbiosis: When Ghetto and Prison Meet and Mesh," *Punishment and Society* 1 (2001): 95–133; Loïc J. D. Wacquant, "From Slavery to Mass Incarceration," *New Left Review* 13 (January-February 2002): 41–60; Loïc J. D. Wacquant, *Punishing the Poor: The Neoliberal Government of Social Insecurity* (Duke University Press, 2009).

23. Castro, "Prostitutes Take Refuge in the Shadows of Skid Row," 2.

24. "The Changing Face of Misery," 54.

25. Cindy I-Fen Cheng, "From Sanctuary to Skid Row," University of Southern California Center for Transpacific Studies, November 18, 2014.

26. Hobson, "Policing Gay LA," 193–94.

27. Wendy Cheng, *The Changs Next Door to the Diazes: Remapping Race in Suburban California* (University of Minnesota Press, 2013); Sides, *L.A. City Limits*.

28. Hanhardt, *Safe Space*, 35–80.

29. Harry R. Brickman, MD, PhD, interviewed by Frances Lomas Feldman in Dr. Brickman's Office, July 9, 1999, Oral History Transcripts, Special Collections Library, University of Southern California, 6.

30. See Proceedings, First National Conference on Asian American Mental Health, San Francisco, April 27-19, 1972; and Spanish-Speaking Conference on Mental Health, Chicago, June 8–10, 1972, Box 3, Subject File "A," Folder 1: Asian American Community Mental Health Training Center—Conferences, Box 3, Royal F. Morales Collection, Library of Congress, Asian Reading Room.

31. "Down-to-Earth Psychiatry Helps in Los Angeles Slums," *The Austin American Statesman*, October 10, 1968, B1.

32. According to one prominent Mexican American psychiatrist, "the training program had been largely constructed from the experience of J. Alfred Cannon, MD, literally the first Fellow in Social and Community Psychiatry at UCLA." "Dr. Cannon helped plan the formal training program funded by the NIMH and was for some years its Assistant Director." See Marvin Karno, "A Career in Social Psychiatry," Box 1, Master of Social Psychiatry Degree Program Revival, 1986–1988, Marvin Karno Professional Papers, Darling Biomedical Library, University of California Los Angeles.

33. Master of Social Psychiatry Program, 1965–1975, Box 1, Folder 1, Marvin Karno Professional Papers, Darling Biomedical Library, University of California Los Angeles.

34. See Proceedings, First National Conference on Asian American Mental Health, San Francisco, April 27-19, 1972; and Spanish-Speaking Conference on Mental Health, Chicago, June 8–10, 1972, Box 3, Subject File "A," Folder 1: Asian American Community Mental Health Training Center—Conferences, Box 3, Royal F. Morales Collection, Library of Congress, Asian Reading Room.

35. Drawing from E. Franklin Frazier, Abram Kardiner, Bertram Karon, and Thomas Pettigrew, mental health workers of color produced several different terms to describe psychic states related to racism. Psychiatrists Cannon and Pouissant

favored "black psyche" while social workers like Filipina American Juanita Tamayo Lott ("Migration of a Mentality," *Social Casework*, 1976) and The Black Task Force of the Council on Social Work Education (1972) preferred the terms "internal colonialism." The term "ghetto mentality" was first applied to Jewish and Catholic communities prior to the 1950s and continued to have currency in popular discussions around poor behavior.

36. My descriptions of the AAMHTC come from Asian American Mental Health Training Center Final Report July 1972—June 1978, Box 2, Subject File "A," Folder 5 Asian American Mental Health Training Center, Royal F. Morales Collection, Library of Congress, Asian Reading Room.

37. SIPA, Inc. Pamphlet, Fall 1984, Subject File "S", Papers Box 15, Search to Involve Pilipino Americans, Royal F. Morales Collection, Library of Congress, Asian Reading Room.

38. County Justice System Subvention Application, Subject File "S", Papers Box 15, Search to Involve Pilipino Americans, Royal F. Morales Collection, Library of Congress, Asian Reading Room, 3.

39. Watase Memo, August 10, 1987, Subject Files "U", Box 1, United Way, Royal F. Morales Collection, Library of Congress, Asian Reading Room.

40. Widener, *Black Arts West*, 224.

41. "Briefing Report: Central City East" (1991), Box 5, Bunker Hill Redevelopment Papers, Special Collections Library, University of Southern California, 1-1.

42. Evelyn Hooker, "The Adjustment of the Male Overt Homosexual," *Journal of Projective Techniques* 21, no. 1 (1957): 18–31. Also see Ronald Bayer, *Homosexuality and American Psychiatry: The Politics of Diagnosis* (Princeton University Press, 1981); Regina Kunzel, "Queer History, Mad History, and the Politics of Health," *American Quarterly* 69, no. 2 (2017): 315–19; Henry Milton, *Departing from Deviance* (University of Chicago Press, 2001).

43. "An Interview with Evelyn Hooker," Laud Humphreys in *Alternative Lifestyles* (n.d.), Box 1, Folder 5, Evelyn Hooker Collection, Charles Young Special Collections Library, University of California at Los Angeles, 194–95.

44. "Mattachine Society Missions and Purposes" (1951), in Will Roscoe, *Radically Gay*, ed. Harry Hay (Beacon Press, 1996), 131–32.

45. Canaday, *The Straight State*; Kunzel, *Criminal Intimacy*; Jennifer Terry, *An American Obsession* (University of Chicago Press, 1999).

46. "An Interview with Evelyn Hooker," 196.

47. Evelyn Hooker, "The Homosexual Community," 1961, Evelyn Hooker Collection, Charles Young Special Collections Library, University of California at Los Angeles, 4.

48. "The Hooker Report," *Homophile Studies* 22, 1969, Box 4, Folder 3, Charles Young Special Collections Library, University of California at Los Angeles.

49. Evelyn Hooker, Lecture on the Task Force on Homosexuality, ONE Program #157, Feb. 7, 1971 (Audio Recording) ONE Archives, University of Southern California.

50. Puar, "Bodies with New Organs," 48–51.

51. Hooker, "The Homosexual Community," 7.

52. "The Hooker Report," 9.

53. Lynn Lilliston, "Help Center for the Gay Community: Clinics and Rap Groups Among Many Services," *Los Angeles Times*, July 6, 1973, Box 1, Folder 11, Board of Directors, Gay and Lesbian Community Services Center Collection, ONE Archives, University of Southern California.

54. Ian Baldwin, "Rethinking the 'Era of Limits,'" *California History* 91, no. 3: 42–59.

55. Lilliston, "Help Center for the Gay Community."

56. Community Advisory Board Meeting, October 8, 1974, Box 1, Folder 12, Board of Directors, Gay and Lesbian Community Services Center Collection, ONE Archives, University of Southern California, 4.

57. Lilian Faderman and Stuart Timmons, *Gay L.A.: A History of Sexual Outlaws, Power Politics, and Lipstick Lesbians* (University of California Press, 2006), 218.

58. Mass Distribution Letter to Supporters from Robert H. Eichberg, PhD, Sept 25, 1977, Box 1, Folder 12, Municipal Elections Committee of Los Angeles, ONE Archives, University of Southern California.

59. Dudley Clendinen and Nagourney, *Out for Good: The Struggle to Build a Gay Rights Movement in America* (Simon and Schuster, 1999); Jane Ward, "Producing 'Pride' in West Hollywood," *Sexualities* 6, no. 1 (2003): 70.

60. Dennis Altman and Robert Wray, "Gay Power/Gay Money," *LA Weekly*, June 25–July 1, 1982, Box 3, Folder 11, Municipal Elections Committee of Los Angeles, ONE Archives, University of Southern California, 8.

61. MECLA formalized support for GLCSC in 1983. See MECLA 1983–1984 Annual Report, Box 1, Folder 1, Municipal Elections Committee of Los Angeles, ONE Archives, University of Southern California.

62. Lewis, "We Are Certain of Our Own Insanity."

63. These observations of inclusion through disavowal of a community's least normative members are indebted to Shah, *Contagious Divides*.

64. I have written about these divisions with Alex Burnett in "One Out Gay Cop."

65. Linda Breakstone, "California Homosexuals' Political Clout at Crossroads," *Los Angeles Herald Examiner*, November 17, 1985, Box 4698, Folder 1, Thomas Bradley Papers, Charles Young Special Collections Library, University of California at Los Angeles.

66. "California Homosexuals' Political Clout at Crossroads."

67. "MECLA Doesn't Speak For Us!," Box 1, Folder 40, Municipal Elections Committee of Los Angeles, ONE Archives, University of Southern California.

68. 12-12-85 Open Forum Notes, Box 1, Folder 29 Municipal Elections Committee of Los Angeles, ONE Archives, University of Southern California, 2.

69. "Gay Alley Patrols Help Police Discourage After-Hours Cruising," *L.A. Edge*, July 27, 1983, Box 1, Folder 3, Gay and Lesbian Police Advisory Task Force Collection, ONE Archives, University of Southern California.

70. "In Cops' Eyes, Gay Community Is A Real Threat," 1978, Box 1, Folder 4, Gay and Lesbian Police Advisory Task Force Collection, ONE Archives, University of Southern California.

71. Ed Davis, "GOP *Can* Be the Party of the People," *Los Angeles Times*, April 22, 1984, Box 3, Folder 8, Municipal Elections Committee of Los Angeles, ONE Archives, University of Southern California.

72. Castro, "Prostitutes Take Refuge in the Shadows of Skid Row."

73. William Julius Wilson, *The Declining Significance of Race* (University of Chicago Press, 1978).

74. Ferguson, *Aberrations in Black*.

75. George L. Kelling and James Q. Wilson, "Broken Windows: The Police and Neighborhood Safety," *The Atlantic*, March 1982, 29–38, quotation from 30.

76. See Ramos, "Pathologizing the Crisis."

77. "Sanity in the Sierra Madre: The Tarahumara Indians," Box 2, Folder 3 Violence Lectures, Louis Jolyon West Papers, Charles Young Special Collections Library, University of California at Los Angeles, 12.

78. "Sanity in the Sierra Madre: The Tarahumara Indians," Box 2, Folder 3 Violence Lectures, Louis Jolyon West Papers, Charles Young Special Collections Library, University of California at Los Angeles, 15.

79. The coalition included the NAACP, the National Organization of Women, the Mexican American Political Association, the Committee Opposing Psychiatric Abuse of Prisoners (COPAP), United Farm Workers Organizing Committee, and the California Prisoners Union.

80. Robert Litman and Louis Jolyon West, "Research on Violence: The Ethical Equation," in *Behavior and Brain Electrical Activity*, ed. N. Burch and H. L. Altshuler (Plenum, n.d.) 525–39.

81. "Changing Face of Misery," Community Redevelopment Agency of Los Angeles, 1988, Box 5, Folder 14, Bunker Hill Redevelopment Papers, Special Collections Library, University of Southern California, 9.

82. Dorothy Townsend, "Dealing with Children Living in Skid Row," *Los Angeles Times*, July 10, 1983, 1.

83. "Changing Face of Misery," 54.

84. "To Build Community," May 1988, Box 5, Folder 11, Bunker Hill Redevelopment Papers, Special Collections Library, University of Southern California, 19.

85. Cannon, "Re-Africanization."

86. George Ramos, "Had Apparent Heart Attack in Zimbabwe: Dr. J. Alfred Cannon; Health Crusader," *Los Angeles Times*, March 11, 1988, http://articles.latimes.com/1988-03-11/news/mn-1168_1_heart-attack.

87. Samuel Kelton Roberts, Jr., *Infectious Fear* (University of North Carolina Press, 2009), 202.

88. Cary Rudman and John Berthelsen, *An Analysis of the California Department of Corrections Planning Process*, California Assembly Office of Research (1991), 6–8.

89. Gilmore, *Golden Gulag*, 91–92.

90. Gilmore, *Golden Gulag*, 91, 111, and Population Reports, https://www.cdcr.ca.gov/Reports_Research/Offender_Information_Services_Branch/Population_Reports.html.

91. Alisa Roth and others call this phenomenon "trans-institutionalization." See Alisa Roth, *Insane* (Basic Books, 2018); L. Schmidt, A. Reinhardt, R. Kane, and D. Olsen, "The Mentally Ill in Nursing Homes," *Archives of General Psychiatry* 34 (1977): 687–91.

92. California's state hospital system, for instance, now only commits patients who qualify under LPS and those considered mentally disordered offenders, patients deemed not guilty by reason of insanity, sexually violent offenders, sexually violent predators, and those deemed incompetent to stand trial.

93. Max Felker-Kantor, *DARE to Say No: Policing and the War on Drugs in Schools* (University of North Carolina Press, 2024).

CHAPTER SIX

1. Mike Royko, "L.A. Bullet Holes Meet Army Specs," *Chicago Tribune*, November 8, 1989, A3.

2. The study team published three volumes on the viability of the medical center as an anti-poverty machine: "Volume I is a summary; Volume II comprises the text of the Master Plan; Volume III contains the appendices." Grants, Box 981, Folder 891, Commonwealth Fund Series 18, Rockefeller Archives Center.

3. Stuart Schrader, *Badges Without Borders: How Global Counterinsurgency Transformed American Policing* (University of California Press, 2019).

4. Section I of the Master Plan Vol. II. (Historical Context—Drew's Community), The Master Plan Study, Master Plan Report, Grants, Box 98, Folder 890 Charles R. Drew Postgraduate Medical School, Commonwealth Fund Series 18, Rockefeller Archives Center, I-6.

5. This chapter builds on the previous chapter's concluding analysis on the biologization of violence. My interpretation of Black men in the 1970s is indebted to Metzl, *The Protest Psychosis* and Kunzel, *Criminal Intimacy*. Metzl argues Black men replaced White women as the preeminent schizophrenic patients of the 1970s. Black men were often used in pharmaceutical advertisements to help psychiatrists and their patients understand how new drugs worked to curb violent tendencies. Kunzel argues that white male prisoners mobilized claims of rape in prison as a way to preserve their public identities as white heterosexual men.

6. Gilmore, *Golden Gulag*.

7. HoSang, *Racial Propositions*, 266.

8. Royko, "L.A. Bullet Holes Meet Army Specs."

9. L. Briggs, *Reproducing Empire*; Daniel Immawahr, *How to Hide an Empire: A History of the Greater United States* (Farrar, Straus, and Giroux, 2019); Man, *Soldiering Through Empire*; Vijay Prashad, *The Darker Nations: A People's History of the Third World* (New Press, 2008).

10. Greg Grandin, *Empire's Workshop: Latin America, the United States, and the Making of An Imperial Republic* (Picador, 2021); Moon-Ho Jung, *Menace to Empire: Anticolonial Solidarities and the Transpacific Origins of the US Security State* (University of California Press, 2023).

11. Felker-Kantor, *Policing Los Angeles*; James Forman, Jr., *Locking Up Our Own: Crime and Punishment in Black America* (Farrar, Straus, and Giroux, 2017); Schrader, *Badges without Borders.*

12. Man, *Soldiering Through Empire.*

13. Gilmore, *Golden Gulag*; Gabriela Soto Laveaga. *Jungle Laboratories: Mexican Peasants, National Projects, and the Making of the Pill* (Duke University Press, 2009).

14. Winant, *The Next Shift.*

15. Gilmore, *Golden Gulag*, 72–74.

16. According to her, "these modes include informal economic structures for the exchange of illegal and legal goods and services; social parenting, especially by women, in extended families of biological and fictive kin; and the redivision of urban space into units controlled by street organizations" (Gilmore, *Golden Gulag*, 74).

17. Booker King and Ismail Jatoi, "The Mobile Army Surgical Hospital (MASH): A Military and Surgical Legacy," *The Journal of the National Medical Association* 97, no. 5 (May 2005): 648–56.

18. Believing that citizens had unwittingly been led to support a white supremacist organization without knowing it, *Monrovia News Post* editor Tony Cimarusti implored citizens who had seen the "Don't Reward Rioting" bumper stickers to "forget it." The Greater Los Angeles Citizen's Council, he argued, had just changed its name from the White Citizen's Council. By revealing to voters that "it is a White supremacist organization," Cimarusti hoped to convince his neighbors that such an association with a racist organization would not be in keeping with supporting a hospital "open to persons of all races and creeds" and an issue aimed at bettering the "general health and welfare of the county." See Editorial, *Monrovia News Post*, June 7, 1966, Martin Luther King, Jr. Hospital 1965–1990, Kenneth Hahn Papers, Huntington Library.

19. "Watts Not Alone in Need for Improved Hospitals," *Downey Leader*, May 23, 1966, Martin Luther King, Jr. Hospital 1965–1990, Kenneth Hahn Papers, Huntington Library.

20. Memo to Chief K. E. Klinger, Forester and Fire Warden, from Kenneth Hahn, September 22, 1966, Paramedic Program 1966–1969, Kenneth Hahn Papers, Huntington Library.

21. Letter from Robert Mazet to Kenneth Hahn, March 8, 1966, Paramedic Program 1966–1969, Kenneth Hahn Papers, Huntington Library.

22. "Robert Kennedy Shot, Killed in Los Angeles," *Newsweek*, June 16, 1968.

23. Matthew L. Edwards, "Pittsburgh's Freedom House Ambulance Service: The Origins of Emergency Medical Services and the Politics of Race and Health," *The Journal of the History of Medicine and Allied Sciences* 74, no. 4 (September, 2019): 441.

24. According to Brian Zink, many pioneers of emergency medicine received their first experience in the ER as "largely unqualified physician provider[s]." As he explains, "a common method of ER staffing ... was to have a nurse assigned to the ER who would assess patients, make triage decisions, and then call an appropriate physician to deliver care. Physicians were not obligated to provide this care." However, "by 1960, most larger hospitals began to staff their ERs with physicians, residents, or medical students.... Since emergency practice was not considered a real occupation for a physician, only those without a regular job were available to be hired." See *Anyone, Anything, Anytime: A History of Emergency Medicine* (Mosby-Elsevier, 2006), 13–14.

25. For a better accounting of how disparate technologies were "sifted, evaluated, and transformed" to create a unified emergency medical system through federal grants and evaluations, see Andrew T. Simpson, "Transporting Lazarus: Physicians, the State, and the Creation of the Modern Paramedic and Ambulance, 1955–1973," *Journal of History of Medicine* 68 (April 2013): 163–97.

26. The heart ambulance project, launched in the summer of 1969, served suburban citizens residing in Hahn's district in the City of Inglewood. The three private hospitals were Daniel Freeman, Centinela, and Hawthorne General, and the pilot deployed ambulances from the McCormick Ambulance Company, a firm targeted by officials to demonstrate how private ambulance standards could be raised.

27. The heart rescue vehicle project, launched in the winter of 1969, served the suburban residents residing within Hahn's district in the City of Carson and was dubbed the "rescue unit" project because it prioritized speed. It was directed by Dr. Michael Criley, director of cardiology at Harbor-UCLA, and involved the publicly funded Harbor General Hospital. As a base station, it used County Fire Engine 36 in Carson.

28. Hahn Recorded Phone Script, December 4, 1969, Paramedic Program 1966–1969, Kenneth Hahn Papers, Huntington Library.

29. Telegram: Heart Rescue Squads, April 22, 1971, Paramedic Program 1971–1972, Kenneth Hahn Papers, Huntington Library.

30. Letter from Fire Chief Deputy Stanley Barlow to Hahn, June 21, 1971, Paramedic Program 1971–1972, Kenneth Hahn Papers, Huntington Library.

31. Report on the Paramedic Committee, Los Angeles Economy and Efficiency Commission, August 1975, Paramedic Program 1975, Kenneth Hahn Papers, Huntington Library, 1-2.

32. Paramedics Press Release, September 8, 1971, Paramedic Program 1971–1972, Kenneth Hahn Papers, Huntington Library, 3.

33. Paramedics Press Release, September 8, 1971, Paramedic Program 1971–1972, Kenneth Hahn Papers, Huntington Library.

34. Ellen Herman, *The Romance of American Psychology: Political Culture in the Age of Experts* (University of California Press, 1995), 201.

35. Lisa Hsiao, "Project 100,000: The Great Society's Answer to Military Manpower Needs in Vietnam," *Vietnam Generation* 1 (Summer 1989).

36. William A. Williams, *Empire as a Way of Life* (Ig Publishing, 2006), 19.

37. Harry Nelson, "South LA Medical School Sets Individual Care as Major Goal: Drew Facility, Teaching Arm of King Hospital, Hopes to Provide Quality Health Services for 400,000 in Area," *Los Angeles Times*, April 5, 1971.

38. Hahn appointed Black physician Dr. Liston Witherhill to serve on the County Paramedic Ambulance Advisory Board. The antipoverty aims of the county's paramedic program were well advertised. See Nelson, "South LA Medical School Sets Individual Care as Major Goal" and "Drew Postgraduate Medical School Maintains Close Ties with UCLA, USC," *UCLA Weekly*, April 19, 1971, Subseries 2 Box 3 Folder 15 Charles R Drew Medical School, John and Mary Markle Fund Series 1, Rockefeller Archives Center, 1.

39. Paramedics Press Release, September 8, 1971, Paramedic Program 1971–1972, Kenneth Hahn Papers, Huntington Library.

40. Paramedics Press Release, September 8, 1971, Paramedic Program 1971–1972, Kenneth Hahn Papers, Huntington Library.

41. "Attention: The King Hospital is a Potential Death Trap," 1972, Martin Luther King, Jr. Hospital 1965–1990, Kenneth Hahn Papers, Huntington Library.

42. A study team hired by the Department of Health, Education, and Welfare and the Commonwealth studied the newly opened King-Drew Center for a year and a half. Their findings associated "the high incidence of accidents and homicides"—the fourth and fifth leading causes of death in the community after cancer, heart disease, and stroke—with the high rate of "drug traffic that exists on the streets . . . housing projects and . . . schools." Section I of the Master Plan Vol. II. (Historical Context), The Master Plan Report, Grants, Box 981, Folder 891, Commonwealth Fund Series 18, Rockefeller Archives Center, I-6.

43. The Medical Center completed the physical expansion of the ER and Trauma Center in 1976. It would take two years to fully accredit the residency program. Memo from Melvin Fleming to John O'Connor Subject: Paramedic Base Station King Hospital, June 30, 1974; and memo from Dan Grindell to William Delgardo, December 22, 1975, Martin Luther King, Jr. Hospital 1965–1990, Kenneth Hahn Papers, Huntington Library.

44. Roxane Arnold, "Proposition 13 Not Racist, Jarvis Declares," *The Los Angeles Times*, June 19, 1978, B13.

45. For more on the use of joint power agreements, see Jenkins, *The Bonds of Inequality*.

46. Lettergram to Deputies from Kenneth Hahn, May 1, 1972, Martin Luther King, Jr. Hospital 1965–1990, Kenneth Hahn Papers, Huntington Library. The lettergram contained a facsimile of Howard Jarvis's "The People Must Know" column in *The Canyon Crier*, March 6, 1972.

47. Fulton, *Reluctant Metropolis*, 280.

48. Robert Shogan, "Prop. 13 Shakes Liberal Leaders," *Los Angeles Times*, June 25, 1978, 1.

49. Shogan, "Prop. 13 Shakes Liberal Leaders."

50. Prepared Speech Notes, March 28, 1976, Box 1, Folder 13 Urban Metro EMS Symposium Los Angeles 1976, James O. Page Collection, Darling Biomedical Library, University of California Los Angeles.

51. Implementation of a Dynamic State EMS System: North Carolina, A Case Study, 1974, Box 1, Folder 1 American Public Health Association 102nd Annual Meeting New Orleans 1974, James O. Page Collection, Darling Biomedical Library, University of California Los Angeles.

52. Crenshaw, "Race, Reform, and Retrenchment," 1342.

53. "The Birth of 'Emergency'" as presented at the New York Association of Fire Chiefs Association Meeting, June 20, 1977, reprinted in *Size Up* 28, no. 4 (November 1977), Box 1, Folder 51 New York State Fire Chiefs Association 1977, James O. Page Collection, Darling Biomedical Library, University of California Los Angeles.

54. "Emergency Medical Services: The Future Now," *Texas Town & City*, April 1976, Box 1, Folder 32 Texas Statewide EMS Conference 1977, James O. Page Collection, Darling Biomedical Library, University of California Los Angeles.

55. Emergency Medicine Public Announcement Pamphlet, "Emergency Medical Service Systems: A Community Challenge," Liberty Mutual Insurance Companies, 1975, Box 1, Folder 6 First National Conference on Medico-Legal Implications of Emergency Medical Services, Washington DC 1975, James O. Page Collection, Darling Biomedical Library, University of California Los Angeles.

56. Prepared Notes, "EMS in Perspective," 1982, Box 4, Folder 19 EMS Today Conference Houston Texas 1982, James O. Page Collection, Darling Biomedical Library, University of California Los Angeles.

57. Paul Jacobs and Janet Clayton, "Is It Enough? LA Trauma Care Stirs Hot Debate," *Los Angeles Times*, March 29, 1981, A1.

58. "Trauma Care in Los Angeles," *Los Angeles Times*, July 16, 1982, D6.

59. Prepared Notes, "Lessons from the South, Part II," 1979, Box 2, Folder 53 INTERPHASE Calgary, Alberta, Canada 1979, James O. Page Collection, Darling Biomedical Library, University of California Los Angeles.

60. Prepared Notes, "CPR—The Present," 1980, Box 3, Folder 4 Conference on Citizen CPR 1980, James O. Page Collection, Darling Biomedical Library, University of California Los Angeles.

61. Richard E. Meyer and Mike Goodman, "Marauders from Inner City Prey on L.A.'s Suburbs," *Los Angeles Times*, July 12, 1981, A1. Black journalists and activists responded to it in James H. Cleaver, "Local Residents Angered by LA Times 'Attack' on Blacks," *Los Angeles Sentinel*, July 16, 1981, A2.

62. James H. Cleaver, "Massive Street Rally Slated Sunday at Victoria & Adams," *Los Angeles Sentinel*, July 16, 1981, A1.

63. "Proposed Health Cuts Hit," *Los Angeles Sentinel*, October 8, 1981, A3.

64. Cleaver, "Massive Street Rally Slated Sunday at Victoria & Adams"; Carl Chamberlain, "LA Times, Drug Abuse Denounced at Mass Rally," *Los Angeles Sentinel*, July 23, 1981, A1.

65. Cleaver, "Local Residents Angered by LA Times 'Attack' on Blacks."

66. Bill Boyarski, "New LA County Budget Cuts Proposed: More Hospital, Neighborhood Health Center Reductions Included," *The Los Angeles Times* (Orange County Edition), April 27, 1982, A5.

67. See Jacobs and Clayton, "Is It Enough?"; Paul Jacobs, "LA County Emergency Care Hit: Trauma Center Plan Gets Hospital Officials' Qualified OK," *Los Angeles Times*, April 1, 1982, A4; "Trauma Care in Los Angeles."

68. Jacobs and Clayton, "Is It Enough?"

69. "Budget Cuts in Health Services—Letters to the Editors," *Los Angeles Times*, July 28, 1981, C4.

70. The final policy language read as follows: "To be eligible to receive non-emergency medical services other than medical services to protect the health of the community (see Policy No. 521) a patient shall be required to provide financial data, execute financial arrangements and to establish program eligibility, where applicable, before non-emergency care is rendered. This process shall include the following minimum requirements: a) signed declaration of personal employment (or) prepaid health plan status; b) provision of acceptable address verification, or a valid Medi-Cal or Medicare card in those cases were no self-pay liability is likely to result; c) assignment of all declared insurance benefits to the County; d) execution of property liens, where applicable; e) application for Medi-Cal where potential eligibility is indicated. Where potential Medi-Cal is not indicated, a reimbursement agreement will be required. Such reimbursement agreement shall cover any amount remaining after all third-party benefits have been exhausted or the patient's liability under the County's Ability-to-Pay Plan if that is less. Advance patient payments may also be deducted." Letter to Melvin J. Fleming, Deputy Director of Hospitals from William A. Delgardo, Administrator; Subject: Treatment Policy Revisions, 1981, Martin Luther King, Jr. Hospital 1965–1990, Kenneth Hahn Papers, Huntington Library.

71. Thomas Scully, interview on "All Things Considered," National Public Radio, September 3, 2003.

72. HoSang, *Racial Propositions*; Cybelle Fox, "Unauthorized Welfare: The Origins of Immigrant Status Restrictions in American Social Policy," *Journal of American History* 102, no. 4 (2016): 1051–74; Kohler-Hausmann, *Getting Tough*; Marchevsky and Theoharis, *Not Working*.

73. Beatrix Hoffman, "Emergency Rooms: The Reluctant Safety Net," in *History and Health Policy in the United States: Putting the Past Back In*, ed. Rosemary Stevens, Charles Rosenberg, and Lawton Burns (Rutgers University Press, 2006), 250–72.

74. Giorgio Agamben, *Homo Sacer: Sovereign Power and Bare Life* (Stanford University Press, 1998).

EPILOGUE

1. Juan Williams, "'Octavia Butler' from *Talk of the Nation*, National Public Radio (May 8, 2000)," in *Conversations with Octavia Butler*, ed. Conseula Francis (University of Mississippi Press, 2020), 168.

2. Larry McCaffery and Jim McMenamin, "'An Interview with Octavia E. Butler' from *Across the Wounded Galaxies: Interviews with Contemporary American Science Fiction Writers*, edited by Larry McCaffery. Urbana: University of Illinois Press, 1990," in Francis, *Conversations with Octavia Butler*, 15.

3. Lisa See, "Interview from *Publishers Weekly* (December 13, 1993)," in Francis, *Conversations with Octavia Butler*, 39; Joan Fry, "'Congratulations! You've Just Won $295,000: An Interview with Octavia Butler' from *Poets & Writers Magazine* (March/April 1997)," in Francis, *Conversations with Octavia Butler*, 125.

4. Marilyn Mehaffy and AnaLouise Keating, "'Radio Imagination': Octavia Butler on the Poetics of Narrative Embodiment' (1997) first published in *MELUS: The Journal of the Society of the Study of the Multi-Ethnic Literature of the United States* 26.1 (Spring 2001)," in Francis, *Conversations with Octavia Butler*, 118–19.

5. Randall Keenan, "'An Interview with Octavia E. Butler' from *Callaloo* 14.2 (1991), 495–504," in Francis, *Conversations with Octavia Butler*, 34.

6. Rosalie G. Harrison, "'Sci-Fi Visions: An Interview with Octavia Butler' from *Equal Opportunity Forum Magazine* (November, 1980)," in Francis, *Conversations with Octavia Butler*, 6; Mehaffy and Keating, "Radio Imagination," 113.

7. Charles Roswell, "'An Interview with Octavia E. Butler' from *Callaloo* 20:1 (1997), 47–66," in Francis, *Conversations with Octavia Butler*, 94.

8. Roswell, "An Interview with Octavia E. Butler," 94.

9. Keenan, "An Interview with Octavia E. Butler," 28.

10. McCaffery and McMenamin, "An Interview with Octavia E. Butler," 21.

11. Fry, "'Congratulations! You've Just Won $295,000," 129.

12. Roswell, "An Interview with Octavia E. Butler," 94.

13. Fry, "'Congratulations! You've Just Won $295,000," 129.

14. Keenan, "An Interview with Octavia E. Butler," 28; Mehaffy and Keating, "Radio Imagination," 107.

15. McCaffery and McMenamin, "An Interview with Octavia E. Butler," 18.

16. Stephen W. Potts, "'We Keep Playing the Same Record': A Conversation with Octavia Butler' from *Science Fiction Studies* 23:3 (1996)," in Francis, *Conversations with Octavia Butler*, 67.

17. McCaffery and McMenamin, "An Interview with Octavia E. Butler," 18.

18. Mehaffy and Keating, "Radio Imagination," 108–9.

19. Potts, "We Keep Playing the Same Record," 70.

20. H. Jerome Jackson, "'Sci-Fi Tales from Octavia Butler:' from *Crisis* (April 1994)," in Francis, *Conversations with Octavia Butler*, 44.

21. Jelani Cobb, "'Interview with Octavia Butler:' from *JelaniCobb.com*, http://jelanicobb.com (accessed in 2005)," in Francis, *Conversations with Octavia Butler*, 55.

22. Jackson, "Sci-Fi Tales from Octavia Butler," 46.

23. Potts, "We Keep Playing the Same Record," 70.

24. Cobb, "Interview with Octavia Butler," 61.

25. Jackson, "Sci-Fi Tales from Octavia Butler," 45.

26. Cobb, "Interview with Octavia Butler," 61.

27. McCaffery and McMenamin, "An Interview with Octavia E. Butler," 14.

28. Potts, "We Keep Playing the Same Record," 68.
29. Jackson, "Sci-Fi Tales from Octavia Butler," 46.
30. Cobb, "Interview with Octavia Butler," 63.
31. Jackson, "Sci-Fi Tales from Octavia Butler," 48.
32. See "Interview from *Publishers Weekly*," 41; Cobb, "Interview with Octavia Butler," 63.
33. Jackson, "Sci-Fi Tales from Octavia Butler," 45.
34. Potts, "We Keep Playing the Same Record," 68.
35. McCaffery and McMenamin, "An Interview with Octavia E. Butler," 20.
36. Conseula Francis, "Introduction," in Francis, *Conversations with Octavia Butler*, xi.

BIBLIOGRAPHY

ARCHIVAL SOURCES

Charles E. Young Special Collections Library, University of California Los Angeles

Thomas Bradley Papers
Augustus Hawkins Papers
Evelyn Hooker Papers
Louis Jolyon West Papers
Los Angeles Olympic Organizing Committee Collection

Darling Biomedical Library, University of California Los Angeles

James O. Page Papers
Marvin Karno, MD Professional Papers

Huntington Library

John Anson Ford Collection
Kenneth Hahn Collection

Library of Congress, Asian Reading Room

Royal F. Morales Papers

National Archives and Records Administration, Lyndon Baines Johnson Presidential Library

Oral Histories Collection
Welfare Records

Ohio Historical Society

William Howard Whitaker Papers

ONE Archives, University of Southern California

Damron's Address Book
Gay and Lesbian Community Services Center Collection
Municipal Elections Committee of Los Angeles Papers
Gay and Lesbian Police Advisory Task Force Papers

Rockefeller Archive Center

Commonwealth Fund Papers
John and Mary Markle Foundation Papers
Charles R. Drew Postgraduate Medical School Papers

Sophia Smith Collection of Women's History, Smith College

Guida West Papers

Special Collections, University of California Santa Barbara

Alicia Escalante Papers

Special Collections Library, University of Southern California

California Social Welfare Collection
Bunker Hill Redevelopment Papers
Los Angeles Riots Collection
Oral History Transcripts

Wisconsin Historical Society

George A. Wiley Papers

NEWSPAPERS AND PERIODICALS

The Atlantic
Austin American Statesman
Chicago Tribune

Fort Lauderdale News and Sun-Sentinel
Jet Magazine
Los Angeles Herald
Los Angeles Sentinel
Los Angeles Times
Monrovia Daily News Post
The Nation
Newsweek
South Bay Daily Breeze
Time Magazine
Washington Post

PRINTED PRIMARY SOURCES

"All Show and No Substance: Proposition HHH First Year Performance Assessment." Los Angeles Community Action Network (LA CAN), November, 2017.

Blake, Elinor and Thomas Bodenheimer. "Closing the Door on the Poor: The Dismantling of California's Public Hospitals." *Health Policy Advisory Center Report* 16 (1975).

Breslow, Lester. "New Partnerships in the Delivery of Services—A Public Health View of Need." *The American Journal of Public Health* 57, no. 7. (July 1967): 1095.

Cannon, J. Alfred. "The Psycho-Social Aspects of Segregation." *Journal of the National Medication Association* 56, no. 2 (1964): 160–63.

Cannon, J. Alfred. "Re-Africanization: The Last Alternative for Black America." *Phylon* 38, no. 2 (Second Quarter, 1977): 203–10.

Cobb, W. Montague. "The Crushing Irony of De Luxe Jim Crow." *Journal of the National Medical Association* 44 (September 1952): 386–87.

Cobb, W. Montague. "Numa P.G. Adams, 1885–1940." *Journal of the National Medical Association* 43, no. 1 (January, 1951): 42–54.

Davis, Milton S., and R. Tranquada. "A Sociological Evaluation of the Watts Neighborhood Health Center." *Medical Care* 7, no. 2 (March-April, 1969): 105–17.

Derthick, Martha. *Policy Making for Social Security*. Washington, DC: Brookings Institute, 1979.

Haynes, M. Alfred. "An Approach to the Teaching of Family Care." *Journal of the American Medical Association* 173, no. 3 (July, 1960): 1340.

Haynes, M. Alfred. "Professionals and the Community Confront Change." *American Journal of Public Health* 60, no. 3 (March 1970): 519.

Haynes, M. Alfred. "Drew Postgraduate Medical School." *California Medicine/The Western Journal of Medicine* 118, no. 4 (April 1973): 80–81.

Haynes, M. Alfred. "The Distribution of Black Physicians in the United States, 1967." *Journal of the National Medical Association* 61, no. 6 (November 1969): 470–73.

Haynes, M. Alfred. "Problems Facing the Negro in Medicine Today." *The Journal of the American Medical Association* 209, no. 7 (August 18, 1969): 1067–69.

Hill, Julius W. "The Golden State Medical Association." *California Medicine* 111, no. 1 (July 1969): 46–49.

Hooker, Evelyn. "The Adjustment of the Male Overt Homosexual." *Journal of Projective Techniques* 21, no. 1 (1957): 18–31.

Jackson, Oscar J., and Waldenese Nixon. "Medicine in the Black Community." *The Western Journal of Medicine* 114, no. 4 (October 1970): 58.

Kelch, Deborah Reidy. *Caring for Medically Indigent Adults in California: A History*. California Healthcare Foundation, June 2005.

Litman, Robert, and Louis Jolyon West. "Research on Violence: The Ethical Equation." In *Behavior and Brain Electrical Activity*, edited by N. Burch and H. L. Altshuler, 525–39. Plenum, n.d.

"Major Milestones: 43 Years of Care and Treatment of the Mentally Ill." California Legislative Analyst's Office, 2000.

Manchanda, Rishi. "Taming the Perfect Storm: Addressing the Impact of Public Health, Housing, and Law Enforcement Policies on Homelessness and Health in South Los Angeles." St. John's Well Child and Family Center, Esperanza Community Housing Corporation, Los Angeles Community Action Network, Strategic Actions for a Just Economy, and Southside Coalition of Community Health Centers, July 2008.

McCone, John. "Violence in the City—An End or a Beginning?" California Governor's Commission on the Los Angeles Riots, December 1965.

Morden, Margaret Gorsuch, and Richard Bigger. "Studies in Local Government, No. 11: Cooperative Health Administration in Metropolitan Los Angeles." Bureau of Governmental Research (University of California Los Angeles), June 1949.

"Office of Economic Opportunity: The Neighborhood Health Center." Washington, DC: US Government Printing Office, 1967.

Peyton, Thomas Roy. "The Negro Specialist and the Negro General Practitioner." *Journal of the National Medical Association* 55, no. 3 (May 1963): 248–50.

Rudman, Cary, and John Berthelsen. *An Analysis of the California Department of Corrections Planning Process*. California Assembly Office of Research, 1991.

Schmidt, Leonard, A. Reinhardt, R. Kane, and D. Olsen. "The Mentally Ill in Nursing Homes." *Archives of General Psychiatry* 34 (1977): 687–91.

Viseltear, Arthur, J. Arnold Kirsch, and Milton Roemer. "Medical Care Administration—Case Study No. 5: The Watts Hospital: Pilot Study." United States Department of Health, Education, and Welfare Public Health Service, September 1969.

Widney, Joseph Pomeroy. *Civilizations and Their Diseases and Rebuilding a Wrecked World Civilization*. Pacific Publishing Company, 1937.

Widney, Joseph Pomeroy. *Race Life and Race Religions*. Pacific Publishing Company, 1936.

Widney, Joseph Pomeroy. *The Three Americas: Their Racial Past and the Dominant Racial Factors of Their Future*. Pacific Publishing Company, 1935.

SECONDARY SOURCES

Abel, Emily K. "'Only the Best Class of Immigration': Public Health Policy Toward Mexicans and Filipinos in Los Angeles, 1910–1940." *The American Journal of Public Health* 94, no. 6 (June 2004): 932–39.

Agamben, Giorgio. *Homo Sacer: Sovereign Power and Bare Life.* Stanford University Press, 1998.

Agee, Christopher Lowen. *The Streets of San Francisco: Policing and the Creation of a Cosmopolitan Liberal Politics, 1950–1972.* University of Chicago Press, 2014.

Alinsky, Saul, with Marion K. Sanders. *The Professional Radical: Conversations with Saul Alinsky.* Harper and Row, 1970.

Amalguer, Tomás. *Racial Faultlines: The Historical Origins of White Supremacy in California* University of California Press, 2009 [1994].

Anderson, Warwick. *Colonial Pathologies: American Tropical Medicine, Race, and Hygiene in the Philippines.* Duke University Press, 2006.

Anderson, Warwick. "Making Global Health History: The Postcolonial Worldliness of Biomedicine." *The Social History of Medicine* 27, no. 2 (2014): 372–84.

Aumoithe, George. "Dismantling the Safety-Net Hospital: The Construction of 'Underutilization' and Scarce Public Hospital Care." *Journal of Urban History* 49, no. 6 (2023): 1282–311.

Avila, Eric. *Popular Culture in the Age of White Flight.* University of California Press, 2006.

Baldoz, Rick. *The Third Asiatic Invasion: Empire and Migration in Filipino America, 1898–1946.* New York University Press, 2011.

Baldwin, Ian. "Rethinking the 'Era of Limits.'" *California History* 91, no. 3: 42–59.

Baldwin, James. *Another Country.* New York: Vintage Books, 1993.

Baldwin, James. *No Name in the Street.* Knopf Doubleday Publishing, 1972.

Baker, Robert B. "The American Medical Association and Race." *American Medical Association Journal of Ethics* 16, no. 6 (2014): 479–88.

Baker, Robert B., Harriet A. Washington, Ololade Olakanmi, Todd L. Savitt, Elizabeth A. Jacobs, Eddie Hoover, and Matthew K. Wynia. "African American Physicians and Organized Medicine, 1846–1968: Origins of a Racial Divide." *Journal of the American Medical Association* 300, no. 3 (2008): 306–13.

Baradaran, Mehrsa. *The Color of Money: Black Banks and the Racial Wealth Gap.* Belknap Press of Harvard University Press, 2017.

Barraclough, Laura. *Making the San Fernando Valley: Rural Landscapes, Urban Development, and White Privilege.* University of Georgia Press, 2010.

Bayers, Ronald. *Homosexuality and American Psychiatry: The Politics of Diagnosis.* Princeton University Press, 1981.

Beam, Myrl. *Gay, Inc.: The Nonprofitization of Queer Politics.* University of Minnesota Press, 2018.

Bell, Derrick A., Jr. "Brown vs. Board of Education and the Interest-Convergence Dilemma." *Harvard Law Review* 93 (January 1980): 518–33.

Bermudez, Rosie. "La Causa de los Pobres: Alicia Escalante's Lived Experience of Poverty." In *Chicana Movidas: New Narratives of Activism and Feminism in the Movement Era*, edited by Dionne Espinoza, Maria Eugenia Cotera, and Maylei Blackwell, 123–37. University of Texas Press, 2018.

Berry, Daina Ramey. *The Price for Their Pound of Flesh: The Value of the Enslaved, from Womb to Grave, in the Building of a Nation*. Beacon Press, 2017.

Biondi, Martha. *The Black Revolution on Campus*. University of California Press, 2012.

Birn, Anne-Emanuelle, and Raul Necochea Lopez. *Peripheral Nerve: Health and Medicine in Cold War Latin America*. Duke University Press, 2020.

Bloom, Josh, and Waldo E. Martin Jr. *Black Against Empire: The History and Politics of the Black Panther Party*. University of California Press, 2016.

Boag, Peter. *Same-Sex Affairs: Constructing and Controlling Homosexuality in the Pacific Northwest*. University of California Press, 2003.

Bonacich, Edna, and Richard Appelbaum. *Behind the Label: Inequality in the Los Angeles Apparel Industry*. University of California Press, 2000.

Bonacich, Edna, Lucie Cheng, and Paul Ong, eds. *The New Asian Immigration in Los Angeles and Global Restructuring*. Temple University Press, 1994.

Bonacich, Edna, Lucie Cheng, Norma Chinchilla, Nora Hamilton, and Paul Ong, eds. *Global Production: The Apparel Industry in the Pacific Rim*. Temple University Press, 1994.

Braun, Lundy. *Breathing Race into the Machine: The Surprising Career of the Spirometer from Plantation to Genetics*. University of Minnesota Press, 2014.

Briggs, Charles. *Incommunicable: Towards Communicative Justice in Health and Medicine*. Duke University Press, 2024.

Briggs, Laura. *How All Politics Became Reproductive Politics: From Welfare Reform to Foreclosure to Trump*. University of California, 2018.

Briggs, Laura. *Reproducing Empire: Race, Sex, Science, and US Imperialism in Puerto Rico*. University of California, 2003.

Brown, Phil. ed., *Mental Health Care and Social Policy*. Routledge, 1985.

Brown, Scot. *Fighting for US: Maulana Karenga, the US Organization, and Black Cultural Nationalism*. New York University Press, 2003.

Cacho, Lisa Marie. *Social Death: Racialized Rightlessness and the Criminalization of the Unprotected*. New York University Press, 2012.

Canaday, Margot. *The Straight State: Sexuality and Citizenship in Twentieth Century America*. Princeton University Press, 2009.

Canaday, Margot. *Queer Career: Sexuality and Work in Modern America*. Princeton University Press, 2023.

Capo, Julio, Jr. *Welcome to Fairyland: Queer Miami before 1940*. University of North Carolina Press, 2017.

Chauncey, George. *Gay New York: Gender, Urban Culture, and the Makings of the Gay Male World, 1890–1940*. Basic Books, 1994.

Chávez-García, Miroslava. *States of Delinquency: Race and Science in the Making of California's Juvenile Justice System*. University of California Press, 2012.

Cheng, Wendy. *The Changs Next Door to the Diazes: Remapping Race in Suburban California*. University of Minnesota Press, 2013.

Chowkwanyun, Merlin. *All Health Politics is Local: Community Battles for Medical Care and Environmental Health*. University of North Carolina Press, 2022.

Clendinen, Dudley, and Adam Nagourney. *Out for Good: The Struggle to Build a Gay Rights Movement in America*. Simon and Schuster, 1999.

Cohen, Cathy J. *Boundaries of Blackness: AIDS and the Breakdown of Black Politics*. University of Chicago Press, 1999.

Cohen, Cathy J. "Punks, Bulldaggers, and Welfare Queens: The Radical Potential of Queer Politics?" *GLQ* 3: 437–65.

Collins, Patricia Hill. *Black Sexual Politics: African Americans, Gender, and the New Racism*. Routledge, 2004.

Connolly, Nathan B. *A World More Concrete: Real Estate and the Remaking of Jim Crow South Florida*. University of Chicago Press, 2014.

Cowie, Jefferson. *Stayin' Alive: The 1970s and the Last Days of the Working Class*. New Press, 2010.

Clouthard, Glenn. *Red Skin, White Masks: Rejecting the Colonial Politics of Recognition*. Minneapolis: University of Minnesota Press, 2014.

Crenshaw, Kimberlé. "Demarginalizing the Intersections of Race and Sex: A Black Feminist Critique of Antidiscrimination Doctrine, Feminist Theory and Antiracist Politics." *University of Chicago Legal Forum* 1989, Issue 1, Article 8: 139–67.

Crenshaw, Kimberlé. "Race, Reform, and Retrenchment." *Harvard Law Review* 101, no. 7 (May 1988): 1331–87.

Curran, Andrew S. *The Anatomy of Blackness: Science and Slavery in an Age of Enlightenment*. Johns Hopkins University Press, 2011.

Davis, Mike. *City of Quartz: Excavating the Future in Los Angeles*. Vintage, 1992.

Dawson, Michael. *Behind the Mule: Race and Class in African-American Politics*. Princeton University Press, 1994.

Dear, Michael, and Jennifer Wolch. *Landscapes of Despair: From Deinstitutionalization to Homelessness*. Princeton University Press, 1987.

Deverell, William. *Whitewashed Adobe: The Rise of Los Angeles and the Re-Making of Its Mexican Past*. University of California Press, 2004.

Dittmer, John. *The Good Doctors: The Medical Committee for Human Rights and the Struggle for Social Justice in Health Care*. University of Mississippi Press, 2009.

Downs, Jim. *Sick from Freedom*. Oxford University Press, 2012.

Doyle, Dennis A. *Psychiatry and Racial Liberalism in Harlem, 1936–1968*. University of Rochester Press, 2016.

Du Bois, W. E. B. *Black Reconstruction in America, 1860–1880*. Harcourt, Bruce and Company, 1935. Reprint, The Free Press, 1998.

Du Bois, W. E. B. *The Souls of Black Folk*. Introduction by Patricia H. Hinchey. Myers Education Press, 2018.

Dudziak, Mary. *Cold War Civil Rights: Race and the Image of American Democracy*. Princeton University Press, 2000.

Eaton, Charlie. *Bankers in the Ivory Tower: The Troubling Rise of Financiers in US Higher Education*. University of Chicago Press, 2022.
Edwards, Matthew L. "Pittsburgh's Freedom House Ambulance Service: The Origins of Emergency Medical Services and the Politics of Race and Health." *The Journal of the History of Medicine and Allied Sciences* 74, no. 4 (September 2019).
Ehrenreich, Barbara. *Nickel and Dimed: On (Not) Getting By in America*. Metropolitan Books, 2001.
Elias, Allison. *The Rise of Corporate Feminism: Women in the American Office, 1960–1990*. Columbia University Press, 2022.
Engel, Jonathan. *Poor People's Medicine: Medicaid and American Charity Care since 1965*. Duke University Press, 2006.
Faderman, Lilian, and Stuart Timmons. *Gay L.A.: A History of Sexual Outlaws, Power Politics, and Lipstick Lesbians*. University of California Press, 2006.
Fanon, Frantz. *Black Skin, White Masks*. Translated by Richard Philcox. Foreword by Kwame Anthony Appiah. New York: Grove Press, 2008.
Farmer, Ashley D. *Remaking Black Power: How Black Women Transformed an Era*. University of North Carolina Press, 2017.
Farmer, Paul. *Pathologies of Power: Health, Human Rights, and the New War on the Poor*. University of California Press, 2005.
Fett, Sharla. *Working Cures: Healing, Health, and Power on Southern Slave Plantations*. University of North Carolina Press, 2002.
Ferguson, Roderick A. *Aberrations in Black: Towards a Queer of Color Critique*. University of Minnesota Press, 2004.
Felker-Kantor, Max. *Policing Los Angeles: Race, Resistance, and the Rise of the LAPD*. University of North Carolina Press, 2018.
Felker-Kantor, Max. *DARE to Say No: Policing and the War on Drugs in Schools*. University of North Carolina Press, 2024.
Fernandez, Johanna. *The Young Lords: A Radical History*. University of North Carolina Press, 2020.
Ferrer, Ada. *Insurgent Cuba: Race, Nation, and Revolution, 1868–1898*. University of North Carolina Press, 1999.
Flamming, Douglas. *Bound for Freedom: Black Los Angeles in Jim Crow America*. University of California Press, 2006.
Flanagan, Richard M. *Mayors and the Challenge of Urban Leadership*. University Press of America, 2004.
Fong, Sarah E. K. "Racial-Settler Capitalism: Character Building and the Accumulation of Land and Labor in the Late Nineteenth Century." *American Indian Culture and Research Journal* 43, no. 2 (2019): 25–48.
Forman, James, Jr. *Locking Up Our Own: Crime and Punishment in Black America*. Farrar, Straus, and Giroux, 2017.
Fox, Cybelle. "Unauthorized Welfare: The Origins of Immigrant Status Restrictions in American Social Policy." *Journal of American History* 102, no. 4 (2016): 1051–74.
Francis, Consuela, ed. *Conversations with Octavia Butler*. University of Mississippi Press, 2020.

Frazier, E. Franklin. *The Black Bourgeoisie: The Rise of a New Middle Class in the United States*. Collier, 1962.
Fulton, William. *Reluctant Metropolis: The Politics of Urban Growth in Los Angeles*. Johns Hopkins University Press, 2001.
Gaines, Kevin. *Uplifting the Race: Black Leadership, Politics, and Culture in the Twentieth Century*. University of North Carolina Press, 1996.
Gamble, Vanessa Northington. *Making a Place for Ourselves: The Black Hospital Movement, 1920–1945*. Oxford University Press, 1995.
Gamble, Vanessa Northington. "'Sisters of a Darker Race': African American Graduates of the Woman's Medical College of Pennsylvania, 1867–1925." *Bulletin of History of Medicine* 95 (2021): 169–97.
Gamble, Vanessa Northington. "Black Autonomy versus White Control: Black Hospitals and the Dilemmas of White Philanthropy, 1920–1940." *Minerva* 35, no. 3 (October 1997): 247–67.
Garcia, Matt. *A World of Its Own: Race, Labor, and Citrus in the Making of Greater Los Angeles, 1900–1970*. University of North Carolina Press, 2002.
Geiger, Jack H. "The First Community Health Center in Mississippi: Communities Empowering Themselves." *The American Journal of Public Health* 106, no. 10 (October 2016): 1738–40.
Gerstle, Gary. *American Crucible: Race and Nation in the Twentieth Century*. Princeton University Press, 2017.
Gerstle, Gary, Nelson Lichtenstein, and Alice O'Connor, eds. *Beyond the New Deal Order: US Politics from the Great Depression to the Great Recession*. University of Pennsylvania Press, 2019.
Georgakas, Dan, and Marvin Surkin. *Detroit, I Do Mind Dying: A Study in Urban Revolution*. South End Press, 1998.
Gil-Raino, Sebastian. *The Remnants of Race Science: UNESCO and Economic Development in the Global South*. Columbia University Press, 2023.
Gilmore, Ruth Wilson. *Abolition Geography: Essays Towards Liberation*. Verso Press, 2022.
Gilmore, Ruth Wilson. *Golden Gulag: Prisons, Surplus, Crisis, and Opposition in Globalizing California*. University of California Press, 2007.
Gill-Peterson, Jules. *Histories of the Transgender Child*. University of Minnesota Press, 2018.
Goldberg, David. *Black Firefighters and the FDNY: The Struggle for Jobs, Justice, and Equity in New York City*. University of North Carolina Press, 2020.
Goldberg, David, and Trevor Griffey. *Black Power at Work: Community Control, Affirmative Action, and the Construction Industry*. Cornell University Press, 2010.
Goldfarb, Lyn, and Alison Sotomayor, dirs. *Bridging the Divide: Tom Bradley and the Politics of Race*. Our L.A., 2016.
Goldstein, Alyosha. *Poverty in Common: The Politics of Community Action During the American Century*. Duke University Press, 2012.
Gómez, Pablo F. "The Circulation of Bodily Knowledge in the Seventeenth-Century Black Spanish Caribbean." *Social History of Medicine* 26, no. 3: 383–402.

Gómez, Pablo F. *The Experiential Caribbean: Creating Knowledge and Healing in the Early Modern Atlantic.* University of North Carolina Press, 2017.

Gómez, Pablo F., and Diego Armus, eds. *The Gray Zones of Medicine: Healers and History in Latin America.* University of Pittsburgh Press, 2021.

Gonaver, Wendy. *The Peculiar Institution and the Making of Modern Psychiatry, 1840–1880.* University of North Carolina Press, 2018.

Grandin, Greg. *Empire's Workshop: Latin America, the United States, and the Making of An Imperial Republic.* Picador, 2021.

Grob, Gerald. *From Asylum to Community: Mental Health Policy in Modern America.* Princeton University Press, 1991.

Grob, Gerald. *The Mad Among Us.* Free Press, 1984.

Grob, Gerald. *Mental Illness and American Society, 1875–1940.* Princeton University Press, 1983.

Grob, Gerald. *Mental Institutions in America: Social Policy to 1875.* Free Press, 1973.

Gutierrez, David. *Walls and Mirrors: Mexican Americans, Mexican Immigrants, and the Politics of Ethnicity.* University of California Press, 1995.

Gutierrez, Elena. *Fertile Matters: The Politics of Mexican-Origin Women's Reproduction.* University of Texas Press, 2014.

Haley, Sarah. *No Mercy Here: Gender, Punishment, and the Making of Jim Crow Modernity.* University of North Carolina Press, 2016.

Hamilton, David. *From New Day to New Deal: American Farm Policy from Hoover to Roosevelt.* University of North Carolina Press, 1991.

Hanhardt, Christina B. "Broken Windows at Blue's." In *Policing the Planet: Why the Policing Crisis Led to Black Lives Matter,* edited by Jordan T. Camp and Christina Heatherton, 41–62. Verso, 2016.

Hanhardt, Christina B. *Safe Space: Gay Neighborhood History and the Politics of Violence.* Duke University Press, 2013.

Hare, Nathan. *The Black Anglo-Saxons.* Collier-MacMillan, 1965.

Harlan, Louis R., ed. *The Booker T. Washington Papers.* Vol. 3. University of Illinois Press, 1974.

Harris, Cheryl I. "Whiteness as Property." *Harvard Law Review* 106, no. 8 (June, 1993): 1710–91.

Harris, LaShawn. *Sex Workers, Psychics, and Number Runners: Black Women in New York City's Underground.* University of Illinois Press, 2016.

Harsin Drager, Emmett. "Early Gender Clinics, Transsexual Etiology, and the Racialized Family." *GLQ* 29, no. 1 (2023): 13–26.

Hartman, Saidiya. *Wayward Lives, Beautiful Experiments: Intimate Histories of Riotous Black Girls, Troublesome Women, and Queer Radicals.* W. W. Norton, 2019.

Haynes, Douglas Melvin. "Policing the Social Boundaries of the American Medical Association, 1847–70." *Journal of History of Medicine and Allied Sciences* 60, no. 2 (2005): 170–95.

Hernandez, Kelly Lytle. *City of Inmates: Conquest, Rebellion, and the Rise of Human Caging in Los Angeles.* University of North Carolina Press, 2017.

Hernandez, Kelly Lytle. *Migra! A History of the U.S. Border Patrol*. University of California Press, 2010.

Higginbotham, Evelyn Brooks. *Righteous Discontent: The Women's Movement in the Black Baptist Church, 1880–1920*. Harvard University Press, 1993.

Herman, Ellen. *The Romance of American Psychology: Political Culture in the Age of Experts*. University of California Press, 1995.

Herschthal, Eric. *The Science of Abolition: How Slaveholders Became the Enemies of Progress*. New Haven: Yale University Press, 2021.

Hicks, Cheryl D. *Talk with You Like A Woman: African American Women, Justice, and Reform in New York, 1890–1935*. University of North Carolina Press, 2010.

Hine, Darlene Clark. "Black Professionals and Race Consciousness: Origins of the Civil Rights Movement, 1890–1950." *The Journal of American History* 89, no. 4 (2003): 1279–94.

Hirsch, Arnold. *Making the Second Ghetto: Race and Housing in Chicago, 1940–1960*. University of Chicago, 2021. Reprint.

Hobson, Emily. "Policing Gay LA." In *The Rising Tide of Color*, edited by Moon-Ho Jung. University of Washington Press, 2014.

Hoffman, Beatrix. *Health Care for Some: Rights and Rationing in the United States Since 1930*. University of Chicago Press, 2012.

Hoffman, Beatrix. "Emergency Rooms: The Reluctant Safety Net." In Stevens, Rosenberg, and Burns, 250–72.

Hogarth, Rana. *Medicalizing Blackness: Making Racial Difference in the Atlantic World, 1780–1840*. University of North Carolina, 2017.

Hondagneu-Sotelo, Pierrette. *Domestica: Immigrant Workers Cleaning and Caring in the Shadows of Affluence*. University of California Press, 2001.

Hondagneu-Sotelo, Pierrette. *Gendered Transitions: Mexican Experiences of Immigration*. University of California Press, 1994.

Hondagneu-Sotelo, Pierrette. *Paradise Transplanted: Migration and the Making of California Gardens*. University of California Press, 2014.

hooks, bell. *We Real Cool*. Routledge, 2004.

HoSang, Daniel Martinez. *Racial Propositions: Ballot Initiatives and the Making of Postwar California*. University of California Press, 2010.

Howard, Clayton. *The Closet and the Cul-De-Sac: The Politics of Sexual Privacy in Northern California*. University of Pennsylvania Press, 2019.

Hsiao, Lisa. "Project 100,000: The Great Society's Answer to Military Manpower Needs in Vietnam." *Vietnam Generation* 1 (Summer 1989).

Immawahr, Daniel. *How to Hide an Empire: A History of the Greater United States*. Farrar, Straus, and Giroux, 2019.

Jenkins, Destin. *The Bonds of Inequality: Debt and the Making of the American City*. University of Chicago Press, 2021.

Johnson, Susan Lee. *Roaring Camp: The Social World of the California Gold Rush*. W. W. Norton, 2001.

Jung, Moon-Ho. *Menace to Empire: Anticolonial Solidarities and the Transpacific Origins of the US Security State*. University of California Press, 2023.

Kahan, Benjamin. *The Book of Minor Perverts: Sexology, Etiology, and the Emergences of Sexuality*. University of Chicago Press, 2019.
Kananoja, Kalle. *Healing Knowledge in Atlantic Africa: Medical Encounters, 1500–1850*. Cambridge University Press, 2021.
Kardiner, Abram, and Lionel Ovesey. *The Mark of Oppression*. W. W. Norton, 1951.
Karuka, Manu. *Empire's Tracks: Indigenous Nations, Chinese Workers, and the Transcontinental Railroad*. University of California Press, 2019.
Katznelson, Ira. *When Affirmative Action Was White: An Untold History of Racial Inequality in Twentieth-Century America*. W. W. Norton, 2005.
Kelley, Robin D. G. *Hammer and Hoe: Alabama Communists During the Great Depression*. University of North Carolina Press, 1990.
King, Tiffany Lethabo. *The Black Shoals: Offshore Formulations of Black and Native Studies*. Duke University Press, 2019.
King, Booker, and Ismail Jatoi. "The Mobile Army Surgical Hospital (MASH): A Military and Surgical Legacy." *The Journal of the National Medical Association* 97, no. 5 (2005): 648–56.
Kohler-Hausmann, Julilly. *Getting Tough: Welfare and Imprisonment in 1970s America*. Princeton University Press, 2017.
Kornbluh, Felicia, and Gwendolyn Mink. *Ensuring Poverty: Welfare Reform in Feminist Perspective*. University of Pennsylvania Press, 2018.
Koshy, Susan. *Sexual Naturalization: Asian Americans and Miscegenation*. Stanford University Press, 2004.
Kunzel, Regina. *Criminal Intimacy: Prison and the Uneven History of Modern American Sexuality*. University of Chicago Press, 2008.
Kunzel, Regina. *In the Shadow of Diagnosis: Psychiatric Power and Queer Life*. University of Chicago Press, 2024.
Kunzel, Regina. "Queer History, Mad History, and the Politics of Health." *American Quarterly* 69, no. 2 (June 2017): 315–19.
Kurashige, Scott. *The Shifting Grounds of Race: Black and Japanese Americans in the Making of Multiethnic Los Angeles*. Princeton University Press, 2008.
Langsley, Donald G. "The Community Mental Health Center: Does It Treat Patients?" *Hospital and Community Psychiatry* 31 (1980): 815–19.
Lee, Erika. *At America's Gates: Chinese Immigration during the Exclusion Era, 1882–1943*. University of North Carolina Press, 2003.
Lee, Robert. *Orientals: Asian Americans in Popular Culture*. Temple University Press, 1999.
Lefkowitz, Bonnie. *Community Health Centers: A Movement and the People Who Made It Happen*. Rutgers University Press, 2007.
LeFlouria, Talitha L. *Chained in Silence: Black Women and Convict Labor in the New South*. University of North Carolina Press, 2016.
Leighton, Jared. "'All of Us are Unapprehended Felons': Gay Liberation, the Black Panther Party, and Intercommunal Efforts Against Police Brutality in the Bay Area." *The Journal of Social History* (2018): 1–26.

Leonard, Karen. *Making Ethnic Choices: California's Punjabi Mexican Americans.* Temple University Press, 1992.

Lewis, A. J. "'We Are Certain of Our Own Insanity': Antipsychiatry and the Gay Liberation Movement, 1968–1980." *Journal of the History of Sexuality* 25, no. 1 (2016): 83–113.

Lew-Williams, Beth. *The Chinese Must Go: Violence, Exclusion, and the Making of the Alien in America.* Harvard University Press, 2021.

Lipsitz, George. *A Life in the Struggle: Ivory Perry and the Culture of Opposition.* Temple University Press, 1995.

Lipsitz, George. "Shattering Silences: Dictions, Contradictions, and Ethnic Studies at the Crossroads." *Kalfou* 7, no. 2 (2020): 222–48.

Lira, Natalie. *Laboratory of Deficiency: Sterilization and Confinement in California, 1900–1950s.* University of California Press, 2022.

Long, Gretchen. "I Studied and Practiced Medicine Without Molestation: African American Doctors in the First Years of Freedom." In *Precarious Prescriptions: Contested Histories of Race and Health in North America,* edited by Laurie B. Green, John McKiernan-Gonzalez, and Martin Summers. University of Minnesota Press, 2014.

Looker, Benjamin. *A Nation of Neighborhoods: Imagining Cities, Communities, and Democracy in Postwar America.* University of Chicago Press, 2015.

Lorde, Audre. *Sister Outsider.* Freedom Crossing Press, 1984.

Lowe, Lisa. *Immigrant Acts: On Asian American Cultural Politics.* Duke University Press, 1996.

Loyd, Jenna. *Health Rights Are Civil Rights: Peace and Justice Activism in Los Angeles, 1963–1978.* University of Minnesota Press, 2014.

Ludmerer, Kenneth. *Learning to Heal: The Development of American Medical Education.* Johns Hopkins University, 1985.

Magliari, Michael. "'A Species of Slavery': The Compromise of 1850, Popular Sovereignty, and the Expansion of Unfree Indian Labor in the American West." *The Journal of American History* 109, no. 3 (December 2022): 518–47.

Man, Simeon. *Soldiering Through Empire: Race and the Making of the Decolonizing Pacific.* University of California Press, 2018.

Manion, Jenn. *Female Husbands: A Trans History.* Cambridge University Press, 2020.

Marable, Manning. *How Capitalism Underdeveloped Black America: Problems in Race, Political Economy, and Society.* South End Press, 2000 [1983].

Marchevsky, Alejandra. "Forging a Brown-Black Movement: Chicana and African American Women Organizing for Welfare Rights in Los Angeles." In *Chicana Movidas: New Narratives of Activism and Feminism in the Movement Era,* edited by Dionne Espinoza, Maria Eugenia Cotera, and Maylei Blackwell, 227–44. University of Texas Press, 2018.

Marchevsky, Alejandra, and Jeanne Theoharis. *Not Working: Latina Immigrants, Low-Wage Jobs, and the Failure of Welfare Reform.* New York University Press, 2006.

Markowitz, Gerald, and David Rosner. *Children, Race, and Power: Kenneth and Mamie Clark's Northside Center*. Routledge, 1996.

Marquez, Bayley. *Plantation Pedagogy: The Violence of Schooling Across Black and Indigenous Space*. University of California Press, 2024.

McAlevey, Jane F. *No Shortcuts: Organizing for Power in the New Gilded Age*. Oxford University Press, 2016.

McAlevey, Jane F. *Rules to Win By: Power and Participation in Union Negotiations*. Oxford University Press, 2023.

McAlevey, Jane F. *Raising Expectations (and Raising Hell): My Decade Fighting for the Labor Movement*. Verso, 2012.

McGirr, Lisa. *Suburban Warriors: The Origins of the New American Right*. Princeton University Press, 2001.

McKee, Guian. *Hospital City, Health Care Nation: Race, Capital, and the Costs of American Health Care*. University of Pennsylvania Press, 2023.

McKiernan-González, John. *Fevered Measures: Public Health and Race at the Texas-Mexico Border, 1848–1942*. Duke University Press, 2012.

McRuer, Robert. "Compulsory Able-Bodiedness and Queer/Disabled Existence." In *The Disability Studies Reader*, edited by Lennard Davis. Routledge, 2006.

McRuer, Robert. *Crip Theory: Cultural Signs of Queerness and Disability*. New York University, 2006.

McQueeney, Kevin. *A City Without Care: 300 Years of Racism, Health Disparities, and Health Care Activism in New Orleans*. University of North Carolina Press, 2023.

McWilliams, Carey. *California: The Great Exception*. University of California Press, 1999.

Mechanic, David, and Gerald Grob. "The Plight of the Mentally Ill in America." In Stevens, Rosenberg, and Burns, *History and Health Policy in the United States*, 240–43.

Melamed, Jodi. *Represent and Destroy: Rationalizing Violence in the New Racial Capitalism*. University of Minnesota Press, 2011.

Metzl, Jonathan M. *The Protest Psychosis: How Schizophrenia Became a Black Disease*. Beacon Press, 2009.

Mendes, Gabriel. *Under the Strain of Color: Harlem's Lafargue Clinic and the Promise of an Anti-Racist Psychiatry*. Cornell University Press, 2015.

Miles, Tiya. *Ties That Bind: The Story of an Afro-Cherokee Family in Slavery and Freedom*. University of California Press, 2015.

Milkman, Ruth. *LA Story: Immigrant Workers and the Future of the US Labor Movement*. Russell Sage Foundation, 2006.

Milkman, Ruth. *Organizing Immigrants: The Challenge for Unions in Contemporary California*. ILR Press, 2000.

Miller, Lynn E., and Richard M. Weiss. "Re-Visiting Black Medical School Extinctions in the Flexner Era." *Journal of History of Medicine and Allied Sciences* 67, no. 2 (2012): 217–43.

Milton, Henry. *Departing from Deviance*. University of Chicago Press, 2001.

Minian, Ana. *Undocumented Lives: The Untold Story of Mexican Migration*. Harvard University Press, 2018.
Mitchell, Michele. *Righteous Propagation: African Americans and the Politics of Racial Destiny After Reconstruction*. University of North Carolina Press, 2004.
Mitchell, Timothy. *Rule of Experts: Egypt, Techno-Politics, Modernity*. Berkeley: University of California Press, 2002.
Molina, Natalia. *Fit to Be Citizens?: Public Health and Race in Los Angeles, 1879–1939*. University of California Press, 2006.
Morgen, Sandra. *Into Our Own Hands: The Women's Health Movement in the United States, 1969–1990*. Rutgers University Press, 2002.
Morrissey, Joseph, Howard Goldman, and Lorraine Klerman. "Cycles of Institutional Reform." In *Mental Health Care and Social Policy*, edited by Phil Brown, 70–98. Routledge, 1985.
Mumford, Kevin. "Untangling Pathology: The Moynihan Report and Homosexual Damage, 1965–1975." *Journal of Policy History* 24, no. 1 (2012): 53–73.
Murch, Donna. *Living for the City: Migration, Education, and the Rise of the Black Panther Party in Oakland*. University of North Carolina Press, 2010.
Murillo, Lina-Maria. "Birth Control, Border Control: The Movement for Contraception in El Paso, Texas, 1936–1940." *Pacific Historical Review* 90, no. 3 (2021): 314–44.
Murphy, Kathleen. "Translating the Vernacular: Indigenous and African Knowledge in the Eighteenth-Century British Atlantic." *Atlantic Studies* 8, no. 1 (2011): 29–48.
Myrdal, Gunnar. *An American Dilemma: The Negro Problem and Modern Democracy*. Harper and Brothers, 1944.
Nadasen, Premilla. *Welfare Warriors: The Welfare Rights Movement in the United States*. Routledge, 2005.
Nelson, Alondra. *Body and Soul: The Black Panther Party and the Fight Against Medical Discrimination*. University of Minnesota Press, 2011.
Ngai, Mae. *Impossible Subjects: Illegal Aliens and the Making of Modern America*. Princeton University Press, 2004.
Nicolaides, Becky. *My Blue Heaven: Life and Politics in the Working-Class Suburbs of Los Angeles, 1920–1965*. University of Chicago Press, 2002.
Nuriddin, Ayah. "Engineering Uplift: Black Eugenics as Black Liberation." In *Nature Remade: Engineering Life, Envisioning Worlds*, edited by Luis Campos, Micael Dietrich, Tiago Saraiva, and Christian Young, 186–201. University of Chicago Press, 2021.
O'Connor, Alice. *Poverty Knowledge: Social Science, Social Policy, and the Poor in Twentieth Century U.S. History*. Princeton University Press, 2001.
O'Donnell, Kelly. "Labors of Love and Marriage." *Bulletin of History of Medicine*, forthcoming.
Okihiro, Gary Y. *Margins and Mainstreams: Asians in American History and Culture*. University of Washington Press, 1994.

Okihiro, Gary Y. *Third World Studies: Theorizing Liberation.* 2nd ed. Duke University Press, 2024.

Omi, Michael, and Howard Winant. *Racial Formation in the United States: From the 1960s to the 1990s.* Routledge, 1994.

Orelick, Annelise. *Storming Caesars Palace: How Black Mothers Fought Their Own War on Poverty.* Beacon, 2005.

Owens, Deirdre Cooper. *Medical Bondage: Race, Gender, and the Origins of American Gynecology.* University of Georgia Press, 2017.

Packard, Randall M. *A History of Global Health: Interventions into the Lives of Other Peoples.* Johns Hopkins University Press, 2016.

Painter, Nell Irving. *The History of White People.* W. W. Norton, 2010.

Paiz, Christian. *The Strikers of Coachella Valley: A Rank-and-File History of the UFW Movement.* University of North Carolina Press, 2022.

Parrenas, Rhacel Salazar. *Servants of Globalization: Migration and Domestic Work.* Stanford University Press, 2015.

Patillo, Mary. *Black Picket Fences: Privilege and Peril Among the Black Middle Class.* University of Chicago Press, 1999.

Pearce, Diana. "The Feminization of Poverty: Women, Work, and Welfare." *The Urban and Social Change Review* 11 (1978): 28–36.

Piven, Frances Fox, and Richard Cloward. "The Weight of the Poor: A Strategy to End Poverty." *New Political Science* 33, no. 3 (September 2011): 272–84. Originally published in *The Nation*, May 2, 1966.

Prashad, Vijay. *The Darker Nations: A People's History of the Third World.* New Press, 2008.

Puar, Jasbir. "Bodies with New Organs." *Social Text* 33, no. 3 (2015): 48–51.

Ramos, Nic John. "Pathologizing the Crisis: Psychiatry, Policing, and Racial Liberalism in the Long Community Mental Health Movement." *Journal of History of Medicine and Allied Sciences* 74, no. 1 (2019): 57–84.

Ramos, Nic John. "Poor Influences and Criminal Locations: Los Angeles' Skid Row, Multicultural Identities, and Normal Homosexuality." *American Quarterly* 72, no. 2 (2019): 541–67.

Ramos, Nic John, and Alex Burnett. "'One Out Gay Cop: Gay Moderates, Proposition 64, and Policing in Early AIDS-Crisis Los Angeles, 1969–1992." *Journal of History of Sexuality* 31, no. 3 (September 2022): 362–93.

Ransby, Barbara. *Ella Baker and the Black Freedom Movement: A Radical Democratic Vision.* University of North Carolina Press, 2003.

Raz, Mical. *Abusive Polices: How the American Child Welfare System Lost Its Way.* University of North Carolina Press, 2020.

Raz, Mical. *What's Wrong with the Poor? Psychiatry, Race, and the War on Poverty.* University of North Carolina Press, 2013.

Reddy, Chandan. *Freedom with Violence: Race, Sexuality, and the US State.* Duke University Press, 2011.

Reverby, Susan. *Examining Tuskegee: The Infamous Syphilis Study and Its Legacy.* University of North Carolina Press, 2009.

Riddell, Adeljiza Sosa. "Chicanas and El Movimiento." *Atzlan* 5, no. 1–2 (1974): 155–65.

Roberts, Alaina E. *I've Been Here All the While: Black Freedom on Native Land.* University of Pennsylvania, 2021.

Roberts, Carolyn. "To Heal and to Harm: Medicine, Knowledge, and Power in the Atlantic Slave Trade." PhD diss., Harvard University, 2017.

Roberts, Dorothy. *Fatal Invention: How Science, Politics, and Big Business Re-Create Race in the Twenty-First Century.* New Press, 2012.

Roberts, Dorothy. *Killing the Black Body: Race, Reproduction, and the Meaning of Liberty.* Vintage, 1998.

Roberts, Dorothy. *Torn Apart: How the Child Welfare System Destroys Black Families.* Basic, 2022.

Roberts, Samuel Kelton, Jr. *Infectious Fear: Politics, Disease, and the Health Effects of Segregation.* University of North Carolina Press, 2009.

Rosenberg, Charles. *The Care of Strangers: The Rise of America's Hospital System.* Johns Hopkins University Press, 1987.

Roth, Alisa. *Insane: America's Criminal Treatment of Mental Illness.* Basic Books, 2018.

Rubio, Philip F. *There's Always Work at the Post Office: African American Postal Workers and the Fight for Jobs, Justice, and Equality.* University of North Carolina Press, 2010.

Rusert, Britt. *Fugitive Science: Empiricism and Freedom in Early African American Culture.* New York University Press, 2017.

Saldaña-Portillo, Maria Josefina. *The Revolutionary Imagination in the Americas and the Age of Development.* Duke University Press, 2003.

Sanchez, George. *Becoming Mexican American: Ethnicity, Culture and Identity in Chicano Los Angeles, 1900–1945.* Oxford University Press, 1993.

Sanchez, George. "'What's Good for Boyle Heights is Good for the Jews: Creating Multiracialism on the Eastside During the 1950s." *American Quarterly* 56, no. 3 (2004): 633–61.

Sanchez, George. *Boyle Heights: How a Los Angeles Neighborhood Became the Future of American Democracy.* Berkeley: University of California Press, 2022.

Sassen, Saskia. *The Global City: New York, London, Tokyo.* Princeton University Press, 1991.

Savitt, Todd. *Medicine and Slavery: The Disease and Care of Blacks in Antebellum Virginia.* University of Illinois Press, 1978.

Schrader, Stuart. *Badges Without Borders: How Global Counterinsurgency Transformed American Policing.* University of California Press, 2019.

Segrest, Mab. "Exalted on the Ward: 'Mary Roberts,' The Georgia State Sanitarium, and the Psychiatry 'Specialty' of Race." *American Quarterly* 66, no. 1: 69–94.

Sell, Zach. *Trouble of the World: Slavery and Empire in the Age of Capital.* University of North Carolina Press, 2021.

Shah, Nayan. *Contagious Divides: Epidemics and Race in San Francisco's Chinatown.* University of California Press, 2001.

Shah, Nayan. *Stranger Intimacy: Contesting Race, Sexuality, and the Law in the North American West*. University of California Press, 2011.

Sides, Josh. *L.A. City Limits: African American Los Angeles from the Great Depression to the Present*. University of California Press, 2003.

Simon, Daniel. "The Creation of the King-Drew Medical Complex and the Politics of Public Memory." PhD diss., University of Hawai'i at Manoa, 2014.

Simpson, Andrew T. *The Medical Metropolis: Health Care and Economic Transformation in Pittsburgh and Houston*. University of Pennsylvania Press, 2019.

Simpson, Andrew T. "Transporting Lazarus: Physicians, the State, and the Creation of the Modern Paramedic and Ambulance, 1955–1973." *Journal of History of Medicine* 68 (April 2013): 163–97.

Singh, Nikhil Pal. *Black Is a Country: Race and the Unfinished Struggle for Democracy*. Harvard University Press, 2004.

Smith, Adam. *The Theory of Moral Sentiments*. Edited by Knud Haakonssen. Cambridge University Press, 2002.

Smith, Adam. *The Wealth of Nations*. Edited by Edwin Cannan. Modern Library, 1994.

Smith, David Barton. *The Power to Heal: Civil Rights, Medicare, and the Struggle to Transform America's Health Care System*. Vanderbilt University Press, 2016.

Smith, Matthew. *The First Resort: The History of Social Psychiatry in the United States*. Columbia University Press, 2023.

Smith, Neil. *Uneven Development: Nature, Capital, and the Production of Space*. University of Georgia Press, 1984.

Smith, Sean Morey, and Christopher D. E. Willoughby. *Medicine and Healing in the Age of Slavery*. Louisiana State University Press, 2021.

Snorton, C. Riley. *Black on Both Sides: A Racial History of Trans Identity*. University of Minnesota Press, 2017.

Somerville, Siobhan. *Queering the Color Line: Race and the Invention of Homosexuality in American Culture*. Duke University Press, 2000.

Sonenshein, Raphael. *Politics in Black and White: Race and Power in Los Angeles*. Princeton University Press, 1994.

Soto Laveaga, Gabriela. *Jungle Laboratories: Mexican Peasants, National Projects, and the Making of the Pill*. Duke University Press, 2009.

Spillers, Hortense. "Mama's Baby, Papa's Maybe: An American Grammar Book." *Diacritics* 17, no. 2 (1987): 64–81.

Starr, Kevin. *Inventing the Dream: California Through the Progressive Era*. Oxford University Press, 1985.

Starr, Paul. *The Social Transformation of American Medicine: The Rise of a Sovereign Profession and the Making of a Vast Industry*. Basic, 1982.

Stern, Alexandra Minna. "Building Boundaries and Blood: Medicalization and Nation-Building on the U.S.-Mexico Border, 1910–1930." *Hispanic American Historical Review* 79, no. 1 (1999): 41–81.

Stern, Alexandra Minna. *Eugenic Nation: Faults and Frontiers of Better Breeding in Modern America*. University of California Press, 2005.

Stevens, Rosemary A. *In Sickness and in Wealth: American Hospitals in the Twentieth Century.* Basic Books, 1989.

Stevens, Rosemary A. "Medical Specialization as American Health Policy: Interweaving Public and Private Roles." In Stevens, Rosenberg, and Burns, *History and Health Policy in the United States,* 49–82.

Stevens, Rosemary, Charles Rosenberg, and Lawton Burns, eds. *History and Health Policy in the United States: Putting the Past Back In.* Rutgers University Press, 2006.

Summers, Martin. *Madness in the City of Magnificent Intentions: A History of Race and Mental Illness in the Nation's Capital.* Oxford University Press, 2019.

Summers, Martin. *Manliness and Its Discontents: The Black Middle Class and the Transformation of Masculinity, 1900–1930.* University of North Carolina Press, 2004.

Summers, Martin. "Psychiatry, Mental Health Care, and the Black Freedom Struggle: Chicago's Woodlawn Mental Health Center." *Journal of American History* 110, no. 2 (September 2023): 282–307.

Sweet, James. *Domingos Alvarez, African Healing, and the Intellectual History of the Atlantic World.* University of North Carolina Press, 2011.

Tani, Karen. *States of Dependency: Welfare, Rights, and American Governance, 1935–1972.* Cambridge University Press, 2016.

Tang, Eric. *Unsettled: Cambodian Refugees in the NYC Hyperghetto.* Temple University Press, 2015.

Taylor, Keeanga-Yamahtta. *Race for Profit: How Banks and the Real Estate Industry Undermined Black Homeownership.* University of North Carolina Press, 2019.

Terry, Jennifer. *An American Obsession.* University of Chicago Press, 1999.

Theoharis, Jeanne. *A More Beautiful and Terrible History: The Uses and Misuses of Civil Rights History.* Beacon Press, 2018.

Thomas, Karen Kruse. *Deluxe Jim Crow: Civil Rights and American Health Policy, 1935–1954.* University of Georgia Press, 2011.

Todd-Breland, Elizabeth. *A Political Education: Black Politics and Education Reform in Chicago Since the 1960s.* University of North Carolina, 2018.

Tomes, Nancy. *Remaking the American Patient: How Madison Avenue and Modern Medicine Turned Patients into Consumers.* University of North Carolina Press, 2016.

Tomes, Nancy. "Patients or Health-care Consumers? Why the History of Contested Terms Matters." In Stevens, Rosenberg, and Burns, *History and Health Policy in the United States,* 83–112.

Trotter, Joe. *Black Milwaukee: The Making of an Industrial Proletariat.* University of Illinois Press, 1985.

Trotter, Joe. *Coal, Class, and Color: Blacks in Southern West Virginia, 1915–1932.* University of Illinois Press, 1990.

Trotter, Joe. *Workers on Arrival: Black Labor in the Making of America.* University of California Press, 2019.

Turner, Kofi-Charu Nat. *Caffie Greene and Black Women Activists: Unsung Women of the Black Liberation Movement.* Routledge, 2021.

Vale, Lawrence. *Purging the Poorest: Public Housing and the Design Politics of Twice-Cleared Communities.* University of Chicago Press, 2013.

Wacquant, Loïc J. D. "Deadly Symbiosis: When Ghetto and Prison Meet and Mesh." *Punishment and Society* 1 (2001): 95–133.

Wacquant, Loïc J. D. "From Slavery to Mass Incarceration." *New Left Review* 13 (January-February 2002): 41–60.

Wacquant, Loïc J. D. *Punishing the Poor: The Neoliberal Government of Social Insecurity.* Duke University Press, 2009.

Waite, Kevin. *West of Slavery: The Southern Drum of a Transcontinental Empire.* University of North Carolina Press, 2021.

Wallace, Isabel. *Not Fit to Stay: Public Health Panics and South Asian Exclusion.* University of Washington Press, 2017.

Ward, Jane. "Producing 'Pride' in West Hollywood." *Sexualities* 6, no. 1 (2003): 65–94.

Ward, Thomas J. *Black Physicians in the Jim Crow South.* University of Arkansas Press, 2003.

Washington, Harriet. *Medical Apartheid: The Dark History of Medical Experimentation on Black Americans from Colonial Times to Present.* Anchor Books, 2006.

Weaver, Karol K. *Medical Revolutionaries: The Enslaved Healers of Eighteenth-Century Saint Domingue.* University of Illinois Press, 2006.

Weiner, Marli, with Mazie Hough. *Sex, Sickness, and Slavery: Illness in the Antebellum South.* University of Illinois Press, 2014.

Weinstein, Debbie. *The Pathological Family: Postwar America and the Rise of Family Therapy.* Cornell University Press, 2013.

White, Richard. *The Middle Ground: Indians, Empires, and Republics in the Great Lakes Region, 1650–1815.* Cambridge University Press, 2010.

Widener, Daniel. *Black Arts West: Culture and Struggle in Postwar Los Angeles.* Duke University Press, 2010.

Wilkerson, Isabel. *The Warmth of Other Suns: The Epic Story of America's Great Migration.* Vintage, 2010.

Williams, William A. *Empire as a Way of Life.* Ig Publishing, 2006.

Willoughby, Christopher D. E. *Masters of Health: Racial Science and Slavery in U.S. Medical Schools.* University of North Carolina Press, 2022.

Willse, Craig. *The Value of Homelessness: Managing Surplus Life in the United States.* University of Minnesota, 2015.

Wilson, William Julius. *The Declining Significance of Race: Blacks and Changing American Institutions.* University of Chicago Press, 1978.

Winant, Gabriel. *The Next Shift: The Fall of Industry and the Rise of Health Care in Rust Belt America.* Harvard University Press, 2021.

Woods, Clyde Adrian. *Development Arrested: Race, Power and the Blues in the Mississippi Delta.* Haymarket, 1998.

Yarbrough, Fay A. *Race and the Cherokee Nation: Sovereignty in the Nineteenth Century.* University of Pennsylvania Press, 2008.

Zink, Brian. *Anyone, Anything, Anytime: A History of Emergency Medicine.* Mosby-Elsevier, 2006.

INDEX

academic medical centers, 7–8, 25, 97. *See also names of centers*
accidents, as health concern, 170, 217
activism and activists, 15, 114, 170, 233; Black, 34, 70, 142, 162; Chicano, 15; community, 65, 80, 87, 139; gay, 3, 201, 208; immigrant rights, 247–48; patient rights, 118–20; welfare rights, 26, 143–44, 146, 156, 159, 164, 167, 181–82. *See also* Black Panther Party; civil rights movement; National Welfare Rights Organization; welfare rights movement
affirmative action, 257, 260
Affordable Care Act (2010), 264
Afro-American Studies Center, UCLA, 139
AIDS crisis, 206
Aid to Needy Children (ANC) Mothers Anonymous, 145, 155, 158–60, 162
alcohol abuse and alcoholism, 127, 170, 214
ambulance services, 217, 225–27, 226*fig.*, 229–31
American Medical Association (AMA): Black physicians excluded from, 9, 77, 79, 99; formation and policies of, 40–41; King-Drew Medical Center and, 65; Medicare/Medicaid and, 121, 275n15; Woman's Auxiliary of, 79
Amnesty (Simpson-Mazzoli Act), 248
ANC Mothers Anonymous, 145, 155, 158–60, 162
Anderson, Gail V., 229
Anglo elites, 13
anti-Blackness, 40, 130

anticapitalism, 16, 138
anticolonial movements, 33
antiracism, 21, 33, 138
antipoverty programs, 81–82, 163; Black capitalism and, 12; citizen participation in, 90, 115, 142; community health clinics and, 16, 73, 87, 110, 114, 121, 142; critiques of, 83, 114, 143, 146; federal, 3, 10, 25, 33, 73, 81–82, 85, 140, 145, 156, 163, 170, 181, 216, 221, 232, 258; gender and, 75, 81, 83, 146, 258; Great Society, 3, 268n6; King-Drew Medical Center and, 2, 26, 74–75, 86, 101, 108, 146; logic of, 115–16, 123, 142; as social control, 113–14, 143, 258; War on Poverty, 121, 231. *See also* culture of poverty theory; welfare
anxiety, 131, 190
apparel industry, 165–66, 180
Asian Americans, 13, 54, 147, 189, 195, 260; activism of, 15, 58; mental health services for, 197–98. *See also* Chinatown
asylum, state. *See* mental health: state hospitals for
asylum without walls, 186, 188
at-risk populations, 119, 133, 190
Avalon Carver Community Service Center, 174, 245

Baldwin, James, 33, 83
Bell, Derrick, 4–5, 21. *See also* interest convergence dilemma
bell hooks, 169

biomedicine, 21, 41, 48, 102; commercialization of, 18–19, 49, 52; development of, 34, 77–78, 92; King-Drew Medical Center and, 74, 100–101
Black capitalism, 12, 138–39, 142, 271n25
Black community: class and political divisions in, 11, 84, 135, 137; as constituency, 68–69; economic development in, 6, 12, 16, 32, 66, 135, 152; gender and sexuality in, 2, 12, 16, 23, 75, 130, 196, 258; health of, 106; Jewish community as model for, 69, 71; leadership of, 4, 6, 11, 15, 21, 65, 68–69, 81, 83, 85, 101, 137, 246; mental wellness in, 111*map*, 134, 196–97; self-determination for, 4, 15, 72, 122. *See also* Black freedom; Black nationalism; Black Power movement
Black Congress, 163
Black freedom, 10–11, 16, 27, 114, 137–38, 142, 149, 164, 256
Black gender, 23, 75, 293n60. *See also* Spillers, Hortense
Black Ghetto (Los Angeles), 13, 14*map*
Black hospital movement, 34
Black identity, 134, 136–37
Black men: as perceived absent fathers, 4, 12, 16, 75, 130, 168–69, 258; as breadwinners, 2, 12, 15, 26, 73, 75, 81, 83, 103, 106–7, 109, 130, 137–38, 142, 146, 149, 152, 164, 169, 232, 256, 258, 264; criminalization and incarceration of, 22, 169, 213; gender and sexuality of, 22, 130, 137, 196, 217–18, 258; health of, 2; Jim Crow and, 75, 83; leadership of, 37, 71, 137; manhood of, 23, 76, 83, 109, 138, 149, 169, 232; unemployment of, 55, 168; violence against, 22. *See also* Black people
Black nationalism, 3, 15, 32, 84, 126, 134; Black capitalism and, 12, 139, 142; community health and, 26, 126, 134, 141; gender and, 138; self-help and, 69–70; visions of, 138, 141–42
Black Panther Party, 138, 143; Black freedom envisioned by, 15, 139, 142, 196; community health and, 139; health clinics of, 141; mental health services and, 141, 295n99

Black people: in California, 13, 31, 54; class status of, 11, 59, 61, 116, 135, 137; as consumers, 32, 37, 66, 116, 139; culture of, 2, 16, 131, 199; health and healing practices of, 9, 30, 38, 40, 48, 74, 102; inclusion of, 4, 6, 12, 20–21, 76; Los Angeles population maps of, 62*map*, 63*map*, 66*map*, 67*map*, 111*map*, 185*map*, 243*map*; migration of, 13, 31, 54–56, 59, 61, 76, 119, 222, 261; policing of, 1–3, 56, 186; as professionals, 10–11, 256; stereotypes of, 4, 12, 16, 19, 75, 130, 196, 218, 258; vulnerability of, 1, 6; young, 4, 12, 16, 55, 83, 85, 133, 136, 218. *See also* Black men; Black women; labor and workers: Black; poverty: Black
Black physicians. *See* physicians, Black
Black Power movement, 15; community health and, 26, 125, 139, 141, 197; rise of, 115, 134, 195. *See also* Black nationalism; Black Panther Party
Black Student Union (BSU), 139
Black women, 157, 258; as activists, 254; as heads of household, 24, 232; health of, 2; labor of, 9, 38, 160, 258; marginalization of, 21–22, 142; as mothers, 12, 17, 24, 75, 130, 160, 178; as physicians, 79; sexuality of, 16, 258; on welfare, 4, 16, 26, 75, 83, 143, 156, 159–60, 162, 170, 248. *See also* Black people; welfare rights movement: Black women in
Booker, Simeon, 36–37
Boyle Heights, 14*map*, 45*map*, 174, 178
Bradley, Tom, 145–49, 181, 188, 191, 194; antipoverty programs and, 74, 82, 182, 184, 187, 192, 195–97, 199, 201, 205, 212, 237, 253, 260; King-Drew Medical Center and, 74, 98, 108, 164, 167, 250, 253, 264; mayoral election of, 15, 172, 173*fig*., 187, 195, 255; multicultural coalition of, 147–48, 164; urban redevelopment and, 152–53, 164–67, 173–75, 178–79, 195, 199–200
breadwinning manhood, 73, 81, 107, 142, 146, 152, 164, 258; Black, 2, 12, 15, 26, 75, 83, 103, 106, 109, 130, 137–38, 149, 169, 232, 256, 264; as policy goal, 50–51, 75,

83, 113, 156, 181; white, 10, 22, 31, 49–51. *See also* Black men: manhood of
Brookins, H. Hartford, 64, 82–84, 285n28
Brown v. Board of Education (1954), 5
Brown, Willie, 55
BSU (Black Student Union), 139
Buggs, John, 59, 61, 65, 84, 286n32
Bunker Hill (Los Angeles): as financial district, 145, 147, 152, 154, 164, 165–66, 172–73, 178–79, 181; redevelopment of, 147, 152–54, 164–65, 173, 178–79, 200*map*
Butler, Octavia: background to, 254; on Black America, 255, 263; on Black freedom and Black nationalism, 256; on capitalism, 253, 257, 262; on community, 256, 263; on gender, 254, 256–57, 263; on kinship, 259–60, 262; on power and oppression, 255, 257, 262–64; on race, 254–58; on racial and sexual liberalism, 253–55, 263; on sociobiology, 257–59; works of, 24, 252–64

California: anti-tax measures in, 18, 97, 218, 230–31, 236–38, 240, 244–45, 250; deinstitutionalization in, 119, 190, 214; hospital system in, 48, 52–53, 56, 96–97, 308n92; racial politics in, 13, 31, 43–44, 54, 64, 119, 260; segregation in, 13, 42–44, 45*map*, 54, 59, 61, 64, 149, 195. *See also* Los Angeles, California; Los Angeles County; *and names of other cities and counties in*
California Advisory Hospital Council, 53, 64–65, 72–73, 80, 87, 90
California Bureau of Hospitals of, 53
California Hospital Association, 53, 66–67
Canaday, Margot, 52, 156
Cannon, J. Alfred, 134, 137, 141, 196; Black nationalism of, 138–39, 142; community mental health work of, 110, 112, 126–27, 132–33, 143–44, 189–90, 197–99, 201–3, 209–10, 213–14; on gender and sexuality, 130–31, 133, 203, 209; at King-Drew Medical Center, 101, 112, 140; research of, 130–34, 201
capitalism, 138–39, 142, 253, 187; Black, 12, 271n25; critiques of, 15, 257, 262; demo-
cratic, 84; free market, 33, 49, 69, 118, 120, 126; global, 7, 17, 24, 150, 216, 220, 223, 236; sexual, 18, 22, 24, 76, 114, 148; white, 271n25. *See also* racial capitalism
carceral state, 22, 119, 126–27, 133, 160, 169, 186–88, 190, 209, 211, 213–14, 218, 260. *See also* policing; prisons
Carter, Alprentice "Bunchy," 139, 141
Carter, Nona, 143
Cartwright, Samuel, 39, 276n30
Castro, Tony, 186, 208
CBOs (Community-based organizations), 132–33, 141, 197–99, 202, 204
Center for the Study of Reduction of Violence (CSRV), 211
Central City Community Mental Health Center, 73, 110, 112, 114, 126, 132–34, 197–99, 202
Central Intelligence Agency (CIA), 2, 73, 84
Charles R. Drew Medical Society. *See* Drew Medical Society
Chicago School, 284–85n22
Chicana Welfare Rights Organization, 163
childcare, 132, 148, 156, 162, 164, 171, 177–78
Chinatown (Los Angeles), 14*map*, 45*map*, 153–54, 165, 174, 179, 198. *See also* Asian Americans
Chowkwanyun, Merlin, 123–24
CIA (Central Intelligence Agency), 2, 73, 84
Cimurusti, Tony, 97, 309n18
citizenship, 5, 44, 52, 59, 113, 115, 213, 248; citizen participation and, 90, 115, 142
civil rights movement: healthcare and, 35–37, 57, 120; legacy of, 21, 54, 116, 125, 142, 157, 202, 217, 257; racial liberalism and, 3, 5
class: health and, 35; race and, 9, 11, 54, 59, 114, 135; sexuality and, 9
Cleaver, Eldridge, 138
Cloward, Richard, 157–58
CMHC (Central City Community Mental Health Center), 73, 110, 112, 114, 126, 132–34, 197–99, 202
Coalition for Economic Survival, 245
Cobb, Montague, 35–36

INDEX · 339

Cohen, Cathy, 22, 187, 293n61
Collins, Patricia Hill, 22, 273n47
Collins, Wendell, 56, 69, 71
colonialism, 34, 84, 108, 110, 125, 139, 198
Commonwealth Foundation, 100, 108, 146, 156, 216, 234
Community-based organizations (CBOs), 132–33, 141, 197–99, 202, 204
community medicine, 26, 75, 101–3, 105–6, 121, 167, 235
community pride campaigns, 15, 184, 195, 199, 201, 205. *See also* gay community: pride campaigns for
Community Redevelopment Agency of Los Angeles (CRA-LA), 147, 152, 154, 165–66, 174, 179, 188, 194, 201
Compton, California, 14*map*, 45*map*, 195, 246
Congress of Racial Equality (CORE), 56
consumerism, 12, 37, 66, 95, 113–15, 117–18, 122, 139, 143, 152, 170, 234, 243, 255
containment and mitigation policy, 186, 188, 192, 193*map*, 194. *See also* Skid Row
Contini, Edgardo, 154
CORE (Congress of Racial Equality), 56
Cornely, Paul, 99–100
County of Los Angeles. *See* Los Angeles County
CRA-LA (Community Redevelopment Agency of Los Angeles), 147, 152, 154, 165–66, 174, 179, 188, 194, 201
Crenshaw (neighborhood), 14*map*, 45*map*, 61, 254
Crenshaw, Kimberlé, 19–21, 116, 240
Criley, Michael, 227, 310n27
crime. *See* gun violence; homicides; prostitution, prostitutes; sex work, sex workers
criminalization: of Black people, 3, 213; of poverty, 24, 161; of sexuality, 3, 16, 24, 258
critical race theory, 4, 19
CSRV (Center for the Study of Reduction of Violence), 211
culture of poverty theory, 16, 20, 73, 75, 81–82, 258; Black family in, 16, 132, 196, 211; Butler's critique of, 256–57; King-Drew Medical Center and, 96; Moynihan and, 196, 232
Cumming, Gordon, 53

Daily News Post (Monrovia), 97, 309n18
Daniels, Ruby, 117
Davis, Mike, 81, 154, 164, 187
Davis, Milton, 125
Dawson, Michael, 11
deindustrialization, 3, 20, 24, 148, 150–51, 191, 222–23. *See also* globalization; service economy
deinstitutionalization, 119, 188–91, 214. *See also* mental health
Democratic Party, 157, 163, 247
deportation, 1, 4, 18, 44, 247
Deverell, Bill, 46
DHEW. *See* US Department of Health, Education, and Welfare
disability, 138, 187, 255
discrimination, 9, 54, 116; in employment, 130, 182, 240; in federal programs, 9–10, 51–52, 272n30; in healthcare, 30, 35, 58, 60, 86–88, 110, 268n6; in housing, 58–59, 61, 116; legal interpretations of, 20, 240
disease: chronic, 92, 214; contagious, 46–47, 92; psychiatric, 39, 128–34, 137–38, 141–42, 187, 189–90, 196–98, 201–3, 205–6, 209–11, 213–14, 217–18, 232, 255–58; venereal, 102. *See also* mental illness
doctoring, 30, 32, 37–38, 68, 77, 79–80
"Don't Reward Rioting" campaign, 97, 224, 309n18
Doyle, Dennis, 129
"Dragons, the," 186, 194, 201, 208
drapetomania, 39–40
Drew Medical School: Allied Health Sciences Center of, 103, 104*fig.*; community medicine at, 75, 101–2, 168, 235; establishment of, 73, 93–94, 97, 100; faculty and administration of, 75, 93, 100–101, 108, 146, 156, 170, 232–33, 253; students at, 104*fig*. *See also* Drew Medical Society; King-Drew Medical Center
Drew Medical Society, 36, 58, 72, 87, 93–94, 96, 100–101
drug abuse, 170, 187, 198, 245–46, 252
Drummett, Clifton, 125

Du Bois, W. E. B., 10–11, 43–44, 81, 135, 277n44, 294n73
Dymally, Mervyn, 83, 98

Egeberg, Roger, 91, 93, 100, 121
Ehrenreich, Barbara, 17
Emergency Medical Treatment and Labor Act (EMTALA), 248
emergency medicine, 6, 18, 97, 215–17, 238, 244, 248, 250–51; development of, 224–27, 229–31, 234–35, 239, 241–42, 246; funding for, 218, 230–31, 240, 242, 245; at King-Drew Medical Center, 27, 232–35, 242–43; military medicine and, 219–20, 222–24, 227, 231–32, 234; politics of, 218–19, 245–47; racialization of, 218–19, 243; trauma care and, 235, 246–49, 264
Emergency! (television show), 238
employment: discrimination in, 130, 182, 240. *See also* labor and workers
EMTALA (Emergency Medical Treatment and Labor Act), 248
entrepreneurship, Black, 10, 32, 68
Escalante, Alicia, 163, 182
ethno-psychiatry, 196, 203
eugenics, 42, 127, 256, 258

Fair Deal, 50
Family Assistance Plan (FAP), 158–59
family life, 12, 75, 130; Black, 2, 16, 81, 83, 105–6, 134, 142, 196, 258; Black mothers and, 17, 24, 160, 178; nuclear, 16, 156, 259, 261; respectable, 26, 76, 114, 142, 198, 253; white, 49–50
Fanon, Frantz, 138–39, 197
FAP (Family Assistance Plan), 158–59
Farmer, Ashley D., 138
federal government, 9, 51–52; civil rights and, 37, 52, 116; healthcare funding by, 3, 9–10, 25, 31, 33, 35–36, 53, 73, 92–94, 110, 113–15, 121, 134, 146, 156–57, 161–63, 170–71, 177–78, 182, 190, 197, 199, 204, 211, 214, 227, 231–32, 238, 244, 248, 264; housing policy of, 3, 54; labor policy of, 50, 145, 156–57. *See also* antipoverty programs: federal; Great Society; US Department of Health, Education, and Welfare; War on Poverty

feminism, 257; Black, 23, 169, 254. *See also* welfare rights movement
feminization of poverty, 148
Ferguson, Rod, 22, 209
Fett, Sharla, 38
financialization, 3, 150–51, 164–66, 179–80, 191, 218, 220, 222, 236
Flexner, Abraham, 41, 77
Florence-Firestone (neighborhood), 14*map*, 45*map*, 63*map*, 163, 171, 176–77
for-profit healthcare system, 1, 18
Frazier, E. Franklin, 81, 137, 285n22, 304n35
Freedman's Hospital, 98
Friedman, Milton, 115
Frye, Marquette, 2

Gamble, Vanessa Northington, 34, 78
Gay and Lesbian Community Services Center (GLCSC), 201, 204–8, 207*fig.*
Gay Liberation Front, 204–5
gays, 195, 201–6, 209–10; as community, 13, 15–16, 21–22, 25, 74, 147, 151, 164, 184–85, 185*map*, 186–90, 256–57; mental health of, 188–90, 195–96; pride campaigns of, 3, 15, 257; respectability of, 22, 187
Geiger, H. Jack, 120–21
gender, 21, 128–31, 143, 196, 258; Black, 75, 293n60; discourses of, 22–23, 79–80, 109, 133–34, 137–38, 142, 146, 152, 156, 256–58, 263; distinctiveness of, 17, 113, 196, 257; labor and, 9, 49, 114, 148, 156; race and, 9, 23, 28, 31, 40, 49, 75, 139, 146; roles of, 16, 40, 83, 157; stability of, 17, 258. *See also* breadwinning manhood; Black men; Black women; heteropatriarchy; patriarchy
GI Bill, 9, 13, 50–51, 195
Gilmore, Ruth Wilson, 21, 187, 218, 223
Giorgi, Elsie, 121–25, 141–42
GLCSC (Gay and Lesbian Community Services Center), 201, 204–8, 207*fig.*
globalization, 3, 20, 24, 147–51, 187, 216, 220, 222, 236; global city and, 2–4, 7, 17–18, 26, 147, 149, 151, 154, 164, 179, 181, 184, 217, 250. *See also* deindustrialization; service economy
Golden State Medical Society, 68, 87

Goldstein, Alyosha, 33, 115, 274n7
Gomez, Pablo, 38
Goodall v. Brite (1933), 47–49, 56, 70
Graf, Walter, 227, 238
Greater Los Angeles Citizen's Council, 309n18
Great Society, 3. *See also* antipoverty programs: federal
Greene, Caffie, 114, 143–44, 163, 298n33
Gregg, Jean, 59, 61
Grindell, Dan, 176–77, 234*fig.*
Grob, Gerald, 118, 127, 190, 290n20, 295n99
gun violence, 6, 18, 27, 215–18, 220, 224, 235, 248

Hahn, Kenneth, 90, 176, 224, 227, 238–39, 250–51; emergency medicine and, 225, 226*fig.*, 228*map*, 229–33, 234*fig.*; King-Drew Medical Center and, 71–72, 91; political career of, 74, 86, 94–95, 108, 229, 231–33
Haley, Sarah, 157
Hall, Charles, 124
Hamilton, Calvin S., 154
Harbor General Hospital (Harbor-UCLA), 46, 57, 64, 96, 175*map*, 227–28, 228*map*, 246, 249*map*
Hargett, James, 68
Harris, Cheryl, 24–25
Hawkins, Augustus, 74, 83–84, 87, 98, 108, 124, 139–40, 142, 253
Haynes, Douglas, 40
Haynes, M. Alfred, 101–3, 102*fig.*, 105–8, 235, 288–89n68; at King-Drew Medical Center, 75, 146, 156, 170, 232–33; research of, 99, 170
healthcare: access to, 3, 19, 35, 52, 54, 58, 60, 103, 107, 120, 143, 146, 159, 161–62, 172, 181–82, 194, 213, 248, 253, 263–65; costs of, 7, 53, 118–19, 121, 142–43, 146, 168, 180, 213, 231, 236, 241, 248; as human right, 146, 162; privatization of, 3, 18, 20, 24, 49, 182, 264. *See also* academic medical centers; biomedicine; emergency medicine; hospitals; mental health; public health
Heart Disease, Cancer, and Stroke Act (1965), 93

Henry, Mary, 143, 245
Herman, Ellen, 232
heteropatriarchy, 2, 22–23, 37, 49, 132, 142
heterosexuality: compulsory, 52, 194–95; as norm, 12, 17, 21, 49–50, 52, 75, 113, 128, 130, 138, 196, 203, 218, 258; policing of, 17, 21–22, 51–52, 143
Hewitt, Ray "Masai," 163
Hicks, Cheryl, 76
Higginbotham, Evelyn Brooks, 11, 76
Hill, Julius, 68, 87
Hill-Burton Hospital Construction Act (1946), 35, 52, 65
Hirsch, Arnold, 54
homelessness, 6, 25–27, 49, 184, 186–92, 194, 198, 205, 209, 211–13, 252
homicides, 170, 217, 235
homophobia, 21–22, 138, 187, 190
homosexuality, 12, 128–30, 187, 203; depathologization of, 201; as mental illness, 196, 198; normality of, 4, 16, 22, 114, 188–89, 195, 201–6, 208–9, 258; policing of, 51, 195; racialization of, 188, 195–96, 209–10, 258; situational, 202. *See also* gays
Hooker, Evelyn, 190, 201–4, 206, 209–10
HoSang, Daniel Martinez, 162, 218
hospitals, 146, 248–49; Black, 32–34, 37, 57, 64–65, 69–72, 77–78, 107; community, 25, 56, 90–91, 224, 227; construction of, 35, 53, 65, 90, 96, 98; costs of, 7, 53, 118–19, 121, 142–43, 168, 180, 213, 231, 236, 241; emergency rooms in, 7, 18, 25, 122, 216, 226, 229, 232–35, 242–43, 243*map*; for-profit, 1, 96, 171–72; locations of, 14*map*, 45 *map*, 66 *map*, 67 *map*, 89 *map*, 111 *map*, 175 *map*, 228 *map*, 243 *map*, 249*map*; private, 1–2, 7, 25, 30–31, 35, 47–48, 54, 56, 65, 71, 90, 93–94, 96, 171–72, 219, 224, 227, 230, 233, 242, 244, 247–50, 264–65; as safety net, 172, 216, 249*map*; segregation in, 9, 34–35, 57; teaching, 8, 25, 30, 35, 42, 53, 56, 58, 92–93, 97, 99, 110, 247. *See also* academic medical centers; public hospitals
Houts, Richard, 227, 230
Howard, Clayton, 52

Howard University, 34, 77, 98–100
Hubert Humphrey Comprehensive Health Clinic, 171, 177–78
Huggins, John, 139
Huh, Paul, 194
hygiene, 42, 77, 113, 128, 244
hypertension, 170

identity politics, 15, 189–93
immigrants, 1, 148, 194, 247–48, 260; deportation of, 4, 18, 44; exploitation of, 20, 166, 211–12; in Los Angeles, 13, 44, 46, 59, 150, 163, 165–66, 211–12; undocumented, 3–4, 19–20
IMPAC (South Central Improvement Action Committee), 140
incarceration, 22, 112, 127, 157, 160, 169, 186–87, 190, 209, 211, 213–14, 260. *See also* carceral state; policing; prisons
interest convergence dilemma, 4–5, 21. *See also* Bell, Derrick

Jarvis, Howard, 236
Jermany, Catherine, 159, 163, 297n25, 298n28
Jim Crow, 3, 9, 13–14, 77, 83; in California, 27, 55, 96; end of, 35, 107, 116; legacy of, 35, 51, 55, 74–75, 98, 112, 164, 261
Johnson, Lyndon B., 10, 35, 81, 142, 216
Joint Power Agreements, 236–37
Jones, Harold, 68
Jones, Jack, 110, 112
Jordan Downs public housing, 156

Kaiser Permanente, 103, 105
Karenga, Ron, 15, 136, 138–39, 141–42, 163, 197, 292n42
Kelling, George, 209–10
Kennedy, Robert F., 225–27
King, Celes, III, 246
King, Martin Luther, Jr. *See* Martin Luther King Jr. Community Hospital; Martin Luther King Jr. General Hospital; King-Drew Medical Center
King-Drew Medical Center, 100–102, 107–9, 112–13, 116, 146, 156, 161–64, 167, 170–71, 215–17, 250; as antipoverty program, 2, 26, 74–75, 86; closure and rebirth of, 264–65; community clinics of, 26, 73, 95, 104–6, 233; emergency medicine at, 6, 18, 27, 97, 232–35, 242–44; establishment of, 1–2, 11, 15, 25, 54, 64, 72–73, 85, 90, 95–96, 145, 224; funding for, 18, 64, 96, 98, 156, 224, 230, 236; health system of, 4, 25–26, 71, 73–74, 94–95, 103, 110, 143–45, 181, 188, 216; leadership of, 6, 26, 64, 71–72, 74–75, 86, 90–91, 94–96, 144, 152, 178, 181, 232–34, 253, 263–64; master plan for, 75, 94, 143–46, 152, 158, 172–73, 181
kinship: alternative, 76, 223, 259–60; patriarchal, 49–50, 146, 257; queer, 257, 259
Klinger, K. E., 225
Knox, Charles, 140
Kurashige, Scott, 58

labor and workers, 7, 19–20, 43–44, 55, 150–51, 166, 222; Black, 9–11, 31, 38, 55, 77, 110, 167, 232; of color, 13, 17, 22, 24, 31, 47, 54, 145, 147–49, 152, 168, 173–74, 181–83, 187, 195, 221, 223, 235, 244, 251, 253–54, 256, 258–60, 262, 265; domestic, 9, 157; forced, 157, 182; informal, 160; low-wage, 17, 26, 147, 173, 183, 217, 235, 260; organized and unionized, 10–11, 42, 51, 54, 65, 157, 245, 265; policies concerning, 50–51, 145, 156–57; service, 3, 148, 187, 236; "throw-away," 260–62; undocumented, 1, 3–4, 148; white, 10, 30, 51, 56, 83, 135, 157, 236; women, 9, 17, 22, 24, 41, 48, 50, 83, 143, 146, 148–49, 156–57, 159–62, 168–69, 180–83, 218, 254, 256–58, 260–61, 263. *See also* deindustrialization; service economy; unemployment; unions; worklessness
LA CAN (Los Angeles Community Action Network), 191
LAC-USC (Los Angeles County General Hospital), 29, 42, 46–47, 57, 64, 66*map*, 96, 175*map*, 228–29, 228*map*, 242–43, 243*map*, 249*map*
Lamont, Robert, 212
Lanterman-Petris-Short (LPS) Act (1967), 190–91, 308n92

LAPD (Los Angeles Police Department), 56, 138, 186, 194, 207–8, 212, 246
Lawson, James, 245
Leighton, Jared, 138
Lewis, Abram J., 205
Lewis, Oscar, 81
Lewis, Tommy, 163
liberalism, liberals. *See* racial liberalism; sexual liberalism
linked fate, 11
Little Tokyo (Los Angeles), 14*map*, 45*map*, 153–54, 165, 174, 179, 201
Long, Gretchen, 40
Lorde, Audre, 23, 138
Los Angeles, California, 7, 17–18, 46, 147, 164–66, 173–75, 178–81, 184, 194–96; Black population in, 62*map*, 63*map*, 66*map*, 67*map*, 111*map*, 185*map*, 243*map*; downtown, 13–14, 61, 98, 145, 152–54, 153*map*, 191, 195, 200*map*, 260; economy of, 3, 28, 30–31, 41, 43, 55, 149, 151, 154–55, 186, 191, 214, 217, 220, 222, 235, 252–53, 257, 261; as global city, 2–4, 26, 149, 151, 154, 217, 250; politics in, 2, 4, 15, 20, 27–28, 74, 81, 84, 108, 114, 145, 154–55, 187–88, 205, 252–53, 255; redevelopment of, 5, 145, 152–54, 182, 188, 191, 200*map*, 201; segregation in, 13, 42–44, 45*map*, 54, 59, 61, 149. *See also* Los Angeles County; *and names of specific neighborhoods*
Los Angeles Community Action Network (LA CAN), 191
Los Angeles County: Board of Supervisors, 1–2, 90, 96, 176, 215, 224–25, 230, 237, 244, 264–65; Department of Charities, 85; Department of Mental Health, 133, 197; health services of, 46–47, 56, 95–96, 108, 170–71, 174, 176–78, 217, 231, 246–48, 250; Human Rights Commission, 84. *See also* public hospitals: in Los Angeles County
Los Angeles County General Hospital (LAC-USC), 29, 42, 46–47, 57, 64, 66*map*, 96, 175*map*, 228–29, 228*map*, 242–43, 243*map*, 249*map*
Los Angeles Herald Examiner, 186
Los Angeles Police Department (LAPD), 56, 138, 186, 194, 207–8, 212, 246
Los Angeles River, 46, 184, 194
Los Angeles Times, 110, 212, 242, 245, 247
LPS (Lanterman-Petris-Short) Act (1967), 190–91, 308n92

Mafundi Arts Institute, 136, 197
Magliari, Michael, 44
Malcolm X, 271n25
Manhood. *See* Black men: manhood of; breadwinning manhood
Manning, John, 95
Marable, Manning, 18
Marlow, Harry, 86
marriage, 12, 44, 49–50, 81, 83, 114, 157, 159, 198, 253, 262
Martin Luther King Jr. General Hospital, 73. *See also* King-Drew Medical Center
Martin Luther King Jr. (MLK) Community Hospital, 265. *See also* King-Drew Medical Center
masculinity. *See* Black men: manhood of; breadwinning manhood
M*A*S*H (television show), 238
master plan study, 146, 156, 163–64, 167, 170, 173, 178
maternal mortality, 106, 170
Mayo Clinic, 48
McCone, John, 2, 73, 80–87, 96–98, 174, 267n3; report of, 73, 81–82, 85–87, 96–97, 267n3
McKibben, Lynn, 247
McQueeney, Kevin, 35
MECLA (Municipal Elections Committee of Los Angeles), 201, 205–6, 208
Medex, 103
Medicaid, 10, 33, 35–36, 64–65, 85–87, 90–94, 107, 113, 116, 121, 171–72, 231, 233, 264–65; creation of, 3, 275n15; funding from, 25, 73–74, 146, 161, 247; impact of, 96, 247; standards for, 88, 89*map*
Medicare, 10, 35–36, 64–65, 90–94, 107, 113, 116, 121, 171–72, 231, 233, 247, 264–65; Black physicians and, 33, 87; creation of, 3, 275n15; funding from, 25, 33, 73–74, 85–87, 146, 161; impact of, 87, 96; standards for, 88, 89*map*
medicine: academic, 8–9, 77, 97; history of, 11, 28, 37–43, 48, 53, 77, 79, 92–93, 118,

127, 194, 215–16, 220–24, 226–27, 229–234, 238–42, 250; organized, 10–11, 41; racialization of, 10, 38–42, 70; social, 103, 120; state, 47; Western, 32, 40. *See also* emergency medicine; military medicine

Mellinkoff, Sherman, 92–93, 100

mental health, 13–4, 118–20, 187–91, 195–99, 209–10, 213–14; of Black people, 111*map*, 130–31, 136–37, 140–44, 217, 246; community-based, 26, 73, 95, 110, 112–14, 117, 126–28, 133, 138, 140–41, 143–44, 152, 201–2, 204–5; deinstitutionalization and, 214; of gays, 188–90, 195, 201–5; policing and, 201, 206–10; state hospitals for, 113, 126–27, 186. *See also* mental illness; *and names of mental health centers*

mental illness, 112, 137–38, 141–42, 187, 196–98, 201–3, 209–11, 213–14, 217–18, 255–58; Black people and, 127, 130–31; criminalization of, 127, 133; discourses of, 39, 128–34, 189–90, 205–6, 232; homosexuality as, 12, 128–30; race and, 128–34, 189–90, 232; in Skid Row, 184, 186, 188, 191

Mid-City (Los Angeles), 14*map*, 29–30, 63*map*

military medicine, 215–16, 219–20, 222–24, 227, 231–32, 234, 238

Milkman, Ruth, 166

Mitchell, Richard G., 154

Mitchell, Timothy, 91

Mobley, Lilian, 143–44

Molina, Natalia, 46, 279n53

Moore, Birdell, 123

Morado, Dolores, 123

Morales, Royal "Uncle Roy," 190, 198–99, 210, 214

Mosse, Hilda, 130–31

Moynihan, Daniel Patrick, 73, 81–82, 196, 232

multiculturalism, 3, 15, 27, 144, 147–49, 164, 179, 184, 186–88, 198, 209, 236

Municipal Elections Committee of Los Angeles (MECLA), 201, 205–6, 208

Myrdal, Gunnar, 81, 284n22

NAACP (National Association for the Advancement of Colored People), 34–35, 37, 246, 260

Nadasen, Premilla, 156, 158–59

National Association for the Advancement of Colored People (NAACP), 34–35, 37, 246, 260

National Institutes of Mental Health (NIMH), 110, 126, 197–99, 202–3, 214, 304n32

National Medical Association (NMA), 12, 32, 34–37, 65, 72, 75, 77, 79–80, 87, 99, 101, 232

National Welfare Rights Organization (NWRO): campaigns of, 158–59, 162–63; dissolution of, 159; establishment of, 145; leadership of, 155–59, 162, 164; strategy of, 156–62. *See also* Tillmon, Johnnie; welfare rights movement

Nelson, Alondra, 211

New Deal, 9, 14, 50–52, 54, 60–61, 83, 156, 195, 260

Newton, Huey, 114, 138–39

NIMH (National Institutes of Mental Health), 110, 126, 197–99, 202–3, 214, 304n32

Nixon, Richard, 271n25

NMA (National Medical Association), 12, 32, 34–37, 65, 72, 75, 77, 79–80, 87, 99, 101, 232

NWRO (National Welfare Rights Organization): campaigns of, 158–59, 162–63; dissolution of, 159; establishment of, 145; leadership of, 155–59, 162, 164; strategy of, 156–62. *See also* Tillmon, Johnnie; welfare rights movement

Obama, Barack, 271n25

Okihiro, Gary, 38, 275n21

Olympics (1984), 184, 186, 209

Page, James O., 238–42, 244

Palladino, Moece, 183

Palm Lanes public housing, 117

paramedics, 103, 225, 227–33, 228*map*, 235, 238–40, 242, 247

Parable of the Sower (Butler), 24, 252–53, 259, 261–63

Park, Robert E., 81, 284n22

Patillo, Mary, 11

patriarchy, 15, 22–23, 40, 49–50, 52, 76, 80, 101, 138, 142, 162, 181–82, 256–57, 263. *See also* breadwinning manhood; heteropatriarchy

Patternists (in Butler's fiction), 255–57, 259

Paul, Henry, 58

Pauper Act (1855), 43, 57, 94, 249*map*, 277n41

Pearce, Diana, 148

Peyton, Thomas, 60

philanthropy, 78, 99–100, 108, 158

physicians, 35, 53, 56–58, 74, 99–100, 108–9; authority of, 118, 126; community medicine and, 26, 105–7, 109; education and training of, 29, 40–41, 72, 76–78, 229–32, 238, 240; female, 40–41, 79–80; specialization of, 78, 80, 87, 105, 229; white, 4, 9–10, 16, 25–26, 29–30, 32, 36–38, 40–41, 48, 64, 68–69, 71, 77–79, 90, 101, 142. *See also* physicians, Black

physicians, Black, 6, 11–12, 25, 32–37, 70–73, 86–87, 98–100, 112, 144, 231–32, 253; activism of, 1, 4, 27, 65, 68, 75, 80, 90–91, 94, 108, 110, 124, 156, 258; class status of, 29, 76, 79, 131, 137; discrimination against, 9–10, 30, 58, 60, 77; economic status of, 4, 10, 30, 68, 92; education and training of, 4, 9, 29, 57–58, 68, 74, 76–78, 108–9; elite, 75, 107, 204; gender and, 2, 16, 79–80, 109; at King-Drew Medical Center, 26, 75, 94, 101, 103, 108–9, 156; leadership of, 4, 74–76, 94, 107–9, 156; number of, 66*map*, 67*map*; professionalism of, 69, 76, 78–80; in Watts, 29–31, 55, 60–61, 63*map*, 63–66, 76, 84–85, 90–91, 94–95, 102–3, 110, 123–24, 126, 136, 140, 145, 152, 159, 163, 173–76, 184, 195, 213, 215, 220, 224, 245–46

Piven, Frances Fox, 157–58

policing, 186–88, 192, 194, 206–9, 210, 258; of Black people, 1–3, 56; funding for, 2, 19, 85, 218, 237, 240, 246; of gender and sexuality, 3, 17, 23, 51–52, 80, 143, 195, 201; militarized, 223; of poverty, 3, 7, 24, 149; of Skid Row, 186, 188, 201; of space, 16, 31, 42, 201; of youth, 133, 136, 214. *See also* carceral state; prisons

political whiteness, 219, 237–44, 250

politicians, 15, 27, 74, 144–47, 230–31, 237–38, 247, 250; Black, 4, 6, 11, 36, 65, 80–85, 87, 90–91, 95, 101, 108, 116, 142, 149–50, 164, 166–67, 245–46, 253; conservative, 18, 20, 97, 219; liberal, 3, 17, 20, 97, 218; white, 2–4, 30–32, 41, 44, 46–47, 72, 81, 85, 90, 97, 117, 161, 218–19, 224, 244–45

politics of respectability, 11, 23, 76, 187, 189, 271n22

Poor People's Movement, 157, 163

poverty, 1–2, 3, 7, 17, 26, 61, 65, 148, 181–82, 214, 216; Black, 4, 12, 30, 32–33, 54, 68, 81, 83, 116, 152, 164; causes of, 16–17, 76, 81, 114–15, 132, 169–70, 211; containment of, 147–49, 173, 210; management of, 18, 148, 170–71, 235–36; as pathology, 16, 75, 112, 123–24, 188; racialization of, 114, 169–70, 218; working, 145, 147–51, 169, 173, 191, 195, 209. *See also* antipoverty programs; culture of poverty theory

Powell, Rodney, 125

Price, Rena, 2

pride campaigns, 15, 184, 195, 199, 201, 205

prisons, 4, 19, 119, 127, 133, 149, 186–88, 190, 204, 213–14, 218, 224, 260, 265. *See also* carceral state; policing

Proposition A (1966), 96–97, 224–25, 230

Proposition 13 (1978), 18, 97, 218, 230–31, 236–38, 240, 244–45, 250

Proposition 14 (1964), 61, 64, 70, 82

prostitution, prostitutes, 127, 184, 186, 194, 201, 203, 208, 209, 212. *See also* sex work, sex workers

psychiatry, 112, 137–38, 140–44, 189–90, 196–98, 201–3, 209–11, 213–14, 217–18, 255–58; Black, 68, 110, 125, 127, 130–34; critiques of, 118, 127, 138, 213; ethno-, 196, 203; history of, 39, 118, 127–34, 187, 205–6, 232; race and, 39, 128–34, 187, 196–98, 232; sexuality and, 39, 128–34, 187, 205–6, 232

psychoanalysis, 118, 129, 132, 213

public health, 46–47, 171–78, 146, 181–82, 217–18, 238, 244–48, 250–51, 260; clinics for, 73, 95, 104–6, 110–14, 120–

21, 138, 141, 148, 163, 167, 170, 189, 194, 231, 243, 264; infrastructure of, 17, 26, 58, 194, 224–25, 227, 229–31, 240–41, 264; policy for, 19, 42, 53, 56–57, 90–91, 101, 108, 121, 167, 196; services of, 31, 42–43, 103, 162, 236
public hospitals, 42–43, 46–49, 56–57, 93–97, 107–8, 171–74, 224, 231–33, 243–45; funding for, 18–19, 25–27, 65, 90, 116, 161, 218, 236, 248, 250, 265; in Los Angeles County, 1, 30, 108, 217, 249, 265; patient experience in, 30, 68, 168; purpose of, 2, 25, 218, 236, 248, 250, 265. *See also names of public hospitals*

queer people of color, 3–4, 16–17, 22–23, 186, 209, 253, 258, 260, 265

race, 9, 21–23, 44, 114, 128–34, 137–39, 141–44, 186–90, 195–98, 201–3, 208–10, 253–58; class and, 11, 54, 59, 135; gender and, 28, 31, 40, 49, 75, 146; health and, 30, 38, 103; medicine and, 30, 38–42, 70; mental health and, 213–14, 217–18, 232; poverty and, 3, 17, 61, 65, 169–70, 218; sexuality and, 3–4, 6, 16–18, 28, 31, 40, 43, 49, 52, 73, 75–76, 113, 146, 148–49, 152, 157, 159–60, 181, 184, 194, 217–18, 250, 263; space and, 13–14, 42, 54, 59, 61, 149, 165. *See also* discrimination; racism; *and "racial" entries*
racial capitalism, 4, 19, 21, 30, 37, 54, 69, 76, 91, 107, 148, 187; discourses of, 142; sexual capitalism and, 18, 22, 24, 114
racial liberalism, 3–5, 16, 19, 21, 114, 253–55; contradictions of, 187; critiques of, 17, 76, 162, 263; discourses of, 32, 149
racial science, 16, 31, 38–40, 42, 48, 128–30, 203, 255, 257, 272n35
racism, 3, 128–31; anti-Black, 40; economic, 2, 82; ending of, 5; institutional, 9, 32, 35, 37, 40–44, 54, 59, 61, 73, 77–78, 82–83, 110, 112, 116, 123, 159, 162, 165–66, 182, 187, 190, 195, 263; new, 22; repackaged, 20; scientific, 4, 12, 16, 31, 38–42, 48, 203, 255, 257, 272n35; structural, 12, 106. *See also* discrimination; race; *and "racial" entries*

Reagan, Ronald, 18, 97, 161, 219, 230, 237, 244, 247–50, 271n25, 298n28
Reconstruction era, 9–10, 34, 71, 77, 127, 135
redlining, 195
regionalization plan, 171–72, 177
Regional Medical Programs (RMPs), 93, 100–101
respectability, politics of, 11, 23, 76, 187, 189
Richmond, Julius, 123, 291n33
Riddell, Adeljiza Sosa, 169
riots. *See* Watts Uprisings (1965)
RMPs (Regional Medical Programs), 93, 100–101
Roberts, Sam, Jr., 213
Robinson, Ruth, 124
Roemer, Milton, 70, 88
Roth, Alisa, 214, 308n91
Rouzan, Joseph, 246
Royko, Mike, 215–16, 219–20

Saldaña-Portillo, María Josefina, 33, 274n7
Sanchez, George, 44
Sanville, Richard, 132
Schabarum, Peter, 219, 237, 244, 247, 250
Schooler, James, 53
Schultze, Charles, 82
Seale, Bobby, 114
segregation, 3, 9, 34–35, 37; de facto, 27, 195; de jure, 55, 64, 77, 116; economic, 1, 18; in education, 5; in healthcare, 9, 30, 57; in housing, 13, 42–44, 45*map*, 54, 59, 61, 82, 149, 195; nationalization of, 13–14, 83. *See also* discrimination; Jim Crow; racism
self-determination, 4, 15, 72, 122, 263
service economy, 3, 7, 148, 150–51, 187, 236. *See also* deindustrialization; globalization
sexism, 20–23, 138, 159, 256, 263
sexual capitalism, 18, 22, 24, 76, 114, 148, 187
sexual liberalism, 3–4, 16, 19, 21, 114; contradictions of, 187; critiques of, 253–55, 263; discourses of, 76, 194
sexuality, 3–4, 6, 9, 16–18, 21–23, 141–44, 148–49, 196, 258; Black, 2, 12, 19, 75, 130; criminalization of, 24, 258; discourses of, 28, 31, 40, 43, 49, 52, 73, 75–76, 109,

sexuality *(continued)*
   113–14, 128–34, 137–39, 146, 152, 157–60, 181, 184–90, 194–95, 198, 201–3, 208–10, 217–18, 250, 253–57, 263; respectable, 76, 114, 219, 250, 253. *See also* race: sexuality and
sex work, sex workers, 55, 160, 186, 194, 201, 203, 208. *See also* prostitution, prostitutes
Shah, Nayan, 113
Shamberger, Wilhelmina, 117
Short-Doyle Act (1957), 119, 126
Simkins v. Cone (1963), 35
Simpson-Mazzoli Act (Amnesty), 248
Skid Row (Los Angeles), 184, 186, 188, 191–92, 194, 208–9, 211–14; demographics of; development of, 200*map*; as "homeless district," 25, 189; policies for, 193*map*; policing of, 201, 206–7; in relation to other neighborhoods, 185*map*, 201
slum clearance, 8, 26, 147, 165, 175
Smith, Neil, 75
sociobiology, 257–59
Somerville, Siobhan, 39, 128
South Central Improvement Action Committee (IMPAC), 140
Southeast Multipurpose Comprehensive Health Clinic, 171
Spellman, Mitchell, 75, 99–102, 108, 146, 156, 232–33, 253
Spillers, Hortense, 23, 75, 293n60
Staples, Robert, 23
Straight state, 51, 143

Taylor, Keeanga-Yamahtta, 57
Taylor, Shirley Spencer, 95
Teen Post, 163
Thomas, Charles, 125, 139, 141, 292n42
Thomas, Karen Kruse, 34
Thompson, Roy L., 95
Tillmon, Johnnie, 155*fig.*; activism of, 143, 145, 155–64, 181, 183; childcare center named for, 171, 178; leadership style of, 158–59, 164
Tomes, Nancy, 114, 118
Tranquada, Robert, 121–26, 141–42
trans people, 3–4, 16–17, 22, 186–87, 203, 205, 209, 253, 258, 260, 265

trauma care, 130–31, 203, 210–11, 223, 235, 238, 249, 264. *See also* emergency medicine
Tucker, Essie (Mrs. Marcus O. Tucker), 80
Tucker, Walter, 110
Turner, Kofi-Charu Nat, 143

UCLA. *See* University of California, Los Angeles
Ujima Village, 140–41, 197
unemployment, 3, 7, 55, 85, 168, 223. *See also* worklessness
unions, 1, 9–10, 51, 54–55, 65, 157, 166, 168, 222, 245, 265. *See also* labor and workers
United Neighborhood Organizations of Watts, 95
University of California, Los Angeles (UCLA): Afro-American Studies Center, 139; community mental health at, 110, 190, 198, 201, 210–11, 292n32; King-Drew Medical Center and, 25, 71, 93–96, 100–101, 130, 168, 232; Medical School, 25, 91, 93, 100, 111*map*, 130, 210–11; Neuro-Psychiatric Institute at, 111*map*, 210. *See also* Harbor General Hospital
University of Southern California (USC), 25–26, 110, 112, 121, 155–56, 161, 164; Black community and, 29, 57, 87, 123–25, 139, 142–43; King-Drew Medical Center and, 73, 87, 93–94, 96, 100–101, 232; Medical School, 29, 42, 73, 91, 93, 100, 111*map*, 210; Multipurpose Neighborhood Health Center (Watts Clinic), 73, 123–25, 127, 134, 139, 142. *See also* Los Angeles County General Hospital
urban development, 2, 7–8, 17, 25, 27–28, 41–42, 145–49, 151–54, 164–65, 173–75, 178–81, 188, 191, 194–95, 200*map*, 201, 204, 209–14, 217, 236, 257; racial capitalism and, 4, 187. *See also* Community Redevelopment Agency of Los Angeles; slum clearance
USC. *See* University of Southern California
US Department of Health, Education, and Welfare (DHEW), 146–48, 156, 170, 216, 227, 232, 234
US Organization (Karenga), 15, 136, 141, 163, 197

Vaughn, Florence, 140
Veneman, John, 142, 295n102
violence, 22, 210–12; domestic, 198; epidemiology of, 258; gun, 6, 18, 27, 215–18, 220, 224, 235, 248; racial, 2, 34, 85, 139, 163; sexual, 253, 260; social, 7, 16, 85, 97, 131, 192, 198, 217, 223, 245

Wagensteen, Owen, 99
Ward, Thomas, 78
War on Poverty, 121, 231. *See also* antipoverty programs: federal
Washington, Booker T., 10–11, 149, 294n73
Waters, Maxine, 245
Watts Chamber of Commerce, 65
Watts Health District, 25, 32–33, 65, 87, 90, 171
Watts Hospital. *See* King-Drew Medical Center
Watts Labor Community Action Committee, 95
Watts (neighborhood), 29–30, 86–88, 90–91, 102–3, 110, 112, 123–24, 173–74, 184, 195, 213, 215; Black population of, 32–37, 55, 60–66, 63*map*, 72–73, 76, 84, 94–95, 98, 100, 126, 136, 140, 145, 152, 159, 163, 176, 220, 224, 245–46; health conditions in, 25, 33, 64, 88, 95, 102–3, 173; poverty in, 2, 11, 32–33, 61, 64–65, 71, 73, 75, 84, 95, 126, 132, 136, 140, 145, 152, 159, 163, 176, 220, 224, 245–46. *See also* King-Drew Medical Center; Watts Health District; Watts Uprisings
Watts Uprisings (1965), 2, 11, 15, 54–55, 65, 68, 72–75, 80–82, 121, 146, 152, 224
Weinberger, Caspar, 177
welfare, 17, 83, 156–57, 160, 232, 236; dependency on, 6, 27, 97, 117, 149, 196; programs for, 85, 161, 182, 218, 260; reform of; women on, 4, 16, 26, 75, 143, 159, 162, 170, 248, 258. *See also* welfare rights movement
welfare rights movement, 15, 26, 143, 145, 159–64, 167, 170, 181–83; Black women in, 143, 146, 156–57, 159–60; goals of, 146, 157–58, 263; healthcare and, 146, 263; King-Drew Medical Center and, 146, 156, 178, 263. *See also* National Welfare Rights Organization
Wertham, Fredric, 130–31
West, Louis Jolyon "Jolly," 210–11
white male patronage principle, 31–32, 37, 39–42, 47, 49, 55
whiteness: as political identity, 219, 250; as property, 10, 24–25, 30; as racial category, 10, 24, 40, 46, 51, 56, 59, 270n19
white people, 15, 44, 46, 60–61, 96–97, 135, 218–19, 224, 236–37, 244, 250; elites of, 31–32, 147, 152, 154, 164–67, 172, 179, 184, 201; flight of, 13, 52, 54; as politicians, 2–4, 30–32, 41, 47, 72, 81, 85, 90, 117, 161, 245; sense of supremacy of, 12, 22–23, 75, 78, 82, 131, 138, 162, 198, 253, 263; as taxpayers, 3–5, 9, 11, 17–19, 24, 56–57, 68, 74–75, 85, 94, 102, 108, 113, 170, 190, 231, 233, 241, 264; as voters, 3–6, 9, 18, 24, 47–48, 64, 85, 100, 117, 149, 223, 230, 238, 247, 260–61, 264; as workers, 7, 10, 30, 43, 51, 56, 83, 157, 166, 222. *See also* physicians, white; whiteness
Widney, Joseph Pomeroy, 41–42, 70, 277n39
Wiley, George, 145, 155*fig.*, 155–59, 162, 164
Williams, William A., 232
Willowbrook Plaza Home Owners Improvement Club, 117
Wilson, James, 209–10
Witherill, Liston, 177, 311n38
Wolch, Jennifer, 186
Wood, Alma, 124
Wood, James, 179
Woods, Clyde Adrian, 148
Work Incentive Program (WIN/WIP), 161, 183
worklessness, 3, 7, 26, 49, 199, 223. *See also* unemployment

Yerby, Alonzo, 94, 101
Yorty, Sam, 74, 81–83, 85, 98

Zante, K. Van, 47–50
Zink, Brian, 310n24

AMERICAN CROSSROADS

Edited by Earl Lewis, George Lipsitz, George Sánchez, Dana Takagi, Laura Briggs, and Nikhil Pal Singh

1. *Border Matters: Remapping American Cultural Studies,* by José David Saldívar
2. *The White Scourge: Mexicans, Blacks, and Poor Whites in Texas Cotton Culture,* by Neil Foley
3. *Indians in the Making: Ethnic Relations and Indian Identities around Puget Sound,* by Alexandra Harmon
4. *Aztlán and Viet Nam: Chicano and Chicana Experiences of the War,* edited by George Mariscal
5. *Immigration and the Political Economy of Home: West Indian Brooklyn and American Indian Minneapolis, 1945–1992,* by Rachel Buff
6. *Epic Encounters: Culture, Media, and U.S. Interests in the Middle East since 1945,* by Melani McAlister
7. *Contagious Divides: Epidemics and Race in San Francisco's Chinatown,* by Nayan Shah
8. *Japanese American Celebration and Conflict: A History of Ethnic Identity and Festival, 1934–1990,* by Lon Kurashige
9. *American Sensations: Class, Empire, and the Production of Popular Culture,* by Shelley Streeby
10. *Colored White: Transcending the Racial Past,* by David R. Roediger
11. *Reproducing Empire: Race, Sex, Science, and U.S. Imperialism in Puerto Rico,* by Laura Briggs
12. *meXicana Encounters: The Making of Social Identities on the Borderlands,* by Rosa Linda Fregoso
13. *Popular Culture in the Age of White Flight: Fear and Fantasy in Suburban Los Angeles,* by Eric Avila
14. *Ties That Bind: The Story of an Afro-Cherokee Family in Slavery and Freedom,* by Tiya Miles
15. *Cultural Moves: African Americans and the Politics of Representation,* by Herman S. Gray
16. *Emancipation Betrayed: The Hidden History of Black Organizing and White Violence in Florida from Reconstruction to the Bloody Election of 1920,* by Paul Ortiz
17. *Eugenic Nation: Faults and Frontiers of Better Breeding in Modern America,* by Alexandra Stern

18. *Audiotopia: Music, Race, and America,* by Josh Kun
19. *Black, Brown, Yellow, and Left: Radical Activism in Los Angeles,* by Laura Pulido
20. *Fit to Be Citizens? Public Health and Race in Los Angeles, 1879–1939,* by Natalia Molina
21. *Golden Gulag: Prisons, Surplus, Crisis, and Opposition in Globalizing California,* by Ruth Wilson Gilmore
22. *Proud to Be an Okie: Cultural Politics, Country Music, and Migration to Southern California,* by Peter La Chapelle
23. *Playing America's Game: Baseball, Latinos, and the Color Line,* by Adrian Burgos, Jr.
24. *The Power of the Zoot: Youth Culture and Resistance during World War II,* by Luis Alvarez
25. *Guantánamo: A Working-Class History between Empire and Revolution,* by Jana K. Lipman
26. *Between Arab and White: Race and Ethnicity in the Early Syrian-American Diaspora,* by Sarah M. A. Gualtieri
27. *Mean Streets: Chicago Youths and the Everyday Struggle for Empowerment in the Multiracial City, 1908–1969,* by Andrew J. Diamond
28. *In Sight of America: Photography and the Development of U.S. Immigration Policy,* by Anna Pegler-Gordon
29. *Migra! A History of the U.S. Border Patrol,* by Kelly Lytle Hernández
30. *Racial Propositions: Ballot Initiatives and the Making of Postwar California,* by Daniel Martinez HoSang
31. *Stranger Intimacy: Contesting Race, Sexuality, and the Law in the North American West,* by Nayan Shah
32. *The Nicest Kids in Town:* American Bandstand, *Rock 'n' Roll, and the Struggle for Civil Rights in 1950s Philadelphia,* by Matthew F. Delmont
33. *Jack Johnson, Rebel Sojourner: Boxing in the Shadow of the Global Color Line,* by Theresa Rundstedler
34. *Pacific Connections: The Making of the US-Canadian Borderlands,* by Kornel Chang
35. *States of Delinquency: Race and Science in the Making of California's Juvenile Justice System,* by Miroslava Chávez-García

36. *Spaces of Conflict, Sounds of Solidarity: Music, Race, and Spatial Entitlement in Los Angeles*, by Gaye Theresa Johnson
37. *Covert Capital: Landscapes of Denial and the Making of U.S. Empire in the Suburbs of Northern Virginia*, by Andrew Friedman
38. *How Race Is Made in America: Immigration, Citizenship, and the Historical Power of Racial Scripts*, by Natalia Molina
39. *We Sell Drugs: The Alchemy of US Empire*, by Suzanna Reiss
40. *Abrazando el Espíritu: Bracero Families Confront the US-Mexico Border*, by Ana Elizabeth Rosas
41. *Houston Bound: Culture and Color in a Jim Crow City*, by Tyina L. Steptoe
42. *Why Busing Failed: Race, Media, and the National Resistance to School Desegregation*, by Matthew F. Delmont
43. *Incarcerating the Crisis: Freedom Struggles and the Rise of the Neoliberal State*, by Jordan T. Camp
44. *Lavender and Red: Liberation and Solidarity in the Gay and Lesbian Left*, by Emily K. Hobson
45. *Flavors of Empire: Food and the Making of Thai America*, by Mark Padoongpatt
46. *The Life of Paper: Letters and a Poetics of Living Beyond Captivity*, by Sharon Luk
47. *Strategies of Segregation: Race, Residence, and the Struggle for Educational Equality*, by David G. García
48. *Soldiering through Empire: Race and the Making of the Decolonizing Pacific*, by Simeon Man
49. *An American Language: The History of Spanish in the United States*, by Rosina Lozano
50. *The Color Line and the Assembly Line: Managing Race in the Ford Empire*, by Elizabeth D. Esch
51. *Confessions of a Radical Chicano Doo-Wop Singer*, by Rubén Funkahuatl Guevara
52. *Empire's Tracks: Indigenous Peoples, Racial Aliens, and the Transcontinental Railroad*, by Manu Karuka

53. *Collisions at the Crossroads: How Place and Mobility Make Race,* by Genevieve Carpio

54. *Charros: How Mexican Cowboys are Remapping Race and American Identity,* by Laura R. Barraclough

55. *Louder and Faster: Pain, Joy, and the Body Politic in Asian American Taiko,* by Deborah Wong

56. *Badges without Borders: How Global Counterinsurgency Transformed American Policing,* by Stuart Schrader

57. *Colonial Migrants at the Heart of Empire: Puerto Rican Workers on U.S. Farms,* by Ismael García Colón

58. *Assimilation: An Alternative History,* by Catherine S. Ramírez

59. *Boyle Heights: How a Los Angeles Neighborhood Became the Future of American Democracy,* by George J. Sánchez

60. *Not Yo' Butterfly: My Long Song of Relocation, Race, Love, and Revolution,* by Nobuko Miyamoto

61. *The Deportation Express: A History of America through Mass Removal,* by Ethan Blue

62. *An Archive of Skin, An Archive of Kin: Disability and Life-Making during Medical Incarceration,* by Adria L. Imada

63. *Menace to Empire: Anticolonial Solidarities and the Transpacific Origins of the US Security State,* by Moon-Ho Jung

64. *Suburban Empire: Cold War Militarization in the US Pacific,* by Lauren Hirshberg

65. *Archipelago of Resettlement: Vietnamese Refugee Settlers across Guam and Israel-Palestine,* by Evyn Lê Espiritu Gandhi

66. *Arise! Global Radicalism in the Era of the Mexican Revolution,* by Christina Heatherton

67. *Resisting Change in Suburbia: Asian Immigrants and Frontier Nostalgia in L.A.,* by James Zarsadiaz

68. *Racial Uncertainties: Mexican Americans, School Desegregation, and the Making of Race in Post–Civil Rights America,* by Danielle R. Olden

69. *Pacific Confluence: Fighting over the Nation in Nineteenth-Century Hawai'i,* by Christen T. Sasaki

70. *Possible Histories: Arab Americans and the Queer Ecology of Peddling,* by Charlotte Karem Albrecht

71. *Indian Wars Everywhere: Colonial Violence and the Shadow Doctrines of Empire,* by Stefan Aune
72. *Plantation Pedagogy: The Violence of Schooling across Black and Indigenous Space,* by Bayley J. Marquez
73. *The Danger Zone Is Everywhere: How Housing Discrimination Harms Health and Steals Wealth,* by George Lipsitz
74. *The Violence of Love: Race, Family, and Adoption in the United States,* by Kit W. Myers
75. *Health as Property: Racial Capitalism and Sexual Liberalism in Los Angeles,* by Nic John Ramos

www.ingramcontent.com/pod-product-compliance
Lightning Source LLC
Chambersburg PA
CBHW021334230426
43666CB00006B/291